Complications in Kidney Transplantation

Fahad Aziz • Sandesh Parajuli
Editors

Complications in Kidney Transplantation

A Case-Based Guide to Management

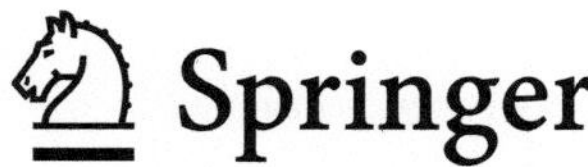 Springer

Editors
Fahad Aziz
University of Wisconsin
Madison, WI, USA

Sandesh Parajuli
Department of Medicine
University of Wisconsin
Madison, WI, USA

ISBN 978-3-031-13571-2   ISBN 978-3-031-13569-9   (eBook)
https://doi.org/10.1007/978-3-031-13569-9

© The Editor(s) (if applicable) and The Author(s), under exclusive license to Springer Nature Switzerland AG 2022
This work is subject to copyright. All rights are solely and exclusively licensed by the Publisher, whether the whole or part of the material is concerned, specifically the rights of translation, reprinting, reuse of illustrations, recitation, broadcasting, reproduction on microfilms or in any other physical way, and transmission or information storage and retrieval, electronic adaptation, computer software, or by similar or dissimilar methodology now known or hereafter developed.
The use of general descriptive names, registered names, trademarks, service marks, etc. in this publication does not imply, even in the absence of a specific statement, that such names are exempt from the relevant protective laws and regulations and therefore free for general use.
The publisher, the authors, and the editors are safe to assume that the advice and information in this book are believed to be true and accurate at the date of publication. Neither the publisher nor the authors or the editors give a warranty, expressed or implied, with respect to the material contained herein or for any errors or omissions that may have been made. The publisher remains neutral with regard to jurisdictional claims in published maps and institutional affiliations.

This Springer imprint is published by the registered company Springer Nature Switzerland AG
The registered company address is: Gewerbestrasse 11, 6330 Cham, Switzerland

Foreword

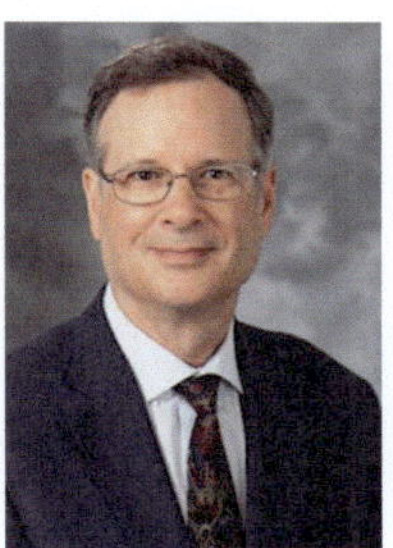

In the United States, it is estimated that more than 200,000 individuals are living with a kidney transplant. Kidney transplantation adds to the quality of life and enhances life expectancy.

This book, focused on kidney transplant recipients, is designed to provide contemporary insights into meeting the clinical challenges that may arise during an individual's transplant journey.

However, for individuals to achieve long-term successful outcomes, close collaboration, and a team-spirit of care including the patient, their families, the transplant surgeons, physicians, coordinators, and many other healthcare providers, is required.

Drs Aziz and Parajuli present the essential aspects of the complex topic of kidney transplantation in a unique style that is easy to follow. Case scenarios are presented for important post-transplant complications. The scenario is followed by a question and answer on the best investigation, the diagnosis, and a discussion of the best treatment option and outcomes.

In this book, that effectively uses narration, various tables and figures, the authors have comprehensively addressed the most important aspects of kidney transplantation that will be a valuable guide to learn all about this miracle therapy.

Dixon B. Kaufman
UW Health Transplant Center
Madison, WI, USA

Ray D. Owen
Division of Transplantation
Department of Surgery
UW School of Medicine and Public Health
Madison, WI, USA

Foreword

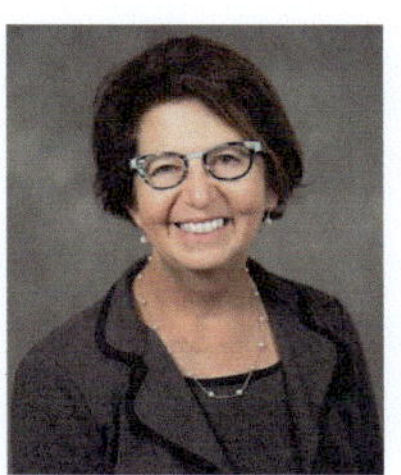

Kidney transplantation remains the treatment of choice for end-stage kidney disease, offering improved survival and quality of life compared to dialysis. Since the first kidney transplant in the United States in 1954, the number of individuals living with a kidney transplant has continued to increase. In the United States alone, there are over 225,000 people living with a functional kidney transplant, with approximately 20,000 new kidney transplants performed annually. Given the increasing number of patients living with a kidney transplant, it is critical that physicians recognize and understand the myriad potential complications of kidney transplantation. Drs Aziz and Parajuli have assembled a practical guide using case-based scenarios to illustrate important post-transplant complications. The pragmatic, evidence-based approach to the diagnosis and management of kidney transplant complications is useful to all health care providers who care for transplant patients.

Lynn M. Schnapp
Department of Medicine
School of Medicine and Public Health
University of Wisconsin-Madison
Madison, WI, USA

Preface

Since the first successful kidney transplant in 1954, the practice and management of kidney transplantation has evolved with time. Kidney transplantation is both a science and an art. Successful kidney transplantation involves multidisciplinary approaches dedicated to providing excellent care and outcomes to patients in need. In our daily clinical practices, we encounter different medical conditions that may not follow the typical presentation, mainly due to multiple other comorbidities and immunosuppressive medications.

To prepare this book, several professionals from various academic institutions in this field shared their experiences based on actual cases or as realistic presentations in a case-based fashion. This book provides an overview and general guide of some common conditions or unique situations among patients pre- and post-kidney transplants, some donor issues, and many more conditions with current literature review.

This is a general guide. Authors have shared their experiences based on their clinical practice. Therefore, management or outcomes presented in these cases may not be applicable in all situations and should be considered individually.

We are grateful to all authors who shared their real-life experiences despite their busy schedules. We hope that these cases will help improve patient care.

This book is dedicated to our patients who we are proud of their struggles and successes.

Madison, WI, USA   Fahad Aziz
Madison, WI, USA   Sandesh Parajuli

Contents

Chapter 1
Obesity in Kidney Transplant Recipients

Adam M. Kressel and Elliot I. Grodstein

Introduction

Overweight (BMI > 25 mg/kg^2) and obese (BMI > 30 mg/kg^2) patients are commonly encountered in clinic and hospital settings each year in the United States and around the world. These patients present with a myriad of pulmonary, cardiac, and metabolic health issues in addition to their increased prevalence of chronic kidney disease [1]. An in-depth understanding of obese patients and their unique risks regarding kidney transplantation is necessary. This chapter presents a case-based scenario and discussion to address some of these topics.

Patient History

A 55-year-old male with end-stage kidney disease (ESKD) has been treated with intermittent hemodialysis three times per week for 2 years. He has type 2 diabetes, hyperlipidemia, coronary artery disease, and a BMI of 37 mg/kg^2. He has been attempting to lose weight recently with a structured diet and exercise plan. He has

A. M. Kressel
Division of Transplant Surgery, Department of Surgery, Northwell Health,
Manhasset, NY, USA
e-mail: AKressel2@northwell.edu

E. I. Grodstein (✉)
Division of Transplant Surgery, Department of Surgery, Northwell Health,
Manhasset, NY, USA

Donald and Barbara Zucker School of Medicine at Hofstra / Northwell Health,
Hempstead, NY, USA
e-mail: egrodstein@northwell.edu

© The Author(s), under exclusive license to Springer Nature
Switzerland AG 2022
F. Aziz, S. Parajuli (eds.), *Complications in Kidney Transplantation*,
https://doi.org/10.1007/978-3-031-13569-9_1

been unable to find a suitable living donor and has remained active on the transplant waiting list.

Question 1

Which of the following statements is true regarding this patient's current and future risks as they relate to kidney transplantation?

A. Given the high likelihood of perioperative complications, the risk of kidney transplantation does not outweigh the risks of continuing hemodialysis.
B. Kidney transplantation in the obese population is associated with an increased incidence of delayed graft function and graft loss.
C. Due to his obesity, this patient is more likely to be transplanted earlier than if he was not obese.
D. This patient is likely to lose weight post-transplant.
E. Since this patient has a BMI > 35, he currently does not qualify for kidney transplantation.

The correct answer is B.

A recently published multi-center retrospective study investigating over 22,000 patients demonstrated an increased incidence of delayed graft function and graft failure for patients with BMI > 35 compared to patients with BMI < 35 without a significant difference in patient mortality [2]. A is incorrect because a survival benefit of transplantation over continuous hemodialysis has been shown in the obese population [3]. C is incorrect because obese patients are unfortunately more likely to have longer waitlist times, not shorter [1]. D is incorrect because most transplanted patients gain weight post-operatively, despite aggressive measures [4]. E is incorrect because though high BMI may exclude a patient from transplant at certain centers, and obesity is not a universal criterion for exclusion from transplantation [1].

Clinical Course

A suitable deceased donor was identified, and the patient was successfully transplanted via standard technique. Prior to discharge, the patient suffered from minor wound dehiscence that was treated non-operatively with local wound care. His postoperative course was complicated by delayed graft function that required 2 weeks of post-transplant hemodialysis, but the graft has since recovered function. On follow-up in the clinic, the patient has been feeling well, tolerating a diet, voiding appropriately, and has laboratory values in the normal range.

Question 2

In the postoperative setting, which of the following is true?

A. Concomitant sleeve gastrectomy and kidney transplant have been unable to consistently decrease post-transplant weight gain.

B. Concomitant sleeve gastrectomy and kidney transplantation have been shown to improve postoperative graft function.
C. There is an increased incidence of wound infection and dehiscence in the obese transplant population.
D. Obesity represents a risk factor for poor recipient survival post-transplant.
E. There is a non-significant increased risk of hospital readmission in obese post-transplant patients.

The correct answer is C.

Peri-operatively, obesity is associated with delayed wound healing and wound complications. Weight gain after transplantation is well described [1, 5], and various techniques to address this have been investigated, including aggressive nutrition/dietary counseling [4] and surgery. One group investigates whether simultaneous transplantation and bariatric surgery provide additional benefit over kidney transplantation alone [6]. With a small sample size, they demonstrated that transplant recipients undergoing simultaneous sleeve gastrectomy significantly decreased their BMI compared to patients undergoing transplant only, but this did not affect the graft function. Therefore, answers A and B are incorrect. Answer D is incorrect. In a meta-analysis covering over 135,000 patients, transplantation was shown to significantly affect graft loss but not overall patient survival [7]. However, there are certainly unmeasured detrimental effects on society due to lost wages, increased hospitalization costs, and nosocomial exposure. Answer E is incorrect as increased length of hospitalization and readmissions within the first year [5] are more common in obese recipients.

Discussion

Obesity is becoming increasingly present in society and impacts transplant patients in various ways. Obese patients are at increased risk of diabetes, cardiovascular disease, metabolic syndrome, and chronic kidney disease. As outlined above, kidney transplantation is beneficial in this population but is associated with unique complications, including a disproportionate frequency of delayed graft function, wound infection, and prolonged hospitalization [8]. With the rise of obesity in the general population, obese kidney transplant donors also confer considerable risk. Fortunately, although the increase in organ utilization from overweight and obese donors—and the concomitant decrease in utilization from normal-weight donors—correlated with delayed graft function, this did not impact graft survival [8].

This trend in organ utilization was studied by Lentine et al., in which the Organ Procurement and Transplantation Network (OPTN) database was evaluated for kidney transplant recipient BMI. The decrease in normal-weight recipients and increase in overweight and obese recipients are easily apparent [9].

Along the same vein, by our evaluation of the OPTN database, there seems to be a consistent increase in utilization from both normal-weight and overweight/obese donors in recent years (Fig. 1.1).

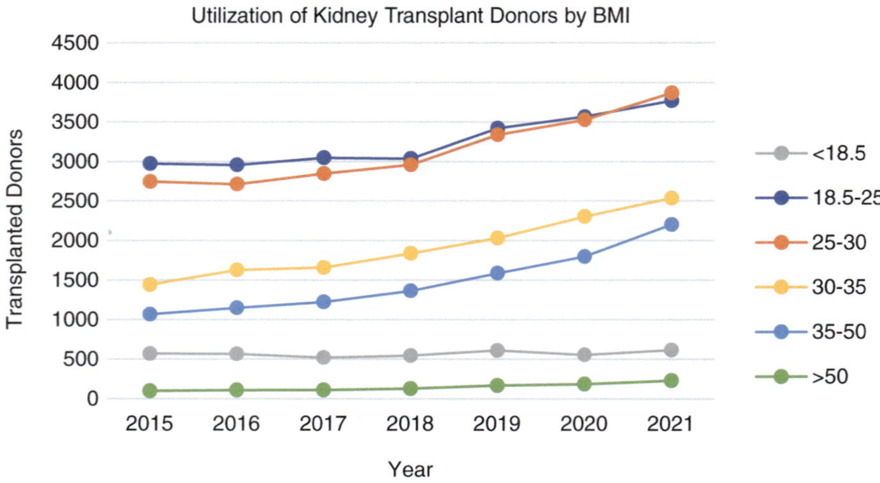

Fig. 1.1 Transplanted Renal Grafts, Stratified by Donor BMI

Certainly, increased organ utilization is beneficial to patients waiting on ever-expanding waitlists. While this may lead to some detrimental outcomes for patients on the extremes of weight, most patients seem to benefit without long-term adverse effects [2]. An in-depth analysis of the benefits of transplantation in the obese population (reduced time on dialysis, increased production, etc.) compared with the costs (increased hospital length of stay, adverse cardiovascular outcomes and interventions, and potential additional services/surgeries related to weight loss) would be valuable.

As referenced earlier, weight gain after transplantation is a well-known phenomenon attributed to increased appetite as a side-effect of medications, generalized well-being, and fewer dietary restrictions [8]. This weight gain can be significant, and numerous weight-loss strategies have been investigated [10]. Beginning with lifestyle modification, patients can enroll in supervised exercise programs, maintain strict glycemic control, and adhere to a healthy diet. Additional pharmacologic options exist but have limited long-term effects given warning compliance [10]. The most aggressive therapy would be surgical, with restrictive and malabsorptive strategies employed [6, 10]. Outcomes remain promising but must be individualized, with additional research needed in this space.

Each year, the number of kidney transplants performed increases, and a growing number of these procedures are performed in overweight and obese patients. This specific population has its inherent risks and surgical challenges, so a thorough understanding of the role of transplantation in obese patients is required to ensure successful outcomes.

References

1. Di Cocco P, et al. Obesity in kidney transplantation. Transpl Int. 2020;33:581–9.
2. Sureshkumar KK, Chopra B, Josephson MA, Shah PB, McGill RL. Recipient obesity and kidney transplant outcomes: a mate-kidney analysis. Am J Kidney Dis. 2021;78:501–510.e1.
3. Glanton CW, Kao TC, Cruess D, Agodoa LYC, Abbott KC. Impact of renal transplantation on survival in end-stage renal disease patients with elevated body mass index. Kidney Int. 2003;63:647–53.
4. Henggeler CK, et al. A randomized controlled trial of an intensive nutrition intervention versus standard nutrition care to avoid excess weight gain after kidney transplantation: the INTENT trial. J Ren Nutr. 2018;28:340–51.
5. Erturk T, Berber I, Cakir U. Effect of obesity on clinical outcomes of kidney transplant patients. Transplant Proc. 2019;51:1093–5.
6. Spaggiari M, et al. Simultaneous robotic kidney transplantation and bariatric surgery for morbidly obese patients with end-stage renal failure. Am J Transplant. 2021;21:1525–34.
7. Hill CJ, et al. Recipient obesity and outcomes after kidney transplantation: a systematic review and meta-analysis. Nephrol Dial Transplant. 2015;30:1403–11.
8. Glicklich D, Mustafa MR. Obesity in kidney transplantation: impact on transplant candidates, recipients, and donors. Cardiol Rev. 2019;27:63–72.
9. Lentine KL, et al. Obesity and kidney transplant candidates: how big is too big for transplantation? Am J Nephrol. 2012;36:575–86.
10. Potluri K, Hou S. Obesity in kidney transplant recipients and candidates. Am J Kidney Dis. 2010;56:143–56.

Chapter 2
Kidney Transplantation in Polycystic Kidney Disease: When to Perform Native Nephrectomies

Christopher J. Little and Steven C. Kim

Introduction

Polycystic kidney disease (PCKD) is a hereditary, multisystem disease involving cystic lesions of the kidneys which can lead to end-stage kidney disease (ESKD), for which kidney transplantation is the treatment of choice [1]. However, a constellation of sequelae such as infection, hemorrhage, flank pain, and massive cystic enlargement can necessitate bilateral native nephrectomies in addition to kidney transplantation [1]. Based on patient and operative considerations, these operations can be staged or performed concurrently [2]. This chapter reviews a clinical case to underscore the indications for bilateral native nephrectomies in PCKD and examine the different strategies for operative timing concerning kidney transplantation.

Patient History

A 52-year-old female with a history of chronic kidney disease (CKD) stage 4 secondary to progressive autosomal dominant polycystic kidney disease presents to the clinic to be evaluated for living donor kidney transplantation from her daughter. She

C. J. Little
Division of Transplantation, Department of Surgery, Emory University School of Medicine, Atlanta, GA, USA

Department of Surgery, University of Washington, Seattle, WA, USA
e-mail: cjlittle@uw.edu

S. C. Kim (✉)
Division of Transplantation, Department of Surgery, Emory University School of Medicine, Atlanta, GA, USA
e-mail: steven.charles.kim@emory.edu

© The Author(s), under exclusive license to Springer Nature Switzerland AG 2022
F. Aziz, S. Parajuli (eds.), *Complications in Kidney Transplantation*,
https://doi.org/10.1007/978-3-031-13569-9_2

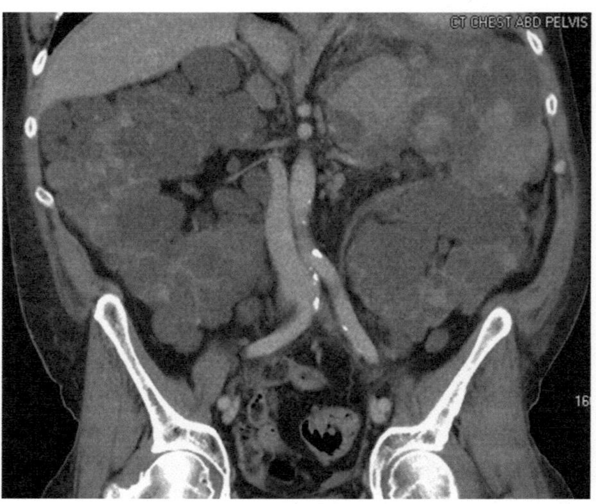

Fig. 2.1 CT scan demonstrating significant bilateral enlargement of polycystic kidneys extending into the pelvis beyond the level of the aortic bifurcation

continues to produce urine and has never required dialysis, though her kidney function has declined with a current eGFR of 20 mL/min per 1.73 m^2. Previously, she was managed with the V2-receptor antagonist, tolvaptan; however, this was discontinued after progressive kidney dysfunction. She describes persistent, dull, bilateral flank pain, which has worsened despite regular use of acetaminophen and tramadol. She is, however, still able to perform her activities of daily living. She reports early satiety, though she continues to have adequate nutritional intake and is maintaining her weight. She does endorse several urinary tract infections (UTI), all of which have been treated outpatient with oral antibiotics. She denies ever having significant hematuria or kidney stones. She does have known hepatic cysts, though her liver function remains normal, and she has no other extrarenal manifestations of her PCKD. Additional past medical history includes hypertension controlled with lisinopril and pregnancy complicated by postpartum hemorrhage requiring several units of blood. She has no prior surgical history. The physical exam is notable for tender, bilateral abdominal masses but is otherwise unremarkable. CT scan reveals massively enlarged bilateral kidneys with multiple large cysts extending beyond the level of the aortic bifurcation (Fig. 2.1).

Question 1

What is the most appropriate next step in management?

A. Kidney transplant alone.
B. Kidney transplant with unilateral native nephrectomy.
C. Kidney transplant with bilateral native nephrectomy.
D. Continue supportive therapy.

The correct answer is C.

This patient has several indications for bilateral native nephrectomies. Given that she is an anticipated kidney transplant recipient, the extension of her bilateral kidney enlargement beyond the level of the aortic bifurcation would likely impede the positioning of the transplanted allograft. Therefore, she would require unilateral native nephrectomy at a minimum to allow for transplantation. However, given that she describes progressive, bilateral flank pain, early satiety, and recurrent UTIs, this patient would benefit from bilateral native nephrectomies to optimize symptomatic relief.

She further asked about the timing of the nephrectomies in her next clinic visit.

Question 2

In what order should the native nephrectomies be performed in relation to her kidney transplant?

A. Before transplant (pre-transplant staging).
B. Simultaneous to transplant.
C. After transplant (post-transplant staging).
D. All are acceptable options.

The correct answer is B.

There are three potential sequences for a kidney transplant and native nephrectomy in the PCKD recipient, each of which has nuanced consideration to be discussed later in this chapter. Concurrent (or simultaneous) nephrectomy refers to removing one or both native kidneys at the time of kidney transplantation, while a staged nephrectomy can be performed before or after the transplant.

Due to her bilateral kidney enlargement encroaching on the heterotopic placement of the kidney allograft, this patient will require pre-transplant or simultaneous native nephrectomy and would not qualify for post-transplant staging. However, given that this patient has an ongoing kidney function, a bilateral native nephrectomy before her planned transplant would require her to start dialysis postoperatively, which necessitates extensive counseling on the morbidities of dialysis access procedures and the disadvantages of initiating hemodialysis. Furthermore, pre-transplant bilateral nephrectomies are associated with higher transfusion requirements that create a potential for allogenic sensitization, placing her at increased risk for allograft rejection [2–4]. This concept is particularly germane in this patient, given her prior sensitizing events of pregnancy and blood product transfusions. Importantly, though she does describe bilateral symptoms and early satiety, she does not yet have significant lifestyle limitations prompting expedited surgical intervention. Based on these factors, simultaneous native nephrectomies at the time of kidney transplant would be the preferred approach for this patient.

Additional Clinical Course

The patient underwent concurrent bilateral native nephrectomies and living donor kidney transplantation without complication. She had immediate allograft function and was discharged from the hospital on postoperative day 4. After recovering from the expected postoperative pain, she reported significant symptomatic relief with the resolution of her flank pain and no experience of early satiety. At follow-up, she demonstrates normal allograft function with an eGFR of 80 mL/min per 1.73 m^2 and serum creatinine of 0.9 mg/dL without evidence of acute rejection.

Discussion

Polycystic kidney disease is a heterogenous hereditary disorder characterized by enlarging cystic lesions within the bilateral kidneys. Autosomal dominant PCKD is the most common subtype with a prevalence of 1 in 1000 live births, while the autosomal recessive form has a prevalence of 1 in 200,000 [5]. Though the autosomal recessive type is typically more severe and diagnosed earlier in life, both forms are variable in onset, multisystem involvement and disease severity. Together, PCKD represents the most common inherited cause of CKD in the USA, with up to half of the patients progressing to ESKD within their lifetime [1, 5]. Consequently, these patients frequently require kidney replacement therapy in the form of dialysis or transplantation.

In addition to functional impairment, PCKD can yield a constellation of sequelae, including hematuria, proteinuria, nephrolithiasis, flank/abdominal pain, infection, and malignancy [1]. Furthermore, the cystic expansion can cause massive kidney enlargement leading to shortness of breath, severe limitation to mobility, and early satiety resulting in poor oral intake and weight loss [1, 5]. Though medical management can slow cyst progression, these downstream manifestations may require surgical intervention, such as endovascular renal artery ablation or nephrectomy, to mitigate morbidity and mortality associated with the disease [1]. Though most patients do not require an operation, indications for unilateral or bilateral native nephrectomy include recurrent infection, suspected malignancy, refractory kidney hemorrhage, persistent pain or mass effect, related ventral hernias, and anticipated kidney transplantation if the native kidneys are large enough to impede on the safe heterotopic placement of the allograft kidney in the pelvis [1].

Importantly, when considering native nephrectomies, operative timing in relation to transplantation must be considered. As mentioned, native nephrectomy in the PCKD recipient can be performed before, during, or after kidney transplantation if indicated. Although no randomized control trial has been conducted to compare outcomes of these approaches, there have been several retrospective studies reported [2].

Pre-transplant nephrectomy is primarily performed for refractory UTIs/pyelonephritis, hematuria, pain, and/or space occupancy, having the advantage of expeditious symptom relief prior to transplant [2]. However, considerable concerns exist involving the physiologic effects of the rendered anephric state, especially in those undergoing a preemptive kidney transplant. These patients are inevitably exposed to the morbidity and mortality of initiating dialysis, as well as the systemic manifestations of kidney disease such as uremia, anemia, fluid dysregulation, electrolyte aberrancies, and heart disease. Though the impact of these effects can be mitigated in anticipated recipients of scheduled, living donor kidneys, many patients will require time on the waitlist prior to kidney transplantation. Further complicating this approach is the increased transfusion requirements associated with the pre-transplant approach, which poses a higher risk of sensitization, described by Grodstein et al. as a significant 16.5% increase in average panel-reactive antibody (PRA) levels after nephrectomy [2–4].

Similar to the pre-transplant approach, simultaneous native nephrectomies are performed for refractory preoperative sequelae or interference with the placement of the kidney allograft [2]. However, in contrast to staged nephrectomies, this strategy involves a single operation rather than two and eliminates the systemic sequelae of anephric physiology and dialysis dependence. Furthermore, the risk of allogenic sensitization associated with pre-transplant nephrectomy is abated with concurrent procedures, thus decreasing waitlist times and mitigating risk for allograft rejection [2]. It is important to note that Grodstein et al. describe a small increased risk of graft thrombosis with simultaneous nephrectomy (4.4%) versus pre-transplant (1.3%) and kidney-alone (0%) recipients; however, a separate meta-analysis of 102 patients revealed no difference in graft thrombosis between the nephrectomized groups [2, 3]. Moreover, there was no association with acute rejection or graft dysfunction, nor was there an increased cumulative risk for major postoperative complications such as bleeding, urine leaks, wound infections, or hernias after simultaneous nephrectomy [2, 4, 6–8]. Though concurrent procedures increase the operative time compared to kidney transplants alone, the cumulative surgical exposure is decreased compared to the staged operations with no increase in length of postoperative hospital stay [2, 8].

There is a paucity of literature describing post-transplant staging, primarily performed for new or worsening symptoms after transplant [9, 10]. However, based on these limited reports, postoperative nephrectomy does not portend worse outcomes, with no significant risk for postoperative complication or allograft compromise [9, 10]. These are important findings given that up to 16% of PCKD patients undergoing kidney transplantation alone progress to unilateral or bilateral native nephrectomy by 10 years of follow-up [3].

To conclude, though pre-and post-transplant staged nephrectomies are considered safe in PCKD recipients, native nephrectomy performed concurrently with kidney transplantation represents an effective operative strategy to efficiently control PCKD sequala while preventing unnecessary exposure to dialysis and mitigating risk for allogenic sensitization. When space occupancy is a primary operative indication, pre-transplant or simultaneous nephrectomy is necessary for placement of the kidney allograft. However, it is important to note that post-transplant nephrectomy is an acceptable strategy for patients with tolerable symptoms at the time of transplant and no dimensional concerns. Regardless of operative timing, some centers are now offering laparoscopic removal of the polycystic native kidneys, demonstrating adequate safety while further decreasing surgical morbidity among these recipients [2, 7, 8]. However, future studies are necessary to further delineate the nuances of each approach; based on the current body of literature, we recommend that timing of native nephrectomy in PCKD patients undergoing kidney transplantation be tailored to the individual recipient based on symptom tolerability and feasibility of transplant.

References

1. Colbert GB, Elrggal ME, Gaur L, Lerma EV. Update and review of adult polycystic kidney disease. Dis Mon. 2020;66(5):100887.
2. Xu J, D'Souza K, Lau NS, Leslie S, Lee T, Yao J, et al. Staged versus concurrent native nephrectomy and renal transplantation in patients with autosomal dominant polycystic kidney disease: a systematic review. Transplant Rev (Orlando). 2021;36:100652.
3. Grodstein EI, Baggett N, Wayne S, Leverson G, D'Alessandro AM, Fernandez LA, et al. An evaluation of the safety and efficacy of simultaneous bilateral nephrectomy and renal transplantation for polycystic kidney disease: a 20-year experience. Transplantation. 2017;101(11):2774–9.
4. Kim JH, Chae SY, Bae HJ, Kim JI, Moon IS, Choi BS, et al. Clinical outcome of simultaneous native nephrectomy and kidney transplantation in patients with autosomal dominant polycystic kidney disease. Transplant Proc. 2016;48(3):840–3.
5. Bergmann C, Guay-Woodford LM, Harris PC, Horie S, Peters DJM, Torres VE. Polycystic kidney disease. Nat Rev Dis Primers. 2018;4(1):50.
6. Veroux M, Zerbo D, Basile G, Gozzo C, Sinagra N, Giaquinta A, et al. Simultaneous native nephrectomy and kidney transplantation in patients with autosomal dominant polycystic kidney disease. PLoS One. 2016;11(6):e0155481.
7. Abrol N, Prieto M. Simultaneous hand-assisted laparoscopic bilateral native nephrectomy and kidney transplantation for patients with large polycystic kidneys. Urology. 2020;146:271–7.
8. Martin AD, Mekeel KL, Castle EP, Vaish SS, Martin GL, Moss AA, et al. Laparoscopic bilateral native nephrectomies with simultaneous kidney transplantation. BJU Int. 2012;110(11 Pt C):E1003–7.
9. Maxeiner A, Bichmann A, Oberländer N, El-Bandar N, Sugünes N, Ralla B, et al. Native nephrectomy before and after renal transplantation in patients with autosomal dominant polycystic kidney disease (ADPKD). J Clin Med. 2019;8(10):1622.
10. Fuller TF, Brennan TV, Feng S, Kang SM, Stock PG, Freise CE. 4 polycystic kidney disease: indications and timing of native nephrectomy relative to kidney transplantation. J Urol. 2005;174(6):2284–8.

Chapter 3
Surgical Challenges in Kidney Re-transplantation

Kevin C. Janek and Jennifer L. Philip

Introduction

For patients that return to dialysis after failed kidney transplantation, re-transplantation is safe, effective, and associated with a substantial mortality benefit compared to long-term dialysis [1]. Subsequent transplants, however, present additional immunologic and technical challenges, which may lead to increased complication rates and shorter graft survival [2, 3]. Here, we focus on the anatomic and surgical considerations in the setting of kidney re-transplant.

Case 1

A 40-year-old man with a history of ESKD due to IgA nephropathy who underwent a deceased donor kidney transplant in the right iliac fossa 7 years ago is seen in the clinic for steadily declining graft function. His eGFR is 20 mL/min per 1.73 m^2 and creatinine is 4.2 mg/dL, and a tunneled dialysis line is placed for initiation of hemodialysis. Allograft biopsy reveals interstitial fibrosis and tubular atrophy, and immunofluorescence staining is strongly positive for IgA and C3 deposits suggestive of recurrent IgA nephropathy. He is otherwise healthy and active and is concerned

K. C. Janek · J. L. Philip (✉)
Department of Surgery, University of Wisconsin-Madison, Madison, WI, USA
e-mail: kjanek@uwhealth.org; philip@surgery.wisc.edu

© The Author(s), under exclusive license to Springer Nature Switzerland AG 2022
F. Aziz, S. Parajuli (eds.), *Complications in Kidney Transplantation*,
https://doi.org/10.1007/978-3-031-13569-9_3

about the effect of dialysis on his lifestyle. He is also referred for consideration of re-transplantation.

Question 1

Which anatomic locations are preferred for repeat renal transplantation?

A. Ipsilateral iliac fossa.
B. Contralateral iliac fossa.
C. Intraperitoneal.
D. A or B.
E. All of the above.

The correct answer is D.

Kidney grafts are routinely placed in the iliac fossa due to the accessibility of the iliac artery and vein for vascular anastomoses and proximity of the bladder for ureteral implantation. For subsequent transplants, the iliac fossa remains the ideal location, and either ipsilateral or contralateral side may be available. Cross-sectional imaging of the abdomen and pelvis should be obtained to look for iliac calcifications other anatomic considerations that favor one side over another. Most second kidney transplants are done on the contralateral side except in selected cases when technically not feasible, and surgical technique proceeds in the standard fashion. Ipsilateral transplantation can be done proximal or distal to the previous anastomosis, and explant is not routinely recommended due to the additional risks. Increased warm ischemia time and blood loss were associated with kidneys placed on the ipsilateral side compared to controls, but there was no significant difference between thrombosis, bleeding, or urological complications [4, 5]. Renal allografts may also be placed intraperitoneal. While this is the typical approach for pediatric recipients of adult kidneys, it is less commonly used in adult recipients. In the setting of re-transplantation, a transperitoneal approach to the iliac vessels via a lower midline incision may be considered. This approach allows for exposure of both iliac vessels via a single incision and allows for more proximal implantation (e.g., on the lower IVC) if distal vascular targets are determined to be unsuitable. However, the transperitoneal approach increases the risk of injury to the intestine or colon, especially in intraperitoneal scar tissue from prior surgery or peritoneal dialysis. Intraperitoneal placement of a renal allograft is associated with a rare risk of allograft torsion [6].

Clinical Course

CT imaging demonstrated patent iliac vessels with minimal calcifications. He underwent living-related kidney transplantation in the contralateral iliac fossa followed by an uncomplicated hospital course.

Case 2

Similar to the previous patient, a 68-year-old man with diabetes mellitus type 2, hypertension, coronary artery disease, peripheral arterial disease, and a history of kidney transplants 15 and 4 years ago is undergoing evaluation for a third kidney transplant. His first renal allograft was from a living-related donor and placed in the right iliac fossa on the right external iliac artery and vein. His first transplant failed due to chronic rejection. At the time of his second transplant, the left iliac artery was considered unusable due to extensive calcifications. His second renal allograft was placed in the right iliac fossa on the common iliac vessels proximal to the failed graft. A CT scan demonstrates extensive calcifications in the bilateral iliac and common femoral arteries; however, it is worse on the left. Transplant nephrectomy is considered.

Question 2

What could be an indication for transplant nephrectomy at the time of re-transplantation?

A. Severe rejection.
B. Graft necrosis.
C. Creates additional space for the new graft.
D. Graft infection.
E. All of the above.

The correct answer is E.

The indications for transplant nephrectomy can range from graft infection, intolerance, severe rejection, or making space for the new graft [7].

Discussion

There are few, if any, absolutes indications for transplant nephrectomy. Thus, the decision regarding transplant nephrectomy should involve an individualized discussion about the risks or benefits. In patients with extensive atherosclerotic risk factors and severe peripheral vascular disease, further workup should be performed to evaluate the adequacy of the iliac blood vessels for allograft implantation. All patients with peripheral arterial disease should be on standard medical therapy of aspirin and a statin unless contraindicated. Iliac arteries with extensive vascular disease are difficult to clamp and have a higher likelihood of injury, including thrombosis and dissection (Fig. 3.1). A non-contrast CT scan of the abdomen and pelvis should be performed and reviewed prior to transplantation.

Surgical times of re-transplant and particularly third and fourth transplants are significantly longer than primary transplants as well as are associated with higher intraoperative complications and blood loss [8]. Given this, these transplants require

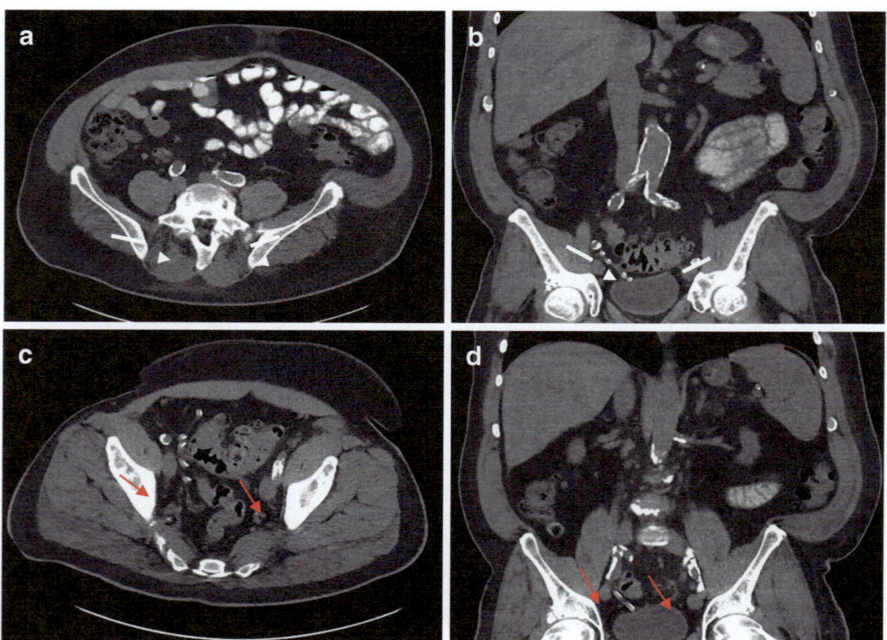

Fig. 3.1 This non-contrasted CT scan of the abdomen and pelvis demonstrates heavily calcified common iliac arteries (**a** and **b**, white arrows) and external iliac arteries (**c** and **d**, red arrows), which are nearly circumferentially diseased. These are not suitable for graft implantation as the vessels lack acceptable tissue quality for vascular anastomosis and compressibility for clamping

surgical teams experienced with re-transplants and allograft nephrectomies. There are several options to manage severe atherosclerosis. When needed, ipsilateral re-transplant is a safe and effective option, even for the third or fourth transplant [4, 8, 9]. This requires additional space for clamping the vessels and the overall size of the kidney. Often in the setting of the third ipsilateral transplant, there is no space in the iliac fossa, and nephrectomy may be indicated with the use of the hilar vessels of the removed kidney to provide vascular inflow and outflow of the new allograft. There are alternative options that would avoid the risks of nephrectomy. Options include interposition grafting of the iliac vessels using donor-harvested iliac artery [10]. Alternatively, intraperitoneal transplantation could be performed, allowing for placement of the renal allograft on the inferior IVC and lower aorta/proximal common iliac artery. Intraperitoneal orthotopic placement has also been described using the splenic vessels for vascular implantation of the graft [8]. For allografts placed higher up on the iliac vessels or in an orthotopic position, the transplant ureter is unlikely to have an appropriate length to reach the bladder for implantation, and ureteral-ureterostomy is typically necessary. This is especially true for living donor kidneys which have shorter length ureters than deceased donor kidneys. Thus, preoperative evaluation of the native ureters is important to consider in potential re-do transplant recipients.

Disclosures Authors have no disclosures.

Funding None.

References

1. Rao PS, Schaubel DE, Wei G, Fenton SSA. Evaluating the survival benefit of kidney retransplantation. Transplantation. 2006;82:669–74.
2. Kainz, A. et al. Waiting time for second kidney transplantation and mortality. CJASN CJN.07620621 (2021). https://doi.org/10.2215/CJN.07620621.
3. Ghadian A, Nourbala MH. Role of renal re-transplantation in ESRD patients. Nephro Urol Mon. 2013;5:721–2.
4. Domagala P, et al. Surgical safety and efficacy of third kidney transplantation in the ipsilateral iliac fossa. Ann Transplant. 2019;24:132–8.
5. Ooms LSS, et al. Kidney retransplantation in the ipsilateral iliac fossa: a surgical challenge: kidney retransplantation in the ipsilateral iliac fossa. Am J Transplant. 2015;15:2947–54.
6. Lucewicz A, et al. Torsion of intraperitoneal kidney transplant: torsion of intraperitoneal kidney transplant. ANZ J Surg. 2012;82:299–302.
7. Fiorentino M, et al. Management of patients with a failed kidney transplant: what should we do? Clin Kidney J. 2021;14:98–106.
8. Lledó-García E, González J, Martínez-Holguín E, Herranz-Amo F, Hernández-Fernández C. Beyond the limits: how to avoid a surgical nightmare in the third and subsequent renal transplantation procedures. Curr Urol Rep. 2020;21:13.
9. Sandal S, Ahn JB, Segev DL, Cantarovich M, McAdams-DeMarco MA. Comparing outcomes of third and fourth kidney transplantation in older and younger patients. Am J Transplant. 2021;21:4023–31.
10. Garcia LE, González J, Serena G, Ciancio G. Arterial reconstruction with donor iliac vessels during kidney transplantation in a patient with severe atherosclerosis. J Vasc Surg Cases Innov Tech. 2019;5:443–6.

Chapter 4
Dual Kidney Transplantation

Riccardo Tamburrini and Alexandra C. Bolognese

Introduction

Dual kidney transplantation (DKT) is the placement of both kidney allografts from a "marginal" deceased donor (MDD) into the same recipient and has developed in response to the continuous organ shortage and increased attention on reducing rates of organ discard [1–3]. Kidneys from MDDs tend to have a lower creatinine clearance due to reduced functional nephron mass, leading to shorter projected allograft survival. Simultaneous transplant of such kidneys, otherwise not appropriate for a single transplant, thereby allows for the expansion of the cadaveric donor pool [4, 5]. This practice was first reported by the University of Maryland and Stanford University in the 1990s and is based on the concept of adequate nephron mass as a predictor of long-term graft outcome [6]. This chapter discusses recipient and donor criteria for consideration for DKT, surgical techniques, and outcomes after DKT. En-bloc transplantation of pediatric dual kidneys is not addressed as it constitutes a separate entity.

Patient History

A 65-year-old man with a body mass index (BMI) of 24 and a history of CKD stage 5 due to hypertension, and diabetes is considered for a kidney transplant. His hypertension and diabetes are medically optimized. He has had no prior abdominal surgeries, and non-contrast computed tomography (CT) of the abdomen and pelvis

R. Tamburrini · A. C. Bolognese (✉)
Division of Transplantation, Department of Surgery, University of Wisconsin–Madison School of Medicine and Public Health, Madison, WI, USA
e-mail: tamburrini@wisc.edu; bolognese@wisc.edu

© The Author(s), under exclusive license to Springer Nature Switzerland AG 2022
F. Aziz, S. Parajuli (eds.), *Complications in Kidney Transplantation*,
https://doi.org/10.1007/978-3-031-13569-9_4

reveals atrophic native kidneys and normal pelvic anatomy with minimal vascular calcifications. Cardiac catheterization reveals mild non-obstructive disease. His panel reactive antibody (PRA) is 0%.

Question 1

Which of the following criteria makes this patient an optimal recipient for consideration of DKT?

A. Low BMI.
B. Advanced age.
C. Normal anatomy.
D. Low immunological risk.
E. All of the above.

The correct answer is E.

All of the above are characteristics of an appropriate recipient for DKT. Many factors go into the decision to transplant kidneys in a dual fashion, including both recipient and donor factors. DKT is the most commonly offered to elderly patients with low immunological risk, conventional anatomy with only mild or moderate vascular calcifications, and normal BMI.

Clinical Course

The above patient is listed for a kidney transplant and gives his consent to be listed for kidneys from donors with kidney donor profile index (KDPI) over 85% and for DKT. A 63-year-old brain-dead donor becomes available. The donor had hypertension of over 10 years' duration and died from a stroke. Terminal creatinine (Cr) was 1.2 mg/dL, and the KDPI is calculated at 88%. The recovery team notes 2 average-sized kidneys with good in situ flush, no gross abnormalities, and single vessels with mild aortic plaque. The kidneys are biopsied, and histologic assessment reveals Remuzzi scores of 5 (right kidney) and 6 (left kidney).

Question 2

How should these kidneys be utilized?

A. These kidneys are most appropriate for dual transplantation in a single recipient.
B. These kidneys are both appropriate for single transplantation in separate recipients.
C. These kidneys are not appropriate for transplantation and should be discarded or used for research.
D. The right kidney should be transplanted, and the left kidney discarded or used for research.

The correct answer is A.

The decision-making process regarding the acceptance and transplantation of marginal organs is complex and varies by center. The KDPI and Remuzzi scores utilize donor characteristics and histologic assessment, respectively, in determining the quality of deceased donor kidneys and can be taken into consideration in making these decisions.

The patient undergoes DKT via a Gibson ("hockey stick") incision, with both kidneys placed on the right iliac vessels via an extraperitoneal approach. His postoperative course is complicated by hyperkalemia and low urine output on postoperative day one. Doppler ultrasound reveals patent vasculature and no evidence of hydronephrosis or peri-transplant collection. He is diagnosed with delayed graft function and requires two additional sessions of hemodialysis postoperatively. He is discharged home on a postoperative day six with increasing urine output and declining serum creatinine and has excellent graft function at 1 year postoperatively.

Discussion

DKT represents a viable avenue for decreasing organ discard rates and expanding the utilization of kidneys from MDDs. This includes donors of advanced age (generally over 60 years); donors with acute kidney injury (rising terminal Cr by at least 50% or 0.3 mg/dL from admission) or chronic kidney disease (glomerular filtration rate less than 60 mL/min/1.73 m^2); donation after circulatory death (DCD) donors; and donors with certain comorbidities including death from stroke. Recipient and donor characteristics, as well as unique technical challenges compared to single kidney transplantation, must be considered to optimize outcomes in DKT.

The current allocation system utilizes KDPI to identify MDDs and estimate projected allograft survival with more granularity than prior systems by summarizing the quality of a deceased donor kidney relative to other kidneys recovered in the prior year [1]. It takes into account clinical and demographic characteristics of the donor, including age, BMI, race/ethnicity, history of hypertension, diabetes, or hepatitis C, cause of death, terminal Cr, and circulatory death donation. While a low KDPI is associated with increased graft quality and expected graft survival, high KDPI kidneys are routinely transplanted with good outcomes when considering recipient history and waitlist times, which vary by center. KDPI helps identify grafts that may be appropriate for DKT when both kidneys are available, thereby providing adequate nephron mass that would not be achieved when transplanted singly. The current allocation system prioritizes recipients willing to undergo dual transplantation of kidneys from a donor with KDPI over 85% in an attempt to maximize organ utilization and decrease discard rates of these organs.

A biopsy-based scoring system developed by Remuzzi et al. helps to discern the likelihood that marginal kidneys will contain adequate nephron mass for good outcomes in the recipient [2]. The Remuzzi score ranges between 0 and 12; four pathologic categories are assessed and given a score between 0 and 3, then totaled for the summative score. The categories evaluated are glomerular sclerosis, tubular atrophy, arterial narrowing, and interstitial fibrosis. Grafts with a score of less than three generally contain adequate functional nephron mass for single transplantation, while scores between 4 and 6 are suitable for DKT such that the sum of total functional nephrons is expected to approach the nephron mass of a single non-marginal kidney. Generally, kidneys with a score above 7 are discarded as functional nephron mass will not be adequate even in DKT, though some centers argue for a summative score of 12 or less as appropriate for DKT [2, 7, 8].

From a technical standpoint, dual transplantation of both donor kidneys can be performed in several ways [9, 10]. One option is a transperitoneal approach, in which a midline incision is made, and the kidneys are then typically placed bilaterally in each iliac fossa. Alternatively, an extraperitoneal approach can be used, as is the most commonly employed in single kidney transplantation. In this case, the kidneys may be placed ipsilaterally, preserving the contralateral side for future retransplant, or bilaterally through two separate extraperitoneal incisions. Generally, in the ipsilateral approach, the right kidney is placed superiorly and laterally with the right renal vein anastomosed via its caval extension to the recipient inferior vena cava or proximal common iliac vein, and an arterial anastomosis is performed between the right renal artery and the common iliac artery. The left kidney is then placed inferiorly and medially with the left renal artery and vein anastomosed to the external iliac vessels (Fig. 4.1). Urinary reconstruction can be performed via separate or conjoined ureteroneocystostomies or by pyeloureterostomy.

Important technical considerations in utilizing any of the above techniques include donor size and anatomy, prior surgical history, and immunologic risk profile. The recipient's pelvis must provide adequate space for the placement of two kidneys without undue tension on anastomoses or compression of vessels. More extensive dissection of the iliac vessels is required for adequate placement, and recipients need to have appropriate non-calcified locations on the vessels for multiple arterial anastomoses and clamp placement. Additionally, with potentially reduced functional nephron mass and graft survival, one must consider smaller and older recipients for kidneys with high combined Remuzzi scores, for whom relative decreased functional nephron mass and years of graft survival may still constitute a positive outcome. Additionally, one must consider the recipient's comorbidities, including cardiac risk profile, as DKT necessarily requires longer operative times due to the additional dissection and anastomotic times. Lastly, DKT theoretically carries a higher immunological risk than a single kidney transplant given the higher nephron mass transplanted, though studies comparing DKT to single transplant have not shown a difference in rates of rejection [2, 5, 11]. However, these data are confounded by elderly and non-sensitized populations generally being preferentially selected for DKT due to perceived increased immunologic risk and is an area for further study.

Outcomes after DKT in appropriately selected recipients are comparable to single kidney transplantation from standard deceased donors with KDPI less than 85% and improved compared to matched criteria single kidney transplantation [11–13]. Delayed graft function (DGF) is seen frequently after DKT with reported rates of 10–30%, not dissimilar to rates reported for single kidney transplantation [2, 5, 11, 14]. Overall, patient and graft survival rates after DKT are also similar [13–15]. In theory, graft thrombosis and urologic complications will increase DKT due to the

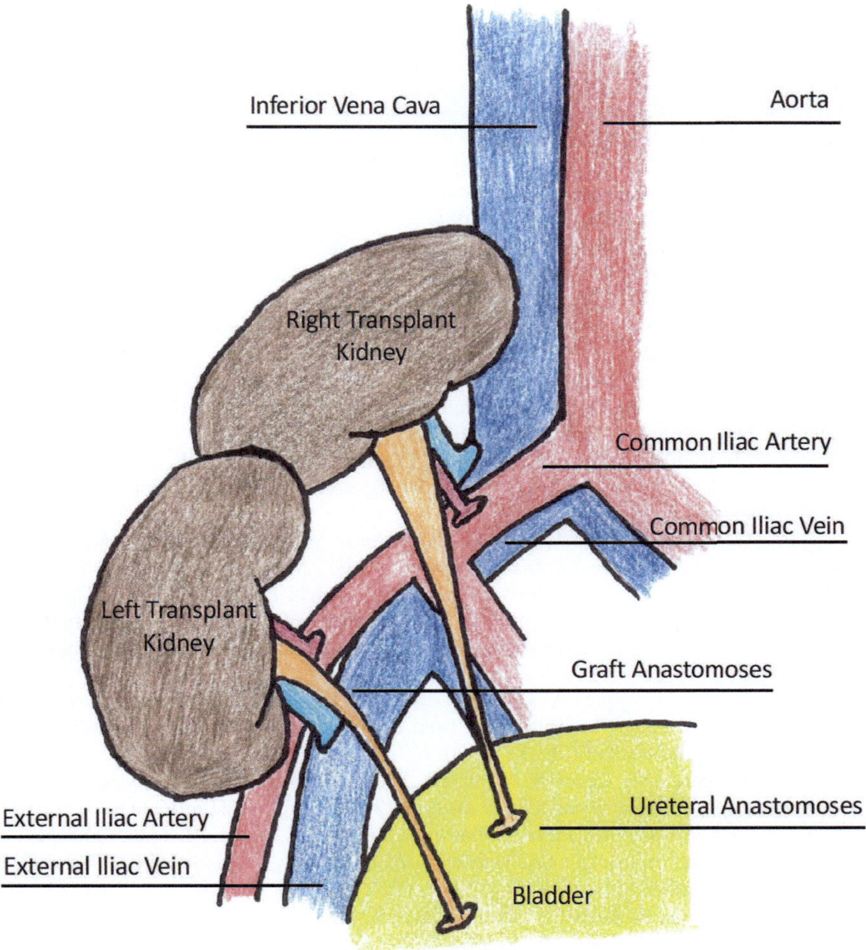

Fig. 4.1 Unilaterally positioned dual kidney allografts. The right kidney is placed superiorly and laterally, with its vessels anastomosed to the recipient inferior IVC/proximal common iliac vein and common iliac artery. After reperfusion, vascular clamps are placed on the external iliac vein and external iliac artery, allowing continued perfusion and drainage of the right kidney. In contrast, the left kidney vessels are anastomosed to the recipient's external iliac vein and artery. Separate ureteroneocystostomies are completed

increased number of anastomoses and increased operative time; however, the available data has not yet demonstrated a significant difference.

Disclosures R. Tamburrini and A. Bolognese report employment with the University of Wisconsin School of Medicine and Public Health.

Funding None.

References

1. Karpinski J, Lajoie G, Cattran D, Fenton S, Zaltzman J, Cardella C, et al. Outcome of kidney transplantation from high-risk donors is determined by both structure and function. Transplantation. 1999;67(8):1162–7.
2. Remuzzi G, Grinyo J, Ruggenenti P, Beatini M, Cole EH, Milford EL, et al. Early experience with dual kidney transplantation in adults using expanded donor criteria. Double kidney transplant group (DKG). J Am Soc Nephrol. 1999;10(12):2591–8.
3. Perico N, Ruggenenti P, Scalamogna M, Remuzzi G. Tackling the shortage of donor kidneys: how to use the best that we have. Am J Nephrol. 2003;23(4):245–59.
4. Lee CM, Carter JT, Weinstein RJ, Pease HM, Scandling JD, Pavalakis M, et al. Dual kidney transplantation: older donors for older recipients11No competing interests declared. J Am Coll Surg. 1999;189(1):82–91.
5. Lu AD, Carter JT, Weinstein RJ, Prapong W, Salvatierra O, Dafoe DC, et al. Excellent outcome in recipients of dual kidney transplants: a report of the first 50 dual kidney transplants at Stanford University. Arch Surg. 1999;134(9):971–5. discussion 5–6
6. Johnson LB, Kuo PC, Dafoe DC, Schweitzer EJ, Alfrey EJ, Klassen DK, et al. Double adult renal allografts: a technique for expansion of the cadaveric kidney donor pool. Surgery. 1996;120(4):580–4.
7. Remuzzi G, Cravedi P, Perna A, Dimitrov BD, Turturro M, Locatelli G, et al. Long-term outcome of renal transplantation from older donors. N Engl J Med. 2006;354(4):343–52.
8. Gandolfini I, Buzio C, Zanelli P, Palmisano A, Cremaschi E, Vaglio A, et al. The kidney donor profile index (KDPI) of marginal donors allocated by standardized pretransplant donor biopsy assessment: distribution and association with graft outcomes. Am J Transplant. 2014;14(11):2515–25.
9. Ekser B, Furian L, Broggiato A, Silvestre C, Pierobon ES, Baldan N, et al. Technical aspects of unilateral dual kidney transplantation from expanded criteria donors: experience of 100 patients. Am J Transplant. 2010;10(9):2000–7.
10. Cocco A, Shahrestani S, Cocco N, Hameed A, Yuen L, Ryan B, et al. Dual kidney transplant techniques: a systematic review. Clin Transpl. 2017;31(8) https://doi.org/10.1111/ctr.13016.
11. Gill J, Cho YW, Danovitch GM, Wilkinson A, Lipshutz G, Pham PT, et al. Outcomes of dual adult kidney transplants in the United States: an analysis of the OPTN/UNOS database. Transplantation. 2008;85(1):62–8.
12. Khalid U, Asderakis A, Rana T, Szabo L, Chavez R, Ilham MA, et al. Dual kidney transplantation offers a valuable source for kidneys with good functional outcome. Transplant Proc. 2016;48(6):1981–5.
13. Lee KW, Park JB, Cha SR, Lee SH, Chung YJ, Yoo H, et al. Dual kidney transplantation offers a safe and effective way to use kidneys from deceased donors older than 70 years. BMC Nephrol. 2020;21(1):3.
14. Lu AD, Carter JT, Weinstein RJ, Stratta RJ, Taylor RJ, Bowers VD, et al. Outcome in recipients of dual kidney transplants: an analysis of the dual registry patients. Transplantation. 2000;69(2):281–5.
15. Moore PS, Farney AC, Sundberg AK, Rohr MS, Hartmann EL, Iskandar SS, et al. Dual kidney transplantation: a case-control comparison with single kidney transplantation from standard and expanded criteria donors. Transplantation. 2007;83(12):1551–6.

Chapter 5
Assessing Risk Before Kidney Transplantation: Does Frailty Matter?

Laura Maursetter

Introduction

There are many factors to consider when determining a patient's eligibility for a kidney transplant. Transplant programs aim to provide patients with the opportunity to improve their quality of life while appropriately assigning the scarce kidney resource most effectively to benefit the population. Contemporary knowledge has evolved to better understand the impact of fragility on the kidney transplant candidacy equation.

Patient History

A 68-year-old male veteran attends a rural dialysis unit three times weekly for the last 1.5 years. He developed ESKD due to urinary retention from severe benign prostatic hypertrophy. Currently, the patient lives alone in his home after his wife died 1 year ago. He enjoys cooking, woodworking, and spending time with his nearby family. He can walk to get his mail at the end of the block, but he no longer uses his stairs for fear of falling (denies ever falling). His family gifted him a house cleaning service every other week, so he no longer performs these tasks.

Given that his kids live nearby, he eats dinner with them most evenings. He is not interested in home dialysis options due to the stress that this burden of care would cause. He has a history of hypertension that has been well controlled for the last 22 years, a colon polyp that was non-dysplastic on a colonoscopy 2 years ago, and a 10-pack year history of tobacco exposure but no current use. He had a myocardial

L. Maursetter (✉)
University of Wisconsin–Madison School of Medicine and Public Health, Madison, WI, USA
e-mail: lmaursetter@medicine.wisc.edu

© The Author(s), under exclusive license to Springer Nature Switzerland AG 2022

F. Aziz, S. Parajuli (eds.), *Complications in Kidney Transplantation*,
https://doi.org/10.1007/978-3-031-13569-9_5

25

infarction 8 years ago with stent placement and denied any symptoms of angina. During his annual interdisciplinary care conference, his candidacy for a kidney transplant was brought up, and you were asked if he should be evaluated.

Question 1
Would you refer him for kidney transplant evaluation?

A. Yes. He does not have any contraindications to transplant.
B. Maybe. I would need more information.
C. No. He is not a candidate for transplant.

The correct answer is B.

This patient has many health concerns that would need further investigation before approval for transplant. Apart from his comorbidities, he has several factors that could signal a decline in functional status, but many of these are situational such as eliminating housework due to family gifts or limited stair ambulation due to living alone. We would need more information before we can assess his candidacy for transplant.

Question 2
Which of the following factors would have the most negative impact on his transplant outcome?

A. Colon polyp.
B. Cardiovascular history.
C. Frailty.
D. Duration of dialysis.
E. Age.

The correct answer is C.

It might come as a surprise that frailty has a more significant impact than the other factors on this list. Many studies have been conducted and confirmed that frailty is an important "vital sign" to consider when making health decisions, including transplantation. One study measured frailty to be associated not only with advanced age but also a lower rate of preemptive transplant, longer duration of delayed graft function, and longer length of hospital stay [1]. Frailty plays such a prominent role that comorbidity only factors into mortality in those who are not frail [2]. This fact should make frailty the initial subject of discussion when a transplant is being considered.

Discussion

Frailty is defined as a decrease in physiologic reserve which limits one's ability to recover from physiological stress [3]. There are five domains thought to be most impacted by frailty (Fig. 5.1), but other areas such as cognition also show an association [4]. Frailty increases a person's vulnerability to health problems, including

Fig. 5.1 The five domains of frailty

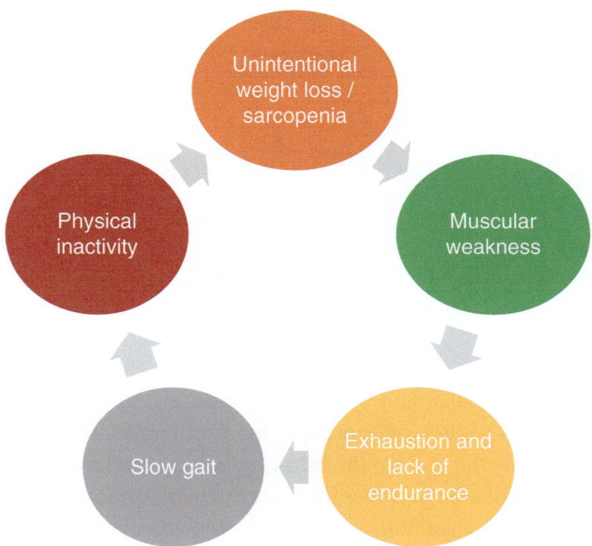

increased dependence on others and increased mortality when exposed to stress [5]. The negative health outcomes associated with this syndrome include a 1.8–2.3 fold increase in mortality, a higher risk of decline of being able to perform activities of daily living, more hospitalizations, physical limitation, falls, and fractures [6].

While the presence of frailty increases with age, comorbid conditions can have an even bigger impact. Kidney disease has a significant relationship with frailty as 15–21% of those with advanced chronic kidney disease (CKD) are frail compared to 3–6% in the general population [7]. This is even more substantial in ESKD, where approximately 73% are found to be frail [8, 9]. Sarcopenia and malnutrition are consistently seen in frail CKD patients. This can stem from the uremic milieu, dietary restrictions needed to control phosphorus, or decreased Vit D analogs which can affect muscle metabolism [10]. Despite the prominence of frailty in the kidney disease population, nephrologists poorly predict frailty. In one study, frailty was misclassified in 36% of dialysis patients by nephrologists [11]. Because nephrologists are the gateway to kidney transplantation and frailty is known to negatively affect this process, proper classification is imperative for patients to have the opportunity to be appropriately referred to transplant.

Among other fields, such as oncology, frailty has become a front-line factor in determining options for therapeutic intervention. This has not been the case in nephrology. Outcomes of patients receiving dialysis have been linked to frailty, but tools to assess the fragility of a patient are not consistently used to determine or advise patients on options for starting or continuing dialysis therapy [12]. Transplant centers have increased their use of frailty tools, but there has been debate about which tool is optimal. At this point, research in frailty has not yielded consistent data, and, as a result, a unified approach to frailty assessment is lacking. Because of the inconsistent approach, there has not been agreement about a level of frailty

Table 5.1 The information asked on a variety of the frequently used tools to measure frailty

Physical	Cognition	Situational	Subjective
Timed walk	Clock drawing	Tasks needing assistance	Exhaustion/fatigue
Weight loss	Mood	Living situation	Weakness
Grip strength	Memory	Mobility aids	Depression
Chair rise			Energy expenditure
Get up and go timed			Health level
Flight of stairs			Independence
Balance testing			

Adapted from frailtyscience.org/frailty-assessment-instruments

where the transplant would be contraindicated [10]. Using the Clinical Frailty Score (CFS) as a screening tool and the Frailty Phenotype assessment for further investigation seems to have the best predictive correlation for kidney transplant outcomes, but this has been met with disagreement among centers [10]. Efficiency, accuracy, equipment availability are all factors to consider when implementing screening tools. That said, determining a unified approach is necessary to be able to consistently assess patients across transplant centers and to be able to compare research outcomes. Table 5.1 was created to provide readers with the type of information gathered by tools to better understand what may be included in the measurement.

Although ESKD tends to worsen frailty, a transplant can improve frailty in the properly selected population [13, 14]. Characteristics of those who benefit most have been difficult to decipher. One study showed that 19.8% of their transplanted population was frail at the time of transplant. Frailty among this group increased at 1 month but improved from baseline by 3 months. This signals that frailty is a factor that maybe reversible [14]. Another study used the Groningen Frailty Indicator (GFI) showed less promise. Most transplant patients (71%) did not change from baseline frailty scores, with 19.3% of non-frail patients becoming frail and 9.7% of frail patients improving to a non-frail status [15]. The determination of which factors are most influential in predicting frailty improvement has not been a conclusive and will require further evaluation.

The reason to proceed with caution in a frail patient is that it can lead to more delayed graft function, longer hospitalization, and more readmissions in addition to increased mortality [16]. Compared to the time of evaluation, those who worsened their frailty scores while on the transplant waitlist had worse outcomes than those who remained stable or improved [16]. Unfortunately, only about 54% of waitlisted candidates remain stable over their wait time [17]. Thus, the KDIGO Pre-Transplant Guidelines have included a recommendation that frailty should be measured at the time of evaluation but also periodically once on the waiting list as it can play a significant role in outcomes [4].

There is limited data about the prolonged effects of frailty after kidney transplantation apart from whether frailty increases or decreases and the graft outcome. For example, frailty has been associated with post-transplant immunosenescence; therefore, a person's level of frailty may need to be taken into consideration post-transplant to properly titrate immunosuppressive medications [16]. Presently, no studies are looking at opportunistic infections in kidney transplant recipients related to the level of frailty. Given the known cognitive impact fragility can have a study of 665 patients aimed to assess cognitive changes over time. This group was followed for 4 years post-transplant, of which 15% were frail at the time of transplant. Initially, there was an improvement in cognition seen among all recipients by 3 months, but at 4 years, cognitive scores were lower among the frail than non-frail recipients [17]. This provides insight into the widespread impact that frailty can have on quality of life factors and is important to uncover for appropriate informed consent before transplant. In addition, data has shown that polypharmacy is present in kidney transplant recipients and is associated with frailty for various reasons. Of the 211 recipients studied, there were 9.4 medications prescribed on average. For those on 10 or more medications, there was 2.5 times the rate of frailty than those who were not even after adjusting for cofounders [18].

While mitigating frailty has not been a focus among the nephrology community, translating work from other fields has shown that frail elderly adults can show improvement. A study of frail elderly adults who underwent high-intensity interval training had a positive impact on frailty in as little as 6 weeks [19]. In addition, programs that aim to incorporate nutritional interventions with rehabilitation improved frailty in patients with hip fractures [20]. This should be a call to action for all areas of nephrology as impacting frailty can improve outcomes in transplant but also in dialysis patients. A variety of studies have looked at various exercise models for CKD patients, both supervised and unsupervised, and have improved frailty [21]. This concept has implications in transplant where the idea of prehabilitation for frail patients prior to transplant could be considered as a part of a requirement for the transplant waitlist [22].

Frailty is a prominent characteristic in the CKD population, making it an important factor in kidney transplant. The impact of frailty on transplant outcomes, which seems to be more important than comorbidities, makes measuring the degree of frailty and identification of patients who are most likely to improve after transplantation of utmost importance. Education and interventions aimed at preventing or improving frailty is important as these efforts are likely to have a positive impact on all kidney disease patients.

References

1. Quint EE, et al. Frailty and kidney transplantation: a systematic review and meta-analysis. Transplant Direct. 2021;7(6):e701.
2. Perez Fernandez M, et al. Comorbidity, frailty, and waitlist mortality among kidney transplant candidates of all ages. Am J Nephrol. 2019;49(2):103–10.
3. Xue QL. The frailty syndrome: definition and natural history. Clin Geriatr Med. 2011;27(1):1–15.
4. Chadban SJ, et al. KDIGO clinical practice guideline on the evaluation and Management of Candidates for kidney transplantation. Transplantation. 2020;104(4S1 Suppl. 1):S11–S103.

5. Rodriguez Manas L, et al. Key messages for a frailty prevention and management policy in Europe from the Advantage Joint Action consortium. J Nutr Health Aging. 2018;22(8):892–7.
6. Vermeiren S, et al. Frailty and the prediction of negative health outcomes: a meta-analysis. J Am Med Dir Assoc. 2016;17(12):1163 e1–1163 e17.
7. Chowdhury R, et al. Frailty and chronic kidney disease: a systematic review. Arch Gerontol Geriatr. 2017;68:135–42.
8. Bao Y, et al. Frailty, dialysis initiation, and mortality in end-stage renal disease. Arch Intern Med. 2012;172(14):1071–7.
9. Tonelli M, et al. Systematic review: kidney transplantation compared with dialysis in clinically relevant outcomes. Am J Transplant. 2011;11(10):2093–109.
10. Wu HHL, Woywodt A, Nixon AC. Frailty and the potential kidney transplant recipient: time for a more holistic assessment? Kidney360. 2020;1(7):685–90.
11. Salter ML, et al. Perceived frailty and measured frailty among adults undergoing hemodialysis: a cross-sectional analysis. BMC Geriatr. 2015;15:52.
12. Sy J, Johansen KL. The impact of frailty on outcomes in dialysis. Curr Opin Nephrol Hypertens. 2017;26(6):537–42.
13. McAdams-DeMarco MA, et al. Frailty and Postkidney transplant health-related quality of life. Transplantation. 2018;102(2):291–9.
14. McAdams-DeMarco MA, et al. Changes in frailty after kidney transplantation. J Am Geriatr Soc. 2015;63(10):2152–7.
15. Quint EE, et al. Transitions in frailty state after kidney transplantation. Langenbeck's Arch Surg. 2020;405(6):843–50.
16. Perez-Saez MJ, et al. Frailty and kidney transplant candidates. Nefrologia (Engl Ed). 2021;41(3):237–43.
17. Chu W, et al. The relationship between depression and frailty in community-dwelling older people: a systematic review and meta-analysis of 84,351 older adults. J Nurs Scholarsh. 2019;51(5):547–59.
18. Kosoku A, et al. Hyperpolypharmacy and frailty in kidney transplant recipients. Transplant Proc. 2022;54:367–73.
19. Losa-Reyna J, et al. Effect of a short multicomponent exercise intervention focused on muscle power in frail and pre frail elderly: a pilot trial. Exp Gerontol. 2019;115:114–21.
20. Inoue T, et al. Undernutrition, sarcopenia, and frailty in fragility hip fracture: advanced strategies for improving clinical outcomes. Nutrients. 2020;12(12):3743.
21. Lorenz EC, et al. Frailty in CKD and transplantation. Kidney Int Rep. 2021;6(9):2270–80.
22. McAdams-DeMarco MA, Chu NM, Segev DL. Frailty and long-term post-kidney transplant outcomes. Curr Transplant Rep. 2019;6(1):45–51.

Chapter 6
A Patient with CFH Mutation

Waleed Zafar and Prince Mohan Anand

Introduction

We present a patient with end-stage kidney disease (ESKD) due to thrombotic microangiopathy (TMA). The case illustrates the importance of early diagnosis and treatment with complement blocking agents. We discuss the use of genetic testing and its value in post-transplant management.

Patient History

A 38-year-old female with end-stage kidney disease (ESKD) on hemodialysis (HD) presented to the transplant clinic for kidney transplant evaluation. She recently moved from another state to stay with her family after being diagnosed with ESKD and starting HD. Her illness had started with a cough, weakness, and some shortness of breath. She was not taking any medications before the symptoms started and started taking an over the counter cough syrup. She attributed her symptoms to depression related to an inability to go out due to the Covid-19 pandemic. She went to an emergency department after her shortness of breath worsened.

W. Zafar
Geisinger Medical Center, Danville, PA, USA
e-mail: wzafar@geisinger.edu

P. M. Anand (✉)
Medical University of South Carolina, Charleston, SC, USA
e-mail: mohanp@musc.edu

© The Author(s), under exclusive license to Springer Nature Switzerland AG 2022

F. Aziz, S. Parajuli (eds.), *Complications in Kidney Transplantation*,
https://doi.org/10.1007/978-3-031-13569-9_6

Per hospital records, the patient was admitted due to a 1 week history of progressive shortness of breath, orthopnea, chills, nausea, multiple episodes of vomiting, diarrhea, productive cough, and new-onset lower extremity edema. There was no rash, joint pains, or fever. At the time of admission, she endorsed the recent use of Ibuprofen but denied excessive or long-term use. She endorsed occasional use of alcohol but denied any drug use. She tested positive for methamphetamines at admission (thought to be from the use of cough syrup). She was never a smoker with no known drug allergies. Family history was significant for hypertension. No significant family history of kidney disease was documented. Her weight was 61.4 kg, and her blood pressure was 150/109 mmHg on admission. Physical exam was remarkable for 2+ lower extremity edema. Labs were significant for metabolic acidosis (pH 7.13), bicarbonate 15 mEq/L, lactate 5.6 mmol/L, sodium 123 mEq/L, potassium 4.2 mEq/L, blood urea nitrogen 51 mg/dL, creatinine 8.3 mg/dL, blood glucose 336 mEq/L, total protein 6.1 g/dL, albumin 2.9 g/dL, normal liver enzymes and CK, white count 12.2 K/mm^3, hemoglobin 7.2 g/dL, platelets 331 K/mm^3, and PTH 656 pg/mL. Pro-BNP was greater than 175,000, with chest X-ray showing pulmonary edema and bilateral pleural effusions. She tested negative for Covid by PCR. Urinalysis was significant for 3+ proteinuria, 3+ hematuria, and 11–20 RBC/hpf. Renal ultrasound showed mildly echogenic kidneys but no hydronephrosis. The hepatitis panel was negative.

Hospital records indicated that she was treated with broad-spectrum antibiotics IV (vancomycin and ceftriaxone) with initial concern for drug-induced endocarditis. Her blood pressure was controlled with amlodipine, carvedilol, and hydralazine. Subsequent workup was negative for ANA, ANCA, anti-GBM, HIV, RA, and SPEP. Serum C3 level was reduced while C4 level was normal. She underwent a kidney biopsy that showed thrombotic microangiopathy (TMA) (Figs. 6.1 and 6.2). In the setting of oliguric AKI, she was started on hemodialysis via a temporary dialysis catheter. She did not receive plasmapheresis.

Fig. 6.1 Kidney biopsy low power (H&E stain)

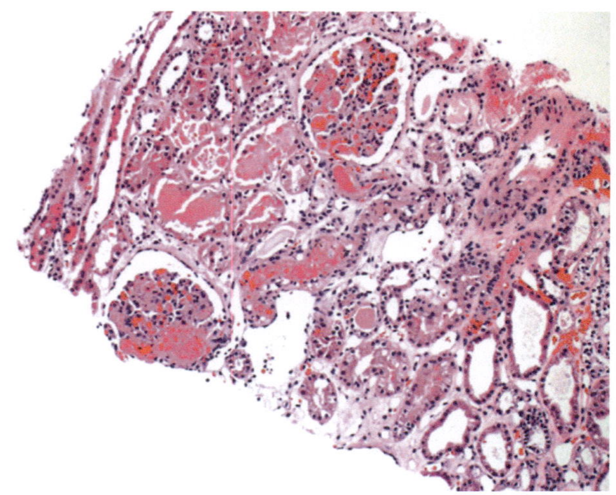

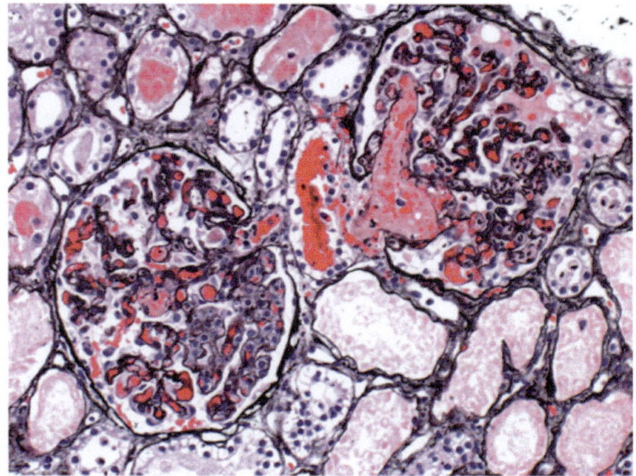

Fig. 6.2 Kidney biopsy high power (Silver+PAS stain)

Question 1

In addition to the above, what other treatment should have been offered?

A. Plasma exchange.
B. Steroids and Mycophenolate mofetil (MMF).
C. Rituximab.
D. Eculizumab.

The correct answer is D.

The patient has activation of the complement pathway with a low C3 level. Her kidney biopsy showed complement-mediated TMA (CM-TMA) [1]. Several studies have shown that early treatment with Eculizumab in CM-TMA can improve renal function [2]. Plasma exchange, mycophenolic acid, and steroids are used with some success in C3 glomerulopathy [3, 4]. Rituximab can be used if an autoantibody activates the complement [5].

Patient Course

A second kidney biopsy performed about 5 months after the onset of initial illness showed thrombotic microangiopathy characterized by fibrinoid necrosis of the glomerular hilar arterioles, mesangiolytic changes, and obliterative edematous intimal thickening of interlobular-sized arteries. Extensive glomerular basement membrane ischemic wrinkling with associated subendothelial lucency was seen on electron microscopy. No immune-complex deposits, fibrillary material, or amyloid were seen. Capillary wall disruption, fibrin deposition, or cellular crescents were not present.

Question 2

Before listing for transplant, what tests/consults will you order?

A. Renal genetic panel.
B. Hematology consult.
C. Complement functional assay.
D. All the above.

The correct answer is D.

You want to ensure genetic testing and complement functional assays are ordered for this patient to find the underlying reason for complement activation.

Subsequent Clinical Course

The patient underwent genetic testing that showed the presence of an autosomal dominant heterozygous pathogenic variant in the CFH gene (CFH: c.3628C > T (p.Arg1210Cys) associated with complement factor H deficiency (decreasing CFH binding to C3b/C3d), a C3 glomerulopathy, putting the patient at risk for CM-TMA [6]. She was evaluated by hematology, and a family history of macular degeneration in her father was noted. Pre-approved eculizumab was obtained, and all the preventative vaccinations were done (Pneumovax, Meningococcal conjugate, and Serogroup B meningococcal vaccines).

Discussion

Factor H is part of the alternative pathway preventing uncontrolled C3 activation and tissue damage [7]. Mutations in the FH gene are associated with age-related macular degeneration, aHUS, and membranoproliferative glomerulonephritis type II (MPGN 2) [7]. aHUS accounts for about 10% of all HUS cases, with 50% progressing to an end-stage renal disease requiring renal replacement therapy [8]. Genetic aHUS accounts for an estimated 60% of all aHUS [9]. As Norris et al. have noted, pathogenic variants in C3, CD46, CFB, CFH, CFHR5, CFI, THBD, or VTN are typically inherited in an autosomal dominant manner with reduced penetrance. DGKE gene-associated variants are usually inherited in an autosomal recessive manner. In contrast, deletions of CFHR3/CFHR1 and CFHR1/CFHR4 are inherited autosomal recessive [9]. It has been suggested that both genetic predisposition and a precipitating event are required to develop sporadic and familial aHUS [8]. In one analysis of 62 patients with CFH gene mutation with aHUS, including 32 patients thought to have familial risk, only 34% had remission (6% complete remission) while 28% progressed to ESKD and 38% died [8]. Genetic abnormalities in complement genes lead to uncontrolled activation of the alternative complement pathway and endothelial damage [6]. Without using complement inhibitor eculizumab, the prognosis for aHUS is poor even after kidney transplantation since there is a high risk of recurrence. Plasmapheresis offers minimal benefits for transplant survival [10, 11]. During Eculizumab therapy, complement activity measurement and disease activity parameters, including haptoglobin and lactate dehydrogenase serum levels and platelet count, are recommended [12].

References

1. Scully M, Cataland S, Coppo P, et al. International working group for thrombotic thrombocytopenic purpura: consensus on the standardization of terminology in thrombotic thrombocytopenic purpura and related thrombotic microangiopathies. J Thromb Haemost. 2017;15:312–22.
2. Menne J, Delmas Y, Fakhouri F, et al. Outcomes in patients with atypical hemolytic uremic syndrome treated with eculizumab in a long term observational study. BMC Nephrol. 2019;20:125.
3. Smith RJH, Appel GB, Blom AM, Cook HT, D'Agati VD, Fakhouri F, et al. C3 glomerulopathy: understanding a rare complement-driven renal disease. Nat Rev Nephrol. 2019;15:129–43.
4. Riedl M, Thorner P, Licht C. C3 glomerulopathy. Pediatr Nephrol. 2017;32:43–57.
5. Sun F, Wang X, Wu W, et al. TMA secondary to SLE: rituximab improves overall but not renal survival. Clin Rheumatol. 2018;37:213–8.
6. Duineveld C, Verhave JC, Berger SP, van de Kar NCAJ, Wetzels JFM. Living donor kidney transplantation in atypical hemolytic uremic syndrome: a case series. Am J Kid Dis. 2017;70(6):770–7.
7. Pickering MC, de Jorge EG, Martinez-Barricarte R, Recalde S, Garcia-Layana A, Rose KL, Moss J, Walport MJ, Cook HT, de Córdoba SR, Botto M. Spontaneous hemolytic uremic syndrome triggered by complement factor H lacking surface recognition domains. J Exp Med. 2007;204(6):1249–56.
8. Noris M, Caprioli J, Bresin E, et al. Relative role of genetic complement abnormalities in sporadic and familial aHUS and their impact on clinical phenotype. Clin J Am Soc Nephrol. 2010;5:1844–59.
9. Noris M, Bresin E, Mele C, Remuzzi G. Genetic atypical hemolytic-uremic syndrome. In: GeneReviews®. Seattle, Seattle (WA): University of Washington; 1993.
10. Legendre CM, Licht C, Muus P, Greenbaum LA, Babu S, Bedrosian C, et al. Terminal complement inhibitor eculizumab in atypical hemolytic-uremic syndrome. N Engl J Med. 2013;368:2169–81.
11. Le Quintrec M, Zuber J, Moulin B, et al. Complement genes strongly predict recurrence and graft outcome in adult renal transplant recipients with atypical hemolytic and uremic syndrome. Am J Transplant. 2013;13(3):663–75.
12. Cugno M, Gualtierott R, Possenti I, et al. Complement functional tests for monitoring eculizumab treatment in patients with atypical hemolytic uremic syndrome. J Thromb Haemost. 2014;12(9):1440–8.

Chapter 7
Deceased Donor with Multiple Arteries

Adam M. Kressel and Elliot I. Grodstein

Introduction

Variations in kidney arterial vasculature have been reported in approximately 20–50% of patients [1, 2]. While short-term complications may be increased in recipients of allografts with altered anatomy, long-term graft and patient outcomes remain comparable [3]. In this case presentation, we describe the surgical management of a deceased donor kidney transplant with an accessory artery and review the current literature.

Patient History

The recipient is a 64-year-old male with a history of hypertension, non-insulin-dependent diabetes, hypothyroidism, cirrhosis without portal hypertension secondary to Hepatitis C, and end-stage kidney disease from polycystic kidney disease. He has been on intermittent hemodialysis for 7 years via an upper extremity arteriovenous fistula and makes little to no urine. At the time of transplant, his body mass

A. M. Kressel
Division of Transplant Surgery, Department of Surgery, Northwell Health, Manhasset, NY, USA
e-mail: AKressel2@northwell.edu

E. I. Grodstein (✉)
Division of Transplant Surgery, Department of Surgery, Northwell Health, Manhasset, NY, USA

Donald and Barbara Zucker School of Medicine at Hofstra / Northwell Health, Hempstead, NY, USA
e-mail: egrodstein@northwell.edu

© The Author(s), under exclusive license to Springer Nature Switzerland AG 2022

F. Aziz, S. Parajuli (eds.), *Complications in Kidney Transplantation*, https://doi.org/10.1007/978-3-031-13569-9_7

"

index was 27.7 kg/m^2 and creatinine was 9.68 mg/dL. The donor organ was a right kidney imported from a 50-year-old male. After verifying all pertinent information, the patient was brought to the operating room for transplantation.

Question 1

What is the most common vascular finding in kidney transplant donors?

A. Single renal artery.
B. Left renal accessory artery.
C. Right renal accessory artery.
D. Bilateral renal accessory arteries.
E. Proximal renal artery branching.

The correct answer is A.

While normal, single artery inflow to each kidney is found in a majority of patients (63.1%), a left accessory renal artery is encountered in 21.9% of patients, a right accessory renal artery is identified in 15.9% of patients, and bilateral accessory arteries found in 4.5% of patients [4]. Additionally, early branching (<2.5 mm from the aorta) is seen in 10.5–13.7% cases [4]. Other studies go further and describe multiple other kidney anatomic variations based on center experience [5]. Understanding the aberrant anatomy of the kidney is imperative given that these are end arteries; inadvertent ligation can cause corresponding kidney ischemia. The draining veins, in contrast, can be ligated without consequence.

Hospital Course

The patient was brought to the operating room, and the donor's kidney was prepared on the back table. Two separate renal arteries were identified emanating from the hilum, one appearing to perfuse mainly the superior pole of the allograft and one perfusing the inferior pole. Both were dissected free from fatty attachments. There was one renal vein and one ureter identified. In the recipient, the transplantation proceeded in the usual fashion. After the venous anastomosis was performed, the right external iliac artery was exposed, and proximal and distal control was obtained. An arteriotomy was performed with a #15 scalpel and completed with a 5 mm vascular punch, and the superior pole artery was anastomosed using a 6–0 proline suture in a running fashion. At this point, the kidney was allowed to re-perfuse to determine the contribution of each donor artery. The lower 1/3 of the kidney remained ischemic, so a separate arterial anastomosis was made for the second artery. The inferior pole renal artery was anastomosed in a similar fashion using 7–0 Prolene suture due to its smaller size. At this point, the kidney appeared to be adequately perfused. The patient tolerated this procedure well and recovered appropriately. Anti-thymocyte globulin was used for induction, furosemide and mannitol were given before the arterial anastomosis, and a double-J ureteral stent was left in place traversing the neoureterocystostomy. The patient recovered well postoperatively and was discharged home 2 days later, no longer requiring hemodialysis.

Question 2

What is the most common postoperative vascular complication of kidney transplant when a graft with multiple arteries is utilized?

A. Anastomotic leak.
B. Renal vein thrombosis.
C. Renal artery thrombosis.
D. Aneurysm.
E. Ischemia.

The correct answer is C.

In patients with single renal arteries, the published rate of renal artery thrombosis is 0.8%, increasing to 4.3% in patients with multiple renal arteries [6]. Renal vein thrombosis is less frequent at 2.1%.

Discussion

Numerous vascular variants are encountered in kidney transplantation [7], each with its management and subsequent complications. The most well-known technique is the Carrel patch (Fig. 7.1), in which a deceased donor artery(ies) is/are removed along with a cuff of the aorta and anastomosed to the recipient, minimizing the manipulation to the actual vessel(s) [8]. Multiple arteries can be re-perfused by using a Carrel patch by sewing in a single "patch" anastomosis. If an artery is inadvertently transected from a Carrell patch (either inadvertently during procurement or purposefully in the case of focal arterial disease), it can either be reimplanted or implanted separately. Small arteries (<2 mm) to the upper pole of the kidney can often be ligated, whereas close consideration needs to be made to reconstruct small arteries to the lower pole of the kidney. These arteries often perfuse the ureter, and ligation can lead to ureteral complications.

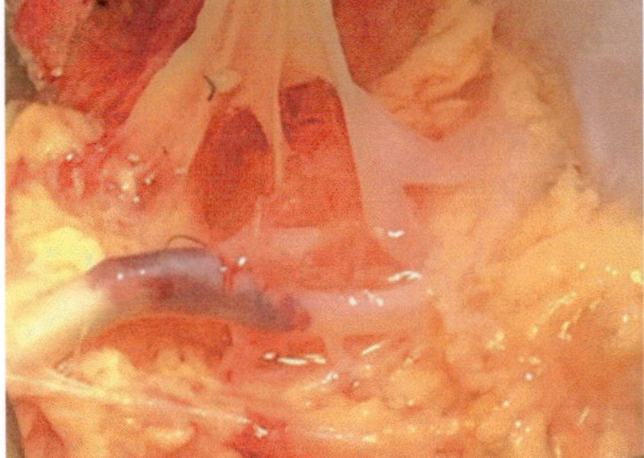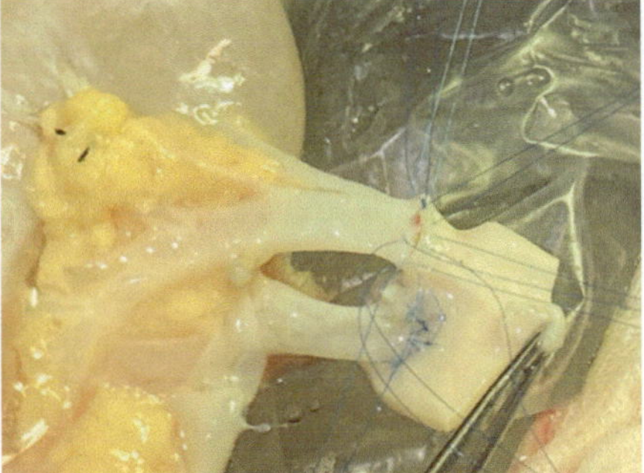

Fig. 7.1 A focally injured renal arterial segment is resected, and the distal artery is reattached onto a Carrel patch in a recipient with atherosclerotic iliac arteries

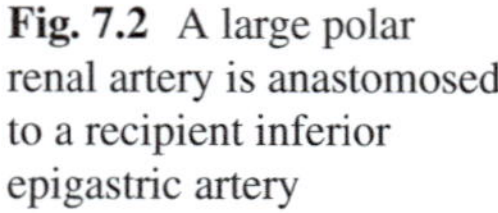

Fig. 7.2 A large polar renal artery is anastomosed to a recipient inferior epigastric artery

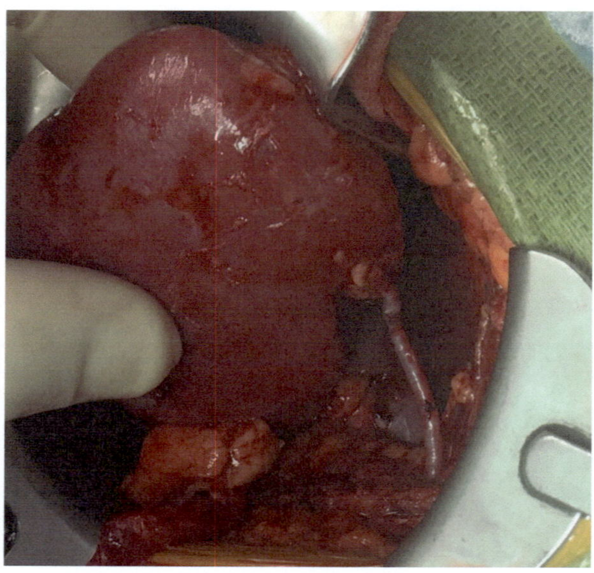

Various end-to-side and end-to-end anastomoses have all been described between the donor vasculature and various recipient blood vessels (e.g., common/external iliac and hypogastric arteries) [9]. In a graft with two renal arteries, the larger of the two can be anastomosed end-to-end to the hypogastric artery with the smaller anastomosed end-to-side in standard fashion to the external iliac artery. Other options for multiple arterial anastomoses are reimplanting a smaller polar renal artery in the main artery in an end-to-side fashion. The inferior epigastric artery can be utilized for aberrant donor anatomy as well (Fig. 7.2), especially if the iliac vessels are heavily calcified with atherosclerotic disease.

A conjoined side-to-side "pants-type" anastomosis can be performed if the donor graft has two similarly sized renal arteries in close proximity. In this case, arteries are reconstructed ex vivo to have a single common lumen, thus obviating the need for two separate arterial anastomoses during transplant. This technique has the added benefit of reducing warm ischemic time. Finally, autogenous recipient autografts or cadaveric/donor allografts can be used to create numerous other combinations for vascular reconstruction to optimize renal arterial inflow.

Of course, a combination of these techniques may be required based on each patient's unique anatomy, with care taken to minimize total ischemic time.

References

1. Recto C, et al. Renal artery variations: a 20.782 kidneys review. Ital J Anat Embryol. 2019;124:153–63.
2. Munnusamy K, et al. Variations in branching pattern of renal artery in kidney donors using CT angiography. J Clin Diagnostic Res. 2016;10:AC01–3.

3. Zorgdrager M, Krikke C, Hofker SH, Leuvenink HGD, Pol RA. Multiple renal arteries in kidney transplantation: a systematic review and meta-analysis. Ann Transplant. 2016;21:469–78.
4. Song WH, et al. Quantitative analysis of renal arterial variations affecting the eligibility of catheter-based renal denervation using multi-detector computed tomography angiography. Sci Rep. 2020;10:1–9.
5. Lorenz EC, et al. Prevalence of renal artery and kidney abnormalities by computed tomography among healthy adults. Clin J Am Soc Nephrol. 2010;5:431–8.
6. Scheuermann U, et al. Influence of multiple donor renal arteries on the outcome and graft survival in deceased donor kidney transplantation. J Clin Med. 2021;10:4395.
7. Watson CJE, Harper SJF. Anatomical variation and its management in transplantation. Am J Transplant. 2015;15:1459–71.
8. Sade RM. Transplantation at 100 years: Alexis carrel, pioneer surgeon. Ann Thorac Surg. 2005;80:2415–8.
9. Novick AC, Magnusson M, Braun WE. Multiple-artery renal transplantation: emphasis on extracorporeal methods of donor arterial reconstruction. J Urol. 1979;122:731–5.

Chapter 8
Donor with a History of Nephrolithiasis

Sam Kant and Sami Alasfar

Introduction

Live donor kidney transplantation is the treatment of choice for patients with end-stage kidney disease. The rigorous live donor evaluation process is meant to protect live donors and provides a systematic way of determining and mitigating any specific risks. Nephrolithiasis, a risk factor for chronic kidney disease, is a problem that is frequently seen in potential live donors and requires detailed workup to ensure there is minimal or no long-term harm to donors.

Patient History

A 32-year-old man with a past medical history of nephrolithiasis is being considered a kidney donor for his wife, who has end-stage kidney disease (ESKD) secondary to anti-glomerular basement membrane disease and is currently on peritoneal dialysis. There is no family history of kidney disease or nephrolithiasis. Regarding the history of nephrolithiasis, he had one episode at the age of 20 years during his time at college, which required a visit to the local emergency room. He subsequently passed the stone spontaneously; however, he did not undergo stone analysis and had no further recurrence. He has a body mass index of 31 kg/m^2. He is a non-smoker and drinks alcohol infrequently (1 unit once a month).

S. Kant (✉) · S. Alasfar
Division of Nephrology, Department of Medicine, The Johns Hopkins University School of Medicine, Baltimore, MD, USA
e-mail: skant1@jhmi.edu; salasfa1@jhu.edu

© The Author(s), under exclusive license to Springer Nature Switzerland AG 2022
F. Aziz, S. Parajuli (eds.), *Complications in Kidney Transplantation*,
https://doi.org/10.1007/978-3-031-13569-9_8

His 5-year risk of developing ESKD as per the kidney failure risk equation is 0.67%. His estimated glomerular filtration rate as per the CKD-EPI creatinine, creatinine-cystatin C, and cystatin C equation is 107/102/100 mL/min/m². CT of the abdomen with intravenous contrast demonstrates the equal size and contrast enhancement of the kidneys with no evidence of stones. Immunogenetic workup reveals a 0/0/1 mismatch at HLA Loci A, B, and DR with negative flow cytometric crossmatch.

Question 1

What is the recommended next step?

A. Proceed with living kidney donation.
B. He is not a candidate for living kidney donation.
C. Proceed with a metabolic workup to identify and mitigate potential abnormalities related to stone formation.
D. Advise further weight loss before being considered for kidney donation.

The correct answer is C.

It is recommended that donors with a previous history of kidney stones undergo a comprehensive evaluation of nephrolithiasis [1]. In addition to a detailed medical and dietary history, laboratory tests such as a biochemical profile, parathyroid hormone (PTH), analysis of current stone, if available, along with metabolic risk profile based on 24-h urine collection (further below) should be completed. Contraindications to donation in the setting of the previous history of nephrolithiasis are further elucidated in the discussion section.

The patient underwent a metabolic workup including a PTH and 24-h urine collection, with results as below:

PTH: 35 pg/mL.
24 urine collection:
Urine volume: 2.7 L.
pH: 6
Sodium: 75 mEq/day.
Calcium: 150 mg/day.
Oxalate: 20 mg/day.
Citrate: 750 mg/day.
Uric acid: 522 mg/day.
Sulfate: 34 mEq/day.
Creatinine: 1600 mg/day.

Question 2

What would be the next step?

A. Decline candidacy for kidney donation.
B. Proceed with kidney donation after education for preventing nephrolithiasis in the future.
C. Genetic testing for cystine stones.
D. Repeat 24-h urine collection.

The correct answer is B.

Discussion

The practice of living donor kidney transplantation continues to grow and now constitutes ~30% of all kidney transplants done in the United States [2]. This has coincided with an increasing prevalence of nephrolithiasis worldwide, with an estimation of lifetime prevalence in men and women being 10% and 7%, respectively [3, 4]. Given the associated risk of developing ESRD, prospective donors with a history of nephrolithiasis or having incidental detection of kidney stones on radiologic imaging have been historically excluded from living kidney donation [5].

Given advances in understanding metabolic risk factors associated with nephrolithiasis and better endourologic techniques, various transplant centers and society guidelines have adopted a less stringent approach to donors with previous nephrolithiasis (symptomatic and asymptomatic). Based on a cohort study of ~2000 living kidney donors who underwent computed tomography (CT), 11% had stones on imaging, with 3% having past symptomatic kidney stones [1]. It has been increasingly recognized that while subjects in the general population with small asymptomatic stones of under 4 mm have a high incidence of future stone events, donors do not have the same risk (23% vs. 2% at 2 years follow-up) [6, 7]. Further, a large matched retrospective cohort study spanning over 8 years of follow-up data demonstrated that donors did not have higher rates of surgical interventions or hospital encounters related to kidney stones than the general population [8].

When it is identified that a prospective donor has a history of previous nephrolithiasis, further assessment may proceed based on the risk of recurrence of stones, along with thorough education regarding potential consequences of stone recurrence post-donation [9]. Patients younger than 40 years of age, with a previous history of frequent/recurrent stones and family history of kidney stones, would be considered to have a high lifetime risk of stone recurrence, while those older than 40 years, with no prior symptoms of kidney stones and/ or with kidney stones less than 15 mm, solitary and unilateral, would be considered low risk [10].

The Kidney Disease Improving Global Outcomes (KDIGO) 2017 clinical practice guidelines on evaluation and care of living kidney donors recommend the following for assessment of this population of prospective donors [9]:

1. Retrieval of information on stone analysis if available.
2. A detailed medical and dietary history with biochemistry panel, PTH (screen for primary hyperparathyroidism), and urinalysis.
3. Review available and/or obtain dedicated imaging studies to ascertain the stone burden.
4. Metabolic testing should consist of one or two 24-h urine collections obtained on a random diet and analyzed at minimum for total volume, pH, calcium, oxalate, uric acid, citrate, sodium, potassium, and creatinine.

Table 8.1 Conditions that may preclude kidney donation in the setting of nephrolithiasis

Bilateral kidney stones
Recurrent/multiple kidney stones
Nephrocalcinosis on radiologic imaging
Recurrent kidney stones despite appropriate treatment
Systemic conditions such as primary or enteric hyperoxaluria, distal renal tubular acidosis, and sarcoidosis
Stone types with high recurrence rates such as cysteine, struvite, and calcium oxalate stones in the setting of inflammatory bowel disease

Patients with a current small single stone <15 mm detected on imaging may be eligible to proceed with a donation if the following conditions are met [11]:

1. No hypercalciuria, hyperuricemia, or metabolic acidosis.
2. No cystinuria or hyperoxaluria.
3. No urinary tract infection.

The presence of bilateral kidney stones, multiple stones, and/or nephrocalcinosis would prevent pursuing donation [11–14]. Prospective donor stone types that have high recurrence rates and are difficult to prevent are also recommended to be excluded from donation; these include (Table 8.1):

1. Cysteine.
2. Struvite.
3. Calcium oxalate stones in the setting of inflammatory bowel disease.
4. Systemic disorders including primary or enteric hyperoxaluria, distal renal tubular acidosis, and sarcoidosis.
5. Recurrent stones despite appropriate treatment.

Once the prospective donor is cleared to proceed with a donation, biochemical indices and metabolic profile based on 24-h urine collection should guide extensive education and strategies to prevent stone recurrence. This should follow various evidence-based guidelines directed at the general population that includes various dietary and pharmacologic interventions [9].

There does not appear to be clear guidance on pursuing ex vivo ureteroscopic removal of stones from explanted donor kidneys before transplantation, but safety and success of the technique for this purpose have been reported [15]. Nephrolithiasis-related adverse events have occurred in recipients of transplants with stone remaining in situ [16].

In conclusion, pursuing kidney donation from donors with a history of nephrolithiasis should be considered to increase the availability of organs for which prolonged waitlist times continue. Careful screening and selection of this donor population are necessary, with many recommended tests to avoid inadvertent harm to both donor and recipient.

Disclosures S. Kant reports employment with the Johns Hopkins University. Sami Alasfar reports employment with the Johns Hopkins University; receiving research funding from CareDx and the World Health Organization (WHO).

Funding None.

References

1. Lorenz EC, Lieske JC, Vrtiska TJ, Krambeck AE, Li X, Bergstralh EJ, Melton LJ, Rule AD. Clinical characteristics of potential kidney donors with asymptomatic kidney stones. Nephrol Dial Transplant [Internet]. 2011;26(8):2695–700.
2. Organ procurement and transplantation network, national data. Accessed 20 Dec 2021. [Internet].
3. Curhan GC. nephrolithiasis. In: Kasper D, et al., editors. Harrison's principles of internal medicine, vol. 19e. New York, NY: McGraw-Hill Education; 2015.
4. Scales CD, Smith AC, Hanley JM, Saigal CS. Prevalence of kidney stones in the United States. Eur Urol [Internet]. 2012;62(1):160–5. Available from: https://www.clinicalkey.es/playcontent/1-s2.0-S0302283812004046
5. El-Zoghby ZM, Lieske JC, Foley RN, Bergstralh EJ, Li X, Melton LJ, Krambeck AE, Rule AD. Urolithiasis and the risk of ESRD. Clin J Am Soc Nephrol [Internet]. 2012;7(9):1409–15. Available from: http://cjasn.asnjournals.org/content/7/9/1409.abstract
6. Rizkala E, Coleman S, Tran C, Isac W, Flechner SM, Goldfarb D, Monga M. Stone disease in living-related renal donors: long-term outcomes for transplant donors and recipients. J Endourol [Internet]. 2013;27(12):152–1524. Available from: https://www.liebertpub.com/doi/abs/10.1089/end.2013.0203
7. Kang HW, Lee SK, Kim WT, Kim Y, Yun S, Lee S, Kim W. Natural history of asymptomatic renal stones and prediction of stone related events. J Urol [Internet]. 2013;189(5):1740–6. Available from: https://www.clinicalkey.es/playcontent/1-s2.0-S0022534712056224
8. Thomas SM, Lam NN, Welk BK, Nguan C, Huang A, Nash DM, Prasad GVR, Knoll GA, Koval JJ, Lentine KL, Kim SJ, Lok CE, Garg AX. Risk of kidney stones with surgical intervention in living kidney donors. Am J Transplant [Internet]. 2013;13(11):2935–44.
9. Lentine K, Kasiske B, Levey A, Adams P, Alberú J, Bakr M, Gallon L, Garvey C, Guleria S, Li P, Segev D, Taler S, Tanabe K, Wright L, Zeier M, Cheung M, Garg A. Summary of kidney disease: improving global outcomes (KDIGO) clinical practice guideline on the evaluation and care of living kidney donors. Transplantation [Internet]. 2017;101(8):1783–92. Available from: http://ovidsp.ovid.com/ovidweb.cgi?T=JS&NEWS=n&CSC=Y&PAGE=fulltext&D=ovft&AN=00007890-201708000-00014
10. Caring for Australians with renal impairment (CARI). The CARI guidelines: Clinical diagnosis of kidney stones. [Internet].
11. Delmonico F. A report of the Amsterdam forum on the care of the live kidney donor: data and medical guidelines. Transplantation [Internet]. 2005;79(6 Suppl):S53–66. Available from: https://www.ncbi.nlm.nih.gov/pubmed/15785361
12. Kälble T, Lucan M, Nicita G, Sells R, Revilla FJB, Wiesel M. EAU guidelines on renal transplantation. Eur Urol [Internet]. 2005;47(2):156–66. https://doi.org/10.1016/j.eururo.2004.02.009.
13. Richardson R, Connelly M, Dipchand C, Garg A, Ghanekar A, Houde I, Johnston O, Mainra R, McCarrell R, Mueller T, Nickerson P, Pippy C, Storsley L, Tinckam K, Wright L, Yilmaz S, Landsberg D. Kidney paired donation protocol for participating donors 2014. Transplantation.

2015;99(10 Suppl. 1):S1–S88. Available from: http://ovidsp.ovid.com/ovidweb.cgi?T=JS&N
EWS=n&CSC=Y&PAGE=fulltext&D=ovft&AN=00007890-201510001-00001

14. AST/ASTS/NATCO/UNOS joint societies work group. Evaluation of the living kidney donor—a consensus document from the AST/ASTS/NATCO/UNOS joint societies work group. [Internet].

15. Olsburgh J, Thomas K, Wong K, Bultitude M, Glass J, Rottenberg G, Silas L, Hilton R, Koffman G. Incidental renal stones in potential live kidney donors: prevalence, assessment and donation, including role of ex vivo ureteroscopy. BJU Int [Internet]. 2013;111(5):784–92. Available from: https://onlinelibrary.wiley.com/doi/abs/10.1111/j.1464-410X.2012.11572.x

16. Strang AM, Lockhart ME, Amling CL, Kolettis PN, Burns JR. Living renal donor allograft lithiasis: a review of stone related morbidity in donors and recipients. J Urol [Internet]. 2008;179(3):832–6. Available from: https://www.clinicalkey.es/playcontent/1-s2.0-S0022534707027528

Chapter 9
Case of Marginal Living Kidney Donor

James Alstott and Maha Mohamed

Introduction

Living kidney donation is the modality of choice for kidney replacement therapy for advanced Chronic Kidney Disease (CKD). While trends for living donation have increased as of 2019, living donor kidney transplants still represent a small part of the total number of kidney transplants performed each year [1]. Because live donation is an altruistic act, which does not provide any direct health benefit to the donor, it is imperative for risks of kidney donation, particularly the risks of subsequent CKD and End-Stage Kidney Disease (ESKD) be minimized by thorough patient selection. Herein we describe a case highlighting relevant and challenging aspects of living donor evaluation.

Case: An Obese Donor with Elevated Blood Pressure

A 55-year-old female presented for a living donor kidney evaluation. She was seeking kidney donation for her husband, who had ESKD due to focal segmental glomerulosclerosis. Her past medical history included obstructive sleep apnea and urinary tract infection when she was younger. She had no prior history of kidney stones, hematuria, or diabetes. However, she had proteinuria and preeclampsia with blood pressure elevated to 140/80 mmHg at the end of her pregnancy. There were no acute deep venous thrombosis or miscarriages in the past. She reported no family history of kidney disease, but her parents had hypertension. She was a former

J. Alstott · M. Mohamed (✉)
Department of Medicine, Division of Nephrology, University of Wisconsin, Madison, WI, USA
e-mail: JAlstott@uwhealth.org; mmohamed2@wisc.edu

© The Author(s), under exclusive license to Springer Nature Switzerland AG 2022

F. Aziz, S. Parajuli (eds.), *Complications in Kidney Transplantation*, https://doi.org/10.1007/978-3-031-13569-9_9

smoker of 20 pack years but quit in 2001. She drank seven or fewer alcoholic drinks per week on average and denied use of any recreational or illicit drug use.

Medications Sertraline, atorvastatin, and occasional use of non-steroidal anti-inflammatory drugs. *Physical examination*: Blood pressure: 141/88 mmHg and heart rate: 69 beats per minute. Estimated body mass index (BMI) 37.03 kg/m^2 as calculated from the following: Height: 5′ 5.67″ (1.668 m). Weight: 227 lb. 1.6 oz. (103 kg). Otherwise, no significant exam findings.

Laboratory Data

Creatinine 0.73 mg/dL, estimated Glomerular Filtration Rate (eGFR): 93 mL/min/1.73 m^2 calculated using CKD-Epi equation without race coefficient. HgA1c 5.5%. Urine microalbumin/creatinine ratio < 5 μg/mg. 24 h urine total: 2129 mL, creatinine clearance: 142 mL/min and urine protein <6.9 mg/dL. Creatinine clearance adjusted for Body Surface Area (BSA) = 116.6 mL/min/1.73 m^2, 24 h urine accuracy = 14.47 mg/kg.

Imaging

CT angiography of the abdomen with and without intravenous contrast (Renal Donor Protocol): RIGHT KIDNEY: Parenchyma: Sub centimeter parapelvic cyst in the lower pole. Right kidney length: 10.0 cm. and kidney volume: 183 mL. LEFT KIDNEY: Kidney length: 10.1 cm. Kidney volume: 181 mL. Both kidneys parenchyma: Normal collecting system: No hydronephrosis or nephrolithiasis. No filling defect on excretion images.

2-Dimensional Echocardiography: Left ventricular size and wall thickness were both normal. Left ventricular ejection fraction 65%. Mild elevated pulmonary artery systolic pressure of 30 mmHg.

In summary, the patient is a middle-aged woman with obesity (BMI 37.0 kg/m^2) and prior preeclampsia who is hypertensive at the time of living donor evaluation but not on anti-hypertensive medications.

Question 1

Which of the following is the most accurate regarding obesity and living kidney donation?

A. Most United States kidney transplant centers exclude living donors with a BMI of > 30.
B. Similar to obesity trends in the general population, an increase in the incidence of obesity has been identified in candidates for living kidney donation in recent decades.

C. Obese kidney donors are more likely to lose weight after kidney donation than individuals with a BMI of 18.5–24.9 kg/m^2.

D. While Black and Hispanic persons have higher rates of ESKD compared to white adults, obesity rates in the United States are similar between these groups.

The correct answer is B.

Population health data shows that obesity has been increasing in the general population over the last 50 years; similarly, obesity among living donors at the time of selection had increased from 8% from 1963–1974 to 26% from 1997–2007. Answer A is incorrect as a survey of transplant centers in the United States (52%) use BMI > 35 kg/m^2 as an exclusion for kidney donation. C is incorrect as a retrospective study of changes in weight post kidney donation found that at 1-year, obese donors had gained a mean of +2.3 ± 0.9 kg ($p < 0.0001$) compared to donors who had a normal BMI whose weight did not change post-donation. D is incorrect as obesity rates in Black and Hispanic adults are higher than in white adults.

Question 2

Regarding her elevated blood pressure, which of the following is not true when providing education and counseling during the visit?

A. She should be advised that an anti-hypertensive medication should be prescribed at the end of the visit to treat essential hypertension.

B. Kidney donation may lead to physiological changes that increase subsequent hypertension risk.

C. If she is Black or Hispanic, there is an increased risk of hypertension after living donation.

D. Medication for the treatment of hypertension is more likely if she has high blood pressure prior to kidney donation than if his blood pressure was within normal limits.

The correct answer is A.

Our donor candidate's clinic blood pressure (BP) was 141/88 mmHg which is elevated for candidate age [2]. A systolic BP (SBP) of >130 or diastolic BP of >80 would be consistent with HTN [3]. Accuracy in the BP measurement should be assessed. Additional ambulatory BP monitoring home and clinic BP values should also be obtained with the average of 2–3 BP measurements obtained on 2–3 separate occasions used to diagnose hypertension (HTN) [4]. Answer A is not true as further BP measurements are necessary to establish a diagnosis of hypertension prior to starting drug treatment. Option B is true as acceleration in the development of hypertension is a concern with kidney donation given the consequent reduction in nephron mass leading to hyperfiltration which may affect the renin–angiotensin–aldosterone system [5]. Indeed, post kidney donation HTN incidence assessed by administrative claims is elevated compared to matched controls from the general population [6]. Additionally, in the United States, similar to HTN trends in the general population, HTN after living donation is more common in certain groups such as Black and Hispanic individuals, which makes answer C an accurate answer [7]. Likewise, answer D is true as pre-donation hypertension is strongly associated (aHR 20.9) for drug-treated HTN after kidney donation [8]. Finally, a study of living donors found that older age (OR 1.09) and increasing BMI (1.12) were associated with the risk of developing HTN after donation [9].

Discussion

Obesity is defined as an abnormal or excessive fat accumulation that may impair health. BMI [weight (kg)/height^2 (meters) = kg/m^2] remains the standard measure for obesity. A BMI of >30.0 is the threshold for the diagnosis of obesity. Obesity is further grouped into three classes: Class I BMI 30–35, Class II BMI 35–40, Class III (severe) BMI > 40. While BMI is easily calculable and widely used to diagnose obesity, BMI is not directly measured by adiposity. Other indirect anthropometric measures such as waist circumference, waist-to-hip, and waist-to-height ratios are inexpensive and can be used to assess central adiposity. In a meta-analysis of over 5 million adults, the risk of eGFR decline, defined as a composite outcome of 40% eGFR decline, eGFR <10 mL/min/1.73 m^2, or the initiation of kidney replacement therapy, was greater with increasing BMI over 25, higher waist circumferences, and higher waist-to-height ratios [10]. Furthermore, multiple studies showed that in the general population, obesity is associated with an increased risk of CKD and ESKD [11–13]. Additionally, obesity in otherwise healthy patients who underwent nephrectomy for non-transplant-related issues was found to develop proteinuria and CKD years later [14].

In the last 50 years, obesity rates nationally and globally have increased markedly. According to the National Health and Nutrition Examination Survey (NHANES) data, the age-adjusted prevalence of obesity was 42.4% of adults in the US in 2017–2018. Similar rates were seen between men and women across all age groups. However, there are notable differences in the rates of obesity by race, with the highest rates in non-Hispanic Black (49.6%) followed by Hispanic (44.8%), non-Hispanic whites (42.2%), and lowest rates in non-Hispanic Asian adults (17.4%) [15].

Obesity has also become increasingly relevant in living kidney donation. Mirroring the high prevalence of obesity in the general population, a retrospective analysis of potential living donors from 2008 to 2012 revealed that 45% of donors had BMI > 30 [16]. Additionally, living donors who were obese at the time of selection had increased from 8% from 1963–1974 to 26% from 1997–2007 [17]. Despite more transplants with obese donors, obesity remains an important consideration in the donor evaluation process. In 2017, a survey analyzing the medical evaluation practices for living donation of the United States transplant programs showed the majority, 52%, of transplant centers excluded donors at BMI threshold of >35, 10% BMI > 30, 3% with BMI threshold of >40%, and 7% of centers had no BMI criteria [18]. Thus, obesity's high prevalence impacts many possible living donors, especially in groups with health disparities disproportionately affected by both CKD and obesity.

Considering risks to the donor, obesity is an area of uncertainty in living donor transplantation candidacy. Traditionally, obesity confers increased surgical morbidity. Obese donors have been found to have longer operative and warm ischemia times [19]. Nevertheless, nephrectomies for living donation with increased

BMI > 30 compared to non-obese donors are not associated with higher short-term surgical morbidity or mortality [20–23].

From a medical perspective, future risk of CKD and particularly progression to ESKD are paramount. Increasing BMI is a risk for incident CKD, but obesity and weight gain increase the risk of diabetes and hypertension, which are the two most common causes of ESKD in the United States [15, 17]. While it may be anticipated that obese donors would be motivated to improve their general health and obesity post kidney donation, research has found that obese donors gain weight post-donation [24]. In the general population, a meta-analysis of almost 5 million people showed a relatively weak association between obesity with future ESKD (hazard ratio per BMI increase of 5 above 30, 1.16; 95% CI, 1.04 to 1.29). However, this was without the additional factor of nephrectomy for donation [25]. Indeed, when analyzing the long-term risk of ESKD in living donors, obese donors compared to non-obese donors had a higher risk for ESKD. Locke et al. found a 7% increase in ESRD risk with each BMI unit increase in BMI above 27 kg/m^2 [26]. Similarly, in a study of 133,824 living kidney donations from 1987 to 2015, for every increase in BMI by a unit of 5, there was a 61% risk of ESKD [27]. It should be noted that the overall ESRD rate for obese donors was still very low (estimated risk of ESKD 20 years after donation 93.9 per 10,000) [26].

An especially germane question to consider when evaluating a living donor with obesity candidacy is whether other mechanisms related directly to obesity impact kidney function and future CKD risk aside from common comorbidities linked to metabolic syndromes such as hypertension and diabetes. Kidney biopsies at the time of implantation from obese donors (who had a normal renal function and no proteinuria) showed subtle changes such as mild arterial hyalinosis and higher glomerular planar surface area [28]. The implications of these morphologic changes are unclear. However, in the short term, elevated pre-donation BMI is associated with impaired kidney compensation defined as eGFR at 1-year post-donation <70% of prior baseline eGFR [29].

Returning to the case where our potential donor has obesity, her BMI is currently 37.0 kg/m^2. Limited retrospective evidence exists that obesity is associated with CKD, ESKD, and post-donation CKD development; therefore, an exclusion for living donation-based solely on her BMI alone is not recommended. Using obesity (especially with BMI in the 30–35 range) in isolation as a rigid exclusion criterion for potential donors on a larger scale would further exacerbate organ shortage and health disparities in kidney transplantation. The currently available data should be used for candidate risk education and informed consent discussion. Particular attention to education and counseling regarding healthy lifestyle choices and means for achieving a healthy weight should be emphasized to mitigate future deleterious health outcomes. Further incorporation of other relevant patient characteristics is needed in this case regarding donation candidacy.

Our donor also had risk factors for hypertension in general given her older age, office elevated systolic blood pressure, and obesity. Additionally, she had a history of preeclampsia with a prior pregnancy which is a risk factor for subsequent hypertension [30]. However, she is currently not on treatment and has no end-organ damage (no albuminuria or left ventricular hypertrophy). She requires further assessment to diagnose hypertension pre-donation, and if diagnosed, she would require guide-line-directed treatment. Her blood pressure is not a contraindication to kidney donation, but she should be informed regarding the risks of post donor nephrectomy hypertension and the need for possible increased drug treatment after donation.

Individuals such as the candidate described in this case who desire to donate a kidney require scrutiny during the living donor evaluation to mitigate future health risks, especially the risk of post-donation ESKD. Studies demonstrated that in well-selected donors and without known risk factors, live kidney donation does not significantly predispose them to develop hypertension and chronic kidney disease post-donation; however, certain risk factors, such as being of African or Hispanic race, obesity, or older age, are associated with higher likelihoods of developing post-donation hypertension. Consistent with the central tenet of the living donation evaluation, an individualized assessment incorporating relevant patient characteristics and consideration of anticipated post-donation life years are paramount. Based on most recent United States statistics, her current life expectancy is 28.5 years [31]. While her estimated GFR and creatinine clearance are at accepted thresholds for donation, her obesity and elevated blood pressure are concerning for increased risk of future CKD and possible other poor health outcomes post-donation. In our case, while an exact risk estimate is difficult to quantify precisely, her lifetime post-donation ESKD risk exceeded the current acceptable evidence risk threshold. The multi-disciplinary transplant committee decided to decline offering living donation after the initial evaluation. 24 h ambulatory blood pressure monitoring for the further assessment of her elevated BP was recommended, and weight loss targeting a BMI of < 35 before reconsidering her for future living donation. Each transplant center has a threshold where post-donation risk becomes prohibitive to kidney donation. While our donor may have been acceptable without obesity and HTN or just one risk factor, the summative risk of her risk factors, in this case, was above our transplant center's acceptable post-donation risk threshold (Fig. 9.1).

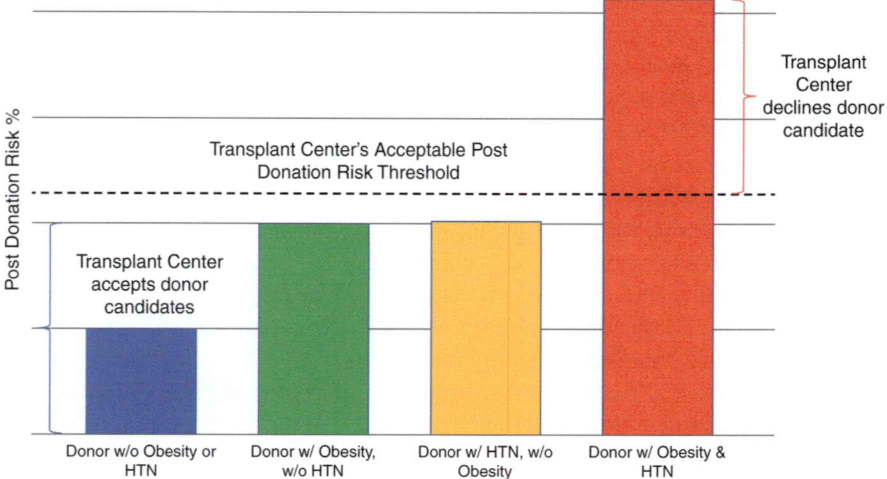

Fig. 9.1 A visual framework for assessing post kidney donation risk. Adapted from Letine et al. [19]

References

1. Hart A, et al. OPTN/SRTR 2019 annual data report: kidney. Am J Transplant. 2021;21(Suppl. 2):21–137.
2. Kovell LC, et al. US hypertension management guidelines: a review of the recent past and recommendations for the future. J Am Heart Assoc. 2015;4(12):e002315.
3. Whelton PK, Carey RM, Aronow WS, et al. 2017 ACC/AHA/AAPA/ABC/ACPM/AGS/APhA/ASH/ASPC/NMA/PCNA guideline for the prevention, detection, evaluation, and management of high blood pressure in adults: a report of the American College of Cardiology/American Heart Association task force on clinical practice guidelines [published correction appears in hypertension. 2018 Jun; 71(6):e140-e144]. Hypertension. 2018;71(6):e13–e115.
4. Huang QF, et al. Ambulatory blood pressure monitoring to diagnose and manage hypertension. Hypertension. 2021;77(2):254–64.
5. Denic A, Glassock RJ, Rule AD. Single-nephron glomerular filtration rate in healthy adults. N Engl J Med. 2017;377(12):1203–4.
6. Garg AX, Prasad GV, Thiessen-Philbrook HR, et al. Cardiovascular disease and hypertension risk in living kidney donors: an analysis of health administrative data in Ontario, Canada. Transplantation. 2008;86:399–406.
7. Rastogi A, et al. Blood pressure and living kidney donors: a clinical perspective. Transplant Direct. 2019;5(10):e488.
8. Lentine KL, Schnitzler MA, Xiao H, et al. Racial variation in medical outcomes among living kidney donors. N Engl J Med. 2010;363(8):724–32.
9. Ibrahim HN, Foley R, Tan L, et al. Long-term consequences of kidney donation. N Engl J Med. 2009;360(5):459–69.
10. Chang AR, Grams ME, Ballew SH, et al. Adiposity and risk of decline in glomerular filtration rate: meta-analysis of individual participant data in a global consortium. BMJ. 2019;364:k5301.
11. Ejerblad E, et al. Obesity and risk for chronic renal failure. J Am Soc Nephrol. 2006;17(6):1695–702.
12. Wang Y, et al. Association between obesity and kidney disease: a systematic review and meta-analysis. Kidney Int. 2008;73(1):19–33.
13. Hsu CY, et al. Body mass index and risk for end-stage renal disease. Ann Intern Med. 2006;144(1):21–8.
14. Praga M, Hernandez E, Herrero JC, et al. Influence of obesity on the appearance of proteinuria and renal insufficiency after unilateral nephrectomy. Kidney Int. 2000;58:2111–8.
15. Hales CM, Carroll MD, Fryar CD, Ogden CL. Prevalence of obesity and severe obesity among adults: United States, 2017–2018. In: NCHS Data Brief, no 360. Hyattsville, MD: National Center for Health Statistics. p. 2020.
16. Sachdeva M, Sunday S, Israel E, et al. Obesity as a barrier to living kidney donation: a center-based analysis. Clin Transpl. 2013;27(6):882–7.
17. Taler SJ, Messersmith EE, Leichtman AB, Gillespie BW, Kew CE, Stegall MD, et al. Demographic, metabolic, and blood pressure characteristics of living kidney donors spanning five decades. Am J Transplant. 2013;13(2):390–8.
18. Garg N, Lentine KL, Inker LA, et al. Metabolic, cardiovascular, and substance use evaluation of living kidney donor candidates: US practices in 2017. Am J Transplant. 2020;20(12):3390–400.
19. Lentine KL, Kasiske BL, Levey AS, et al. KDIGO clinical practice guideline on the evaluation and Care of Living Kidney Donors. Transplantation. 2017;101(8S Suppl 1):S1–S109.
20. Heimbach JK, Taler SJ, Prieto M, et al. Obesity in living kidney donors: clinical characteristics and outcomes in the era of laparoscopic donor nephrectomy. Am J Transplant. 2005;5(5):1057–64. https://doi.org/10.1111/j.1600-6143.2005.00791.x.
21. Unger LW, Feka J, Sabler P, et al. High BMI and male sex as risk factor for increased short-term renal impairment in living kidney donors - retrospective analysis of 289 consecutive cases. Int J Surg. 2017;46:172–7.
22. Schussler L, Khetan P, Peacock M, et al. Is obesity a contraindication for kidney donation? Surg Endosc. 2020;34(10):4632–7.

23. Segev DL, Muzaale AD, Caffo BS, et al. Perioperative mortality and long-term survival following live kidney donation. JAMA. 2010;303(10):959–66.
24. Bugeja A, Harris S, Ernst J, Burns KD, Knoll G, Clark EG. Changes in body weight before and after kidney donation. Can J Kidney Health Dis. 2019;6:2054358119847203.
25. Grams ME, Sang Y, Levey AS, et al. Kidney-failure risk projection for the living kidney-donor candidate. N Engl J Med. 2016;374(5):411–21.
26. Locke JE, Reed RD, Massie A, et al. Obesity increases the risk of end-stage renal disease among living kidney donors. Kidney Int. 2017;91(3):699–703.
27. Massie AB, Muzaale AD, Luo X, et al. Quantifying post donation risk of ESRD in living kidney donors. J Am Soc Nephrol. 2017;28(9):2749–55.
28. Rea DJ, Heimbach JK, Grande JP, et al. Glomerular volume and renal histology in obese and non-obese living kidney donors. Kidney Int. 2006;70(9):1636–41.
29. Shinoda K, Morita S, Akita H, et al. Pre-donation BMI and preserved kidney volume can predict the cohort with unfavorable renal functional compensation at 1-year after kidney donation. BMC Nephrol. 2019;20:46.
30. Garovic VD, August P. Preeclampsia and the future risk of hypertension: the pregnant evidence. Curr Hypertens Rep. 2013;15(2):114–21.
31. Arias E, Tejada-Vera B, Ahmad F. Provisional life expectancy estimates for January through June, 2020.Vital statistics rapid release; no 10. National Center for Health Statistics: Hyattsville, MD; 2021.

Chapter 10
Living Kidney Donor with Family History of Kidney Disease

Gurmukteshwar Singh and Prince Mohan Anand

Introduction

We present the case of a young male who donated a kidney to his mother after a full donor evaluation. He subsequently developed worsening kidney function and had a kidney biopsy and genetic testing, culminating in a diagnosis of autosomal dominant tubulointerstitial kidney disease from a *UMOD* gene mutation. We highlight the importance of genetic testing during the evaluation of donors with a family history of kidney disease.

Patient History

A man in his 20s was evaluated for paired exchange kidney donation. He had wanted to donate his kidney to his mother but could not due to the high titer of donor-specific antibodies. He had no known past medical problems. His serum creatinine was 1.0 mg/dL and 24-h urine creatinine clearance 126 mL/min. The urinary evaluation was normal, without proteinuria, pyuria, or hematuria. His mother had a history of hypertension and gout. She had been diagnosed with

G. Singh
Geisinger Medical Center, Danville, PA, USA
e-mail: gsingh3@geisinger.edu

P. M. Anand (✉)
Medical University of South Carolina, Charleston, SC, USA
e-mail: mohanp@musc.edu

© The Author(s), under exclusive license to Springer Nature Switzerland AG 2022
F. Aziz, S. Parajuli (eds.), *Complications in Kidney Transplantation*,
https://doi.org/10.1007/978-3-031-13569-9_10

non-proteinuric chronic kidney disease (CKD) in her 30s. Her serological workup, serum protein electrophoresis, and kidney ultrasound had been normal. As a shared decision, she and her nephrologist had not pursued a kidney biopsy, believing it would be of low yield given the lack of proteinuria and normal urine sediment. Her kidney function had continued to decline, culminating in end-stage kidney disease (ESKD) and transplant listing in her late-40s.

Question 1
In addition to routine pre-transplant evaluation, what other testing should be pursued before accepting this male as a kidney donor?

A. Serologic workup for autoimmune disease.
B. Genetic testing.
C. Kidney biopsy.
D. No further testing is necessary.

The correct answer is B.
The risk of post-donation ESKD is almost two-fold greater in donors with a first-degree relationship to the recipient [1]. Given the unclear etiology of his mother's early-onset CKD, pre-donation testing for genetic kidney diseases should be pursued. Given that his mother's CKD was non-proteinuric, with normal urinary sediment, the chances of autoimmune disease are low. Moreover, his normal kidney function and urinary evaluation would also argue against ongoing autoimmune pathology. A kidney biopsy is unlikely to be high yield given that he currently has normal kidney function. Even if he has genetic kidney disease, it may be too early to manifest enough features for a conclusive diagnosis.

Patient Course

Unfortunately, this patient was evaluated more than a decade ago, before the widespread availability of genetic testing or awareness of ESKD risk in relatives of recipients. He was accepted for paired exchange kidney donation and underwent laparoscopic left donor nephrectomy with paired exchange kidney transplantation. After kidney donation, his serum creatinine stabilized around 1.7 mg/dL. He then stopped seeing nephrology. A nephrology evaluation was requested about 5 years later as he had developed progressive CKD and gout. His serum creatinine was now close to 2.5 mg/dL. His younger sister had also been diagnosed with stage 4 CKD. A kidney biopsy (Fig. 10.1) was performed, and he was referred for genetic testing.

Fig. 10.1 Kidney biopsy

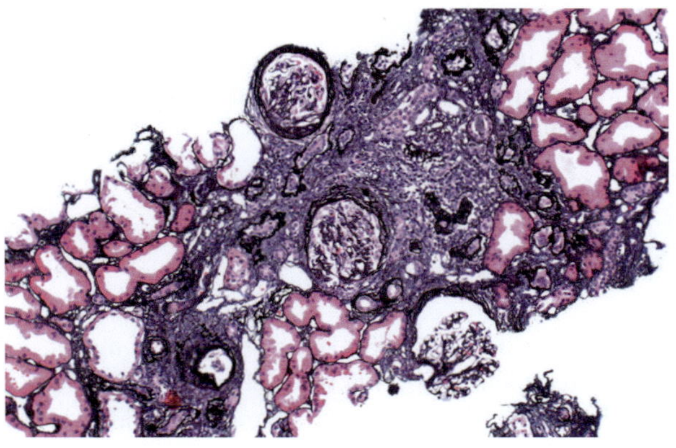

Question 2

Given this patient's clinical course and biopsy findings, what is the most likely underlying cause of progressive kidney disease for him and his mother?

A. Drug-induced interstitial nephritis.
B. Focal segmental glomerulosclerosis.
C. *UMOD* gene mutation.
D. Thrombotic microangiopathy.

The correct answer is C.

The kidney biopsy showed interstitial infiltration by mononuclear cells, global focal glomerulosclerosis, arteriosclerosis, tubular atrophy, and interstitial fibrosis. Tubular basement membrane showed rupture with interstitial Tamm-Horsfall protein extravasation and associated mononuclear cell infiltration. No glomerular tuft collapse or ischemic changes was seen, making focal segmental glomerulosclerosis or thrombotic microangiopathy unlikely. This picture is consistent with interstitial nephritis. The most likely diagnosis is an autosomal dominant tubulointerstitial kidney disease in the absence of offending drug exposure and a strong family history of early-onset progressive CKD. The most common cause of this entity is uromodulin-associated kidney disease due to UMOD gene mutation. This diagnosis is also supported by early-onset gout in our patient and his family [2]. Genetic testing of all three affected family members confirmed a likely pathogenic variant in the *UMOD* gene (c.377 G > A p.C126Y).

Subsequent Clinical Course

The patient's CKD continued to progress, and he was listed for kidney transplantation 8 years after donating his kidney. He has now undergone successful deceased donor kidney transplantation and is clinically stable. The recipient of his donated kidney had a complicated course with episodes of acute cellular rejection versus interstitial nephritis, requiring intensified immunosuppression and culminating in BK virus nephropathy. The recipient became dialysis dependent about 6 years after transplantation.

Discussion

Post-kidney donation ESKD risk is greater in first-degree biological relatives of kidney recipients [1]. This risk gets magnified even further as the biological relationship gets closer. The risk among identical twins is almost 10-fold that among parents or siblings [3]. Conversely, the risk of allograft failure is higher if the recipient is related to the donor, most pronounced in Black recipients [4]. In view of these findings, Kidney Disease Improving Global Outcomes (KDIGO) clinical practice guidelines now recommend genetic history and appropriate testing as a part of donor evaluation [5]. Practical algorithms to work through this decision-making about genetic testing in donors remain elusive.

Recently, a group comprising nephrologists from multiple US centers have shared a proposed framework to guide decisions about genetic testing in living kidney donor candidates [6]. Obtaining a thorough family history of kidney disease is critical. If a family history is present, or there are clinical clues suggestive of glomerular diseases (such as focal segmental glomerulosclerosis or Alport syndrome) or other genetic kidney diseases (such as multiple cysts in the kidneys), genetic testing should be considered prior to kidney donation [6]. Operationalizing such algorithms as part of routine kidney donor evaluation in transplant centers would prevent living kidney donation from high-risk patients such as ours. Moreover, as genetic and target-based therapies are developed, this may allow opportunities for early identification and treatment of genetic kidney diseases [6].

Nephrologists should make concerted efforts to familiarize themselves with the methodology and interpretation of genetic testing. This includes understanding inheritance patterns, genomic testing types, variant significance analysis, and phenotype evaluation to develop a final action plan. Given the lack of detailed genetic curricula in current nephrology training, incorporating genetic counselors, molecular pathologists, and geneticists into transplant evaluation plans might be a prudent course [7]. In one such collaboration at the University of Iowa, genetic panel-based testing was performed on six negative controls, four transplant candidates with presumed genetic kidney disease, and six related potential donors. Based on the results, one potential donor was excluded. The genetic risk could be ruled out in four potential donors. Overall, genetic testing allowed efficient and cost-effective donor risk stratification [8].

Our patient and his family illustrate the characteristic presentation of the autosomal dominant tubulointerstitial disease as recognized over the past decade: progressive non-proteinuric CKD with bland urinary sediment and unremarkable imaging. Of the three forms identified, mutations in the UMOD gene are the most common and frequently associated with early-onset gout. Had he been evaluated in recent years, the systematic evaluation would have ruled him out as a kidney donor. Furthermore, he and his sister would have been diagnosed much earlier, allowing early attempts at therapeutic options like blood pressure control, allopurinol, angiotensin-converting enzyme inhibitors, enrollment in randomized trials, and plans for early transplantation [2]. Other common hereditary genetic diseases amenable to similar benefits with pre-donation genetic testing include cystic kidney disease, collagen IV mutations, and APOL1 nephropathy [9, 10].

Biological relatives of patients with kidney disease are at higher risk for developing ESKD after kidney donation. Appropriate pre-donation genetic testing in collaboration with geneticists should be a routine part of donor risk stratification. This may also allow for the early identification of genetic kidney diseases.

References

1. Massie AB, Muzaale AD, Luo X, Chow EKH, Locke JE, Nguyen AQ, Henderson ML, Snyder JJ, Segev DL. Quantifying postdonation risk of ESRD in living kidney donors. J Am Soc Nephrol. 2017;28:2749–55.
2. Bleyer AJ, Hart PS, Kmoch S. Hereditary interstitial kidney disease. Semin Nephrol. 2010;30:366–73.
3. Wainright JL, Robinson AM, Wilk AR, Klassen DK, Cherikh WS, Stewart DE. Risk of ESRD in prior living kidney donors. Am J Transplant. 2018;18:1129–39.
4. Husain SA, King KL, Sanichar N, Crew RJ, Schold JD, Mohan S. Association between donor-recipient biological relationship and allograft outcomes after living donor kidney transplant. JAMA Netw Open. 2021;4:e215718.
5. Lentine KL, Kasiske BL, Levey AS, Adams PL, Alberú J, Bakr MA, Gallon L, Garvey CA, Guleria S, Li PK, Segev DL, Taler SJ, Tanabe K, Wright L, Zeier MG, Cheung M, Garg AX. KDIGO clinical practice guideline on the evaluation and care of living kidney donors. Transplantation. 2017;101:S1–S109.
6. Tantisattamo E, Reddy UG, Ichii H, Ferrey AJ, Dafoe DC, Ioannou N, Xie J, Pitman TR, Hendricks E, Eguchi N, Kalantar-Zadeh K. Is it time to utilize genetic testing for living kidney donor evaluation? Nephron. 2021;146:1–7.
7. Cocchi E, Nestor JG, Gharavi AG. Clinical genetic screening in adult patients with kidney disease. Clin J Am Soc Nephrol. 2020;15:1497–510.
8. Thomas CP, Mansilla MA, Sompallae R, Mason SO, Nishimura CJ, Kimble MJ, Campbell CA, Kwitek AE, Darbro BW, Stewart ZA, Smith RJH. Screening of living kidney donors for genetic diseases using a comprehensive genetic testing strategy. Am J Transplant. 2017;17:401–10.
9. Cornec-Le Gall E, Chebib FT, Madsen CD, Senum SR, Heyer CM, Lanpher BC, Patterson MC, Albright RC, Yu AS, Torres VE, Harris PC. The value of genetic testing in polycystic kidney diseases illustrated by a family with PKD2 and COL4A1 mutations. Am J Kidney Dis. 2018;72:302–8.
10. Neugut YD, Mohan S, Gharavi AG, Kiryluk K. Cases in precision medicine: APOL1 and genetic testing in the evaluation of chronic kidney disease and potential transplant. Ann Intern Med. 2019;171:659–64.

Chapter 11
Kidney Grafts with Evidence
of Microthrombi in Glomerular Capillaries

Sonali N. de Chickera and Shaifali Sandal

Introduction

Microvascular thrombi (MT) are a relatively uncommon histologic finding in procurement biopsies prior to kidney transplantation (KT). Here, we report our center's experience accepting two kidney allografts from a donor with procurement biopsy demonstrating MT. We also discuss the evidence supporting using such organs, clinical considerations, post-transplant monitoring, and our favorable recipient outcomes.

Case

A 51-year-old donor was pronounced brain dead after a traumatic fall. They were found to have had a massive cerebral hematoma with multiple bilateral segmental and subsegmental pulmonary emboli. Their only significant past medical history was anxiety, depression, and 20-pack-year smoking history. The donor did have a history of high-risk behavior; however, nucleic acid amplification testing for HIV,

S. N. de Chickera
Division of Nephrology, Department of Medicine, University of Western Ontario,
London, ON, Canada

S. Sandal (✉)
Research Institute of the McGill University Health Centre, Montreal, QC, Canada

Division of Nephrology, Department of Medicine, McGill University Health Centre,
Montreal, QC, Canada

Royal Victoria Hospital Glen Site, Montreal, QC, Canada
e-mail: shaifali.sandal@mcgill.ca

© The Author(s), under exclusive license to Springer Nature
Switzerland AG 2022
F. Aziz, S. Parajuli (eds.), *Complications in Kidney Transplantation*,
https://doi.org/10.1007/978-3-031-13569-9_11

hepatitis B, and C was negative. The only prescribed medications they were taking included methylphenidate and duloxetine.

5 days after admission, procurement of their organs was planned. Both kidneys demonstrated excellent structure and function. Ultrasonography did not show any abnormalities. Terminal creatinine was 0.76 mg/dL, eGFR was 92, and urinalysis was only positive for hematuria thought to be due to Foley catheter-related trauma. The electrolytes, liver function tests, and bilirubin remained within normal limits. However, the hemoglobin declined from 13.3 g/dL at admission to 7.2 g/dL at the time of procurement; similarly, platelets decreased from 177 to 111×10^9/L. PT and PTT were elevated with a peak of 92 and 120, respectively, and declined after that. Fibrinogen was 523 mg/dL (normal 200–400 mg/dL).

Upon procurement, both kidneys were noted to have mild petechiae on gross examination, and procurement biopsies were pursued. The biopsy sample had over 300 glomeruli, of which 5–10% were globally sclerosed. Less than 5% of the glomeruli contained thrombi in their capillaries. In addition, the biopsy demonstrated mild arteriosclerosis but no other abnormalities. The immunofluorescence was positive for fibrinogen. Of note, no thrombosis was noted in the renal arteries or renal veins. All other provincial transplant centers turned down these kidneys, so our center accepted both for two recipients.

Question 1
What are the possible causes of glomerular capillary microthrombi in this donor?

A. Lupus nephritis.
B. Brain injury.
C. Atypical hemolytic uremic syndrome.
D. B and C.

The correct answer is B.

MT can be seen in patients' organs who die of brain injury, including the kidneys. The most common cause of glomerular MT is DIC, and other potential causes are summarized in Table 11.1. MT can also be seen with an atypical hemolytic uremic syndrome, including acute kidney injury, thrombocytopenia, and microangiopathic hemolytic anemia. While this donor was anemic and thrombocytopenic,

Table 11.1 Potential causes of thrombi in pre-implantation biopsies of donor graft

Cause	Laboratory parameters in donor
Disseminated intravascular coagulation	Low platelet count, elevated levels of a fibrin-related marker, prolonged PT, low fibrinogen level, increased D-dimer
Heparin-induced thrombocytopenia	Recent heparin exposure and no global coagulation abnormalities, except increased D-dimer. If available, positive heparin-PF4 antibodies
Thrombotic microangiopathies	Microangiopathic hemolytic anemia, thrombocytopenia, schistocytes on the peripheral blood smear, normal coagulation testing, normal D-dimer
Iatrogenic	No coagulation abnormalities and normal platelet count

the platelets declined then stabilized after that, and there was no laboratory evidence of hemolytic anemia as evidenced by the normal bilirubin. Also, the biopsy was not suggestive of the renal-limited hemolytic uremic syndrome, making answers C and D incorrect. Finally, although electron microscopy was not performed, the biopsy demonstrated the absence of immune deposits on immunofluorescence with no mesangial changes to suggest lupus nephritis. This makes answer A incorrect.

After discussion and consideration, it was planned to transplant each of the two renal allografts into two different recipients. The first recipient was a 72-year-old male patient with end-stage kidney disease on hemodialysis secondary to a previously failed kidney transplant due to antibody-mediated rejection. His past medical history was significant for coronary artery disease, hypertension, and ischemic cardiomyopathy (baseline ejection fraction of 40–45%), requiring an implantable cardioverter-defibrillator. There were 5/6 HLA mismatches (HLA-A: 2/2, -B:2/2, and -DR: 1/2), and this recipient's calculated panel reactive antibody was 53%. The second recipient was a 31-year-old male with end-stage kidney disease due to IgA nephropathy and was on peritoneal dialysis. He had no other significant past medical history. This patient had 6/6 HLA mismatches (HLA-A: 2/2, -B: 2/2, and -DR: 2/2) and a calculated panel reactive antibody of 66%. Both patients received alemtuzumab and methylprednisolone for induction, and their maintenance regimens consisted of long-acting tacrolimus and mycophenolate sodium.

Question 2

Given the finding of glomerular capillary microthrombi in the procurement donor biopsy, which of the following statements is correct?

A. Microthrombi in glomerular capillaries portend a poor long-term graft survival.
B. The recipients are at a greater risk of developing disseminated intravascular coagulation post-transplantation.
C. Post-transplant biopsies will demonstrate residual or no microthrombi.
D. The recipients should be given anticoagulation post-transplantation to help clear existing microthrombi and prevent the ongoing microthrombi formation.

The correct answer is C.

Nearly all post-transplant biopsies demonstrate complete resolution of the fibrin thrombi by one 1-month, even where 100% of the glomeruli are involved. Evidence suggests that transplanting kidneys from deceased donors with MT is a safe practice, and long-term outcomes are excellent and comparable to grafts from donors with no MT; thus, A is incorrect. Answer B is incorrect since evidence suggests the resolution of DIC post-KT in most cases. Lastly, there is no empiric evidence to suggest the need for anticoagulation in our recipients since this donor allograft biopsy demonstrated less than 5% of glomerular capillary MT. The recipient's fibrinolysis system can clear MT from the transplanted graft; thus, the response D is not correct either.

Clinical Course

Following transplantation, the first recipient had immediate graft function. His hospital course was complicated by acute-on-chronic heart failure that was managed medically. 1 year later, his creatinine was stable in the 1.4–1.6 mg/dL range. The second recipient developed delayed graft function requiring resumption of dialysis. A post-transplant biopsy on postoperative day 12 showed mild-moderate acute tubular necrosis, no evidence of T cell or antibody-mediated rejection, and medial and intimal thickening of the arteries with no documented MT. Unfortunately, his course was complicated by obstructive nephropathy and recurrent episodes of acute kidney injury. He had a repeat biopsy 3-months post-transplant demonstrating collapsing focal segmental glomerulosclerosis that responded to plasma exchange. 1 year later, his creatinine was stable in the 2.3–2.6 mg/dL range. Ultimately, these cases demonstrate that in the right clinical situation, the use of grafts with biopsy evidence of MT has no significant impact outside of the perioperative period, consistent with the literature thus far.

Discussion

MT is a relatively uncommon histologic finding in procurement biopsies prior to kidney transplant, and potential causes are summarized in Table 11.1. MT in procured biopsies is associated with disseminated intravascular coagulation (DIC) and rarely heparin-induced thrombocytopenia or thrombotic microangiopathy. Depending on the etiology, these thrombi are usually composed of fibrin and occasionally platelets, and rarely, cases of foreign particles, such as particles from surgical gloves, have been described [1].

DIC is a condition in which blood clots form and block small blood vessels. There is no specific marker of DIC; however, scoring systems have been developed and validated for its diagnosis, which relies on platelet count, prolonged PT, and low fibrinogen [2]. Nearly 30–50% of patients with traumatic brain injury develop DIC [3]. This could be due to the up-regulation of proinflammatory mediators and upregulated host immunological responses in irreversible central nervous system injury [4]. However, it is important to note that not all patients with laboratory evidence of DIC will develop glomerular MT. In a cohort of 169 donors with clinical DIC, 38 had pre-implantation biopsies, and MT was only described in four (10.5%) of these biopsies [5]. In another study that reviewed either a pre-implantation or postreperfusion biopsy from 618 grafts, MT was present in only 9.9% of the biopsies [6].

Classifying Severity

To examine the extent of MT in pre-implantation biopsies, the initial suggestion was to classify based on the number of glomeruli involved; mild with <25%, moderate with 25–50%, or severe with >50% of glomeruli involved [7]. It has been argued that simply mentioning the percentage of glomeruli with MT cannot adequately capture the extent of donor organ pathology [8]. In 2015, a Banff working group for the interpretation of pre-implantation kidney biopsies recommended evaluating MT in the most severely affected glomerulus and grade it as mild (<10%), moderate (10–25%), and severe (>25%) based on the percentage of capillaries occluded [9].

Outcomes

An abstract from 1978 that evaluated donor kidneys with histologic evidence of thrombosis suggested that recipients of grafts with MT were more likely to experience short-term allograft failure [10]. Poor preservation is speculated to have played a role [11]. Since DIC is the leading cause of MT in the graft, following this, transplant centers hesitated to accept allografts from donors with DIC. After that, small retrospective series and multiple case reports reported 30–60% incidence of delayed graft function and 3–13% incidence of primary non-function in recipients of grafts where the donor had DIC [3]. Long-term outcomes were excellent and comparable to those from donors with no DIC; [5, 11–13] most, however, did not have procurement biopsy data. To highlight one recent propensity-matched study of 169 recipients of transplants from donors with DIC, history of donor DIC was not associated with primary non-function, delayed graft function, and 5-and 10-year graft function and survival [5].

Focusing on studies where donor biopsies were performed at the time of KT, and they demonstrated MT, results have been encouraging [3, 6–9]. One center examined 230 consecutive pre-anastomotic donor kidney biopsies and found eight (3.5%) that demonstrated MT [7]. They reported a higher risk of delayed graft function with MT; 63% versus 29% of other cases with no MT. The authors reported a relative risk of 2.6 for delayed graft function. Long-term outcomes, however, were good. Next, in a series of 28 KTs that were performed where the donor biopsy showed evidence of MT, authors reported only one patient as having primary non-function, and eight had deaths with functioning graft within 3 years of follow-up [8]. Also, the Banff working group analysis reported that the presence of MT was not significantly associated with either slow or delayed graft function [9]. Lastly, in the largest reported cohort of 61 KTs where donor graft biopsies (either pre-implantation or post-perfusion) demonstrated MT, outcomes were compared with a control group of 557 with no MT [6]. Although delayed graft function rates were higher (49%) when compared with KTs where biopsy demonstrated no MT (39%), this was not statistically different [6]. Primary non-function was noted in 3 cases of MT but were similar as well. Also, 1-year graft function, acute rejection, and graft survival were similar. Overall, this suggests grafts that demonstrate MT have an excellent long-term prognosis.

There are likely donor, recipient, and other allograft factors which are important in determining the outcome of KT where procurement biopsies demonstrated MT independent of MT. Rarely MT in the donor graft has been associated with thrombocytopenia, hemolytic anemia, and transient DIC in the recipient immediately post-transplant [11, 12]. No other adverse outcomes have been reported.

Follow-Up Biopsies

In the above-mentioned studies, while not everyone had a follow-up biopsy, in nearly all cases, no residual MT was described [7, 8]. Even when the donor had acute renal failure and renal biopsy showed 100% of the glomeruli containing fibrin thrombi, one center reported that post-transplant biopsies showed complete resolution of the fibrin thrombi [3]. Batra and colleagues reported their findings from a cohort of 61 KTs where graft biopsies (either pre-implantation or post-perfusion) demonstrated MT, 52 patients had 1-month protocol biopsy; [6] all but two biopsies (4%) showed complete resolution of MT. For some, 1-year protocol biopsies were pursued, and none demonstrated MT. The authors compared findings of 1-year biopsies with a control cohort that had no MT at the time of procurement. The prevalence of moderate to severe interstitial fibrosis and tubular atrophy, the percentage of globally sclerotic glomeruli, and the presence of transplant glomerulopathy were not different. However, the MT group had more intimal arteritis than the control group. Overall, this suggests that the recipient's fibrinolysis system can clear MT from the donor allograft, thus minimizing the impact of donor-derived MT on allograft outcome [6, 8, 11].

Therapeutic Strategies

One center reported their clinical experience using ex vivo thrombolysis before KT in grafts with evidence of MT [14]. In 14 grafts where the initial wedge biopsy demonstrated >50% thrombosed glomeruli, grafts were treated with pulsatile perfusion using a solution that contained 200 mg of Alteplase for 12–16 h. The authors repeated another biopsy and reported a reduction in thrombosed glomeruli from 50% to 23%. Although the cold ischemia time increased, after KT, 10 patients had immediate graft function, 3 had delayed graft function, and 1 had primary nonfunction. Others have suggested that anticoagulation in cases with confirmed extensive fibrin thrombi be considered [3].

Conclusion

In conclusion, evidence suggests that transplanting kidneys from grafts with biopsy evidence of MT is a safe practice, provided that graft function is otherwise good. Some have suggested excluding cases with evidence of extensive coagulative or cortical necrosis [3, 6]. In most cases, the MT resolves by 1-month, and long-term outcomes are good, as pictorially depicted in Fig. 11.1.

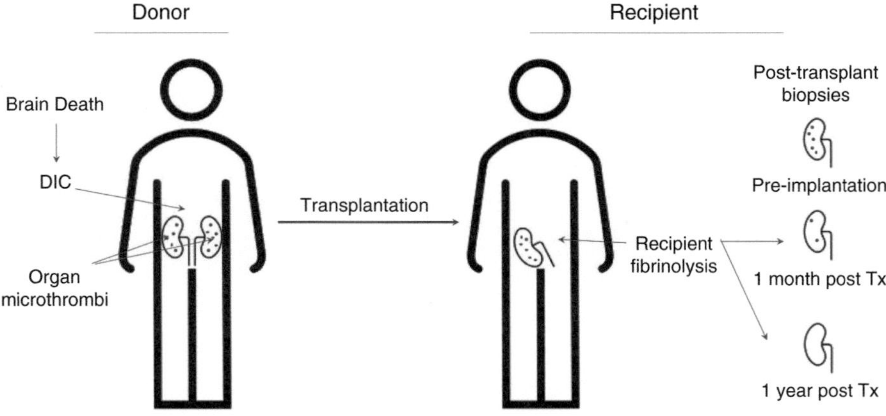

Fig. 11.1 Postulated mechanisms of microthrombi in donor grafts and clearance post-kidney transplantation in the recipient. *DIC* disseminated intravascular coagulation, *Tx* transplant

References

1. Guarrera JV, Nasr SH, Reverte CM, Samstein B, Brown T, Balachandran V, et al. Microscopic intrarenal particles after pulsatile machine preservation do not adversely affect outcomes after renal transplantation. Transplant Proc. 2006;38(10):3384–7.
2. Taylor FB Jr, Toh CH, Hoots WK, Wada H, Levi M. Towards definition, clinical and laboratory criteria, and a scoring system for disseminated intravascular coagulation. Thromb Haemost. 2001;86(5):1327–30.
3. Soares KC, Arend LJ, Lonze BE, Desai NM, Alachkar N, Naqvi F, et al. Successful renal transplantation of deceased donor kidneys with 100% glomerular fibrin thrombi and acute renal failure due to disseminated intravascular coagulation. Transplantation. 2017;101(6):1134–8.
4. Takada M, Nadeau KC, Hancock WW, Mackenzie HS, Shaw GD, Waaga AM, et al. Effects of explosive brain death on cytokine activation of peripheral organs in the rat. Transplantation. 1998;65(12):1533–42.
5. Garrouste C, Baudenon J, Gatault P, Pereira B, Etienne I, Thierry A, et al. No impact of disseminated intravascular coagulation in kidney donors on long-term kidney transplantation outcome: a multicenter propensity-matched study. Am J Transplant. 2019;19(2):448–56.
6. Batra RK, Heilman RL, Smith ML, Thomas LF, Khamash HA, Katariya NN, et al. Rapid resolution of donor-derived glomerular fibrin thrombi after deceased donor kidney transplantation. Am J Transplant. 2016;16(3):1015–20.
7. McCall SJ, Tuttle-Newhall JE, Howell DN, Fields TA. Prognostic significance of microvascular thrombosis in donor kidney allograft biopsies. Transplantation. 2003;75(11):1847–52.
8. Sood P, Randhawa PS, Mehta R, Hariharan S, Tevar AD. Donor kidney microthrombi and outcomes of kidney transplant: a single-center experience. Clin Transpl. 2015;29(5):434–8.
9. Liapis H, Gaut JP, Klein C, Bagnasco S, Kraus E, Farris AB 3rd, et al. Banff histopathological consensus criteria for preimplantation kidney biopsies. Am J Transplant. 2017;17(1):140–50.
10. Meyers AMLJ, Disler PB, et al. Donor disseminated intravascular coagulation (DIC), intraglomerular fibrin deposition, and subsequent graft function. Kidney Int. 1978;13(432):412–4.
11. Pastural M, Barrou B, Delcourt A, Bitker MO, Ourahma S, Richard F. Successful kidney transplantation using organs from a donor with disseminated intravascular coagulation and impaired renal function: case report and review of the literature. Nephrol Dial Transplant. 2001;16(2):412–5.

12. Bennett WM, Hansen KS, Houghton DC, McEvoy KM. Disseminated intravascular coagulation (DIC) in a kidney donor associated with transient recipient DIC. Am J Transplant. 2005;5(2):412–4.
13. Wang CJ, Shafique S, McCullagh J, Diederich DA, Winklhofer FT, Wetmore JB. Implications of donor disseminated intravascular coagulation on kidney allograft recipients. Clin J Am Soc Nephrol. 2011;6(5):1160–7.
14. Nghiem DD, Olson PR, Sureshkumar KK. Role of pulsatile perfusion with tissue plasminogen activator in deceased donor kidneys with extensive glomerular thrombosis. Transplant Proc. 2009;41(1):29–31.

Chapter 12
Arterial Dissections: Challenges in Recognition, Repair, and Reconstruction

Christopher C. Stahl and Juan S. Danobeitia

Introduction

Arterial dissections are rare but constitute a potentially devastating complication of renal transplantation. These can occur acutely in the operative setting or manifest later in the postoperative phase. Both surgeons and clinicians must have a high index of suspicion, and prompt recognition and management are essential in preventing graft injury and/or loss. Here we present the case of a 68-year-old male presenting with an intraoperative dissection of the external iliac artery and discuss the most relevant clinical characteristics, diagnostic methodology, and basic principles of management for arterial dissections in both the acute and postoperative setting.

Patient History

A 68-year-old man with end-stage kidney disease (ESKD) secondary to calcineurin inhibitor toxicity presented to the hospital for potential deceased donor kidney transplantation. His medical history was significant for a liver transplant 20 years prior and numerous vascular comorbidities, including coronary artery disease (CAD) (drug-eluting stents × 2), bilateral carotid artery and vertebral artery stenoses, transient ischemic attack, peripheral arterial disease, hypertension, hyperlipidemia, and a 45 pack-year smoking history (quit smoking 6 months before

C. C. Stahl · J. S. Danobeitia (✉)
Division of Transplantation, Department of Surgery, University of Wisconsin School of Medicine and Public Health, Madison, WI, USA
e-mail: cstahl@uwhealth.org; dano@surgery.wisc.edu

© The Author(s), under exclusive license to Springer Nature Switzerland AG 2022

F. Aziz, S. Parajuli (eds.), *Complications in Kidney Transplantation*,
https://doi.org/10.1007/978-3-031-13569-9_12

presentation). A preoperative computed tomography (CT) scan demonstrated calcified iliac arteries bilaterally.

The patient was listed for a kidney transplant, and an ABO compatible, deceased donor kidney with a kidney donor profile index of 72% left donor kidney with single vessels became available. He was admitted for a planned deceased donor renal transplant to the left iliac fossa with basiliximab induction. The operation was started using a standard technique; however, after the venous and arterial anastomoses were completed and clamps removed, poor kidney reperfusion was noted. The kidney appeared dark and ischemic, and although there was an apparently palpable pulse in the renal artery and donor iliac artery, intraoperative Doppler evaluation demonstrated an acute decrease in the inflow at the level of the proximal external iliac artery.

Question 1

What is the most likely cause for the poor reperfusion of the graft?

A. Venous thrombosis.
B. Technical error at the arterial anastomosis.
C. Extrarenal arterial spasm.
D. Arterial dissection.
E. Hyperacute rejection.

The correct answer is D.

The presentation consisting of immediate ischemia cyanosis to the graft in conjunction with the decreased distal flow to the iliac artery is suggestive of arterial dissection. In the setting of a patient with severe vascular disease, it may be the result of an occlusive intimal injury at the proximal clamp site. An engorged, tense, hyperemic, and pulsatile kidney with diffuse capsular bleeding indicates venous outflow obstruction and possible thrombosis. Extrarenal arterial spasm is a common occurrence and usually results from mechanical trauma and excessive traction on the renal artery during organ procurement or at the time of implantation. This situation may present as a soft kidney upon reperfusion with mild segmental or patchy discoloration that reverts upon rewarming the graft and, in some cases, application of topical vasodilators to the artery. Hyperacute rejection can also manifest as an edematous, flaccid, and cyanotic kidney on reperfusion but is a very rare event in the era of modern tissue typing and crossmatching techniques.

Hospital Course

The arterial anastomosis was immediately taken down in the operating room. No clot was identified, but after extending the arteriotomy, there appeared to be a dissection from the posterior plaque in the left common iliac artery. The kidney was explanted and flushed with cold preservation solution. Vascular surgery was consulted intraoperatively, and an extensive endarterectomy of the left common and external iliac artery was performed with the adequate restoration of arterial flow. The arteriotomy was closed with a patch of bovine pericardium, and the kidney was reimplanted in the usual fashion, with the arterial anastomosis performed in the center of the pericardial patch. The graft showed excellent reperfusion, and the rest of the case was completed in the usual fashion.

Question 2

Many arterial complications are identified in the postoperative, rather than the intra-operative, period. Which of the following scenarios is most consistent with a postoperative arterial thrombosis caused by a dissection flap?

A. Acute onset of flank pain, oliguria, and hematuria.
B. A rapid decline in urine output and renal function with loss of ipsilateral femoral pulses.
C. Increase in creatinine, fever, and pain around the transplanted kidney.
D. Ipsilateral leg swelling and calf pain followed by loss of graft function.
E. Hypotension, tachycardia, decreased urine output, and decreasing hemoglobin level.

The correct answer is B.

The most common presentation of any postoperative arterial inflow complication is an acute reduction in previously robust urine output with an increasing serum creatinine level. Arterial thrombosis or infarction is usually painless due to denervation of the kidney during recovery and manifests only by the rapid decline of graft function in a previously working kidney. Concomitant loss of pulses in the ipsilateral extremity should raise concern for dissection of the iliac vessels and secondary thrombus formation. The diagnosis is made by ultrasound or prompt surgical exploration. Acute onset of flank pain along with oliguria and hematuria is accompanied by graft enlargement and rupture and is usually indicative of renal vein thrombosis. Progressive edema of the ipsilateral leg to the transplant, along with a gradual decline in renal function, is consistent with deep venous thrombosis with proximal iliofemoral extension. Finally, oliguria can be caused by factors unrelated to graft function, such as the acute postoperative bleed in option E. This can cause decreased urine output by decreased renal perfusion or mass effect from a hematoma leading to ureteral or venous obstruction.

Further Clinical Course

The patient had appropriate urine output immediately after surgery that continued to improve until the time of discharge, but a slowly decreasing creatinine level was consistent with slow graft function. He was discharged on postoperative day 4 with a creatinine of 4.28 mg/dL and eventually reached a baseline creatinine of 1.6–1.7 mg/dL.

Discussion

Vascular complications following kidney transplantation are rare (~2–3%) but can be devastating and often lead to graft loss. Arterial complications are the major cause of graft loss in the early postoperative period and are usually caused by errors in surgical technique, including torsion or kinking of the anastomosis or arterial wall dissection from failure to incorporate intima into the suture line at the anastomosis or clamp injuries [1]. Arterial dissections may occur at the level of the anastomosis, recipient common or external iliac arteries, or rarely, the donor renal artery itself [2, 3].

Arterial dissection can be diagnosed early (intraoperatively) or late (postoperatively). Following graft reperfusion, the kidney should turn pink, be firm, and appear homogeneously perfused shortly after blood flow has been restored. A flaccid, cyanotic, mottled, or poorly perfused kidney is the reason for concern. In this situation, the surgeon should start by actively searching for the cause by palpating pulses at the level of the anastomosis, renal artery, and iliac arteries both proximally and distally. Prompt evaluation of the vessels and renal parenchyma with a Doppler probe and/or on-table intraoperative ultrasound can be a very helpful adjunct. Intraoperative signs of dissection include signs of poor arterial flow to the kidney such as weak or absent pulses, mottling, purple discoloration, an abrupt change in doppler signals in an artery, or circular, dark brown discoloration of the arterial wall suggesting an arterial hematoma.

Management can be difficult, and the decision of whether to revise the arterial anastomosis or to proceed with graft explantation followed by cold preservation must be made (Fig. 12.1). Factors going into this decision process include the location of the dissection relative to the anastomosis, the timing of diagnosis, cold ischemic time, the need to administer intravenous contrast and/or heparin, the overall condition of the patient and the renal allograft, and the availability of vascular grafts and angiography resources.

If the decision is made to revise the anastomosis in situ, the patient should first be heparinized. The inflow vessel is then controlled proximally and distally, and the anastomosis is taken down and explored. The transplant artery is then flushed with cold heparinized crystalloid solution, and the renal vein clamped. Careful inspection of the donor and recipient vessels is then performed. Technical errors at the anastomosis should be revised, verifying that the donor's vessel is fully patent with fresh edges and ensuring the inclusion of all layers of the arterial wall with each bite of the new anastomosis. More complex repairs with the kidney left in situ will likely lead to unacceptably long warm ischemic times and should be discouraged. If the injury is extensive or not amenable to in situ repair, the graft must then be explanted and flushed with cold preservation solution as outlined in the vignette.

In rare situations with extensive damage to recipient vasculature, dissections at a clamping site are likely to require endarterectomy, with or without patch angioplasty. Consultation with vascular surgery is advised for these cases. Interposition grafts may be needed to reconstruct the damaged segment, and grafts may be

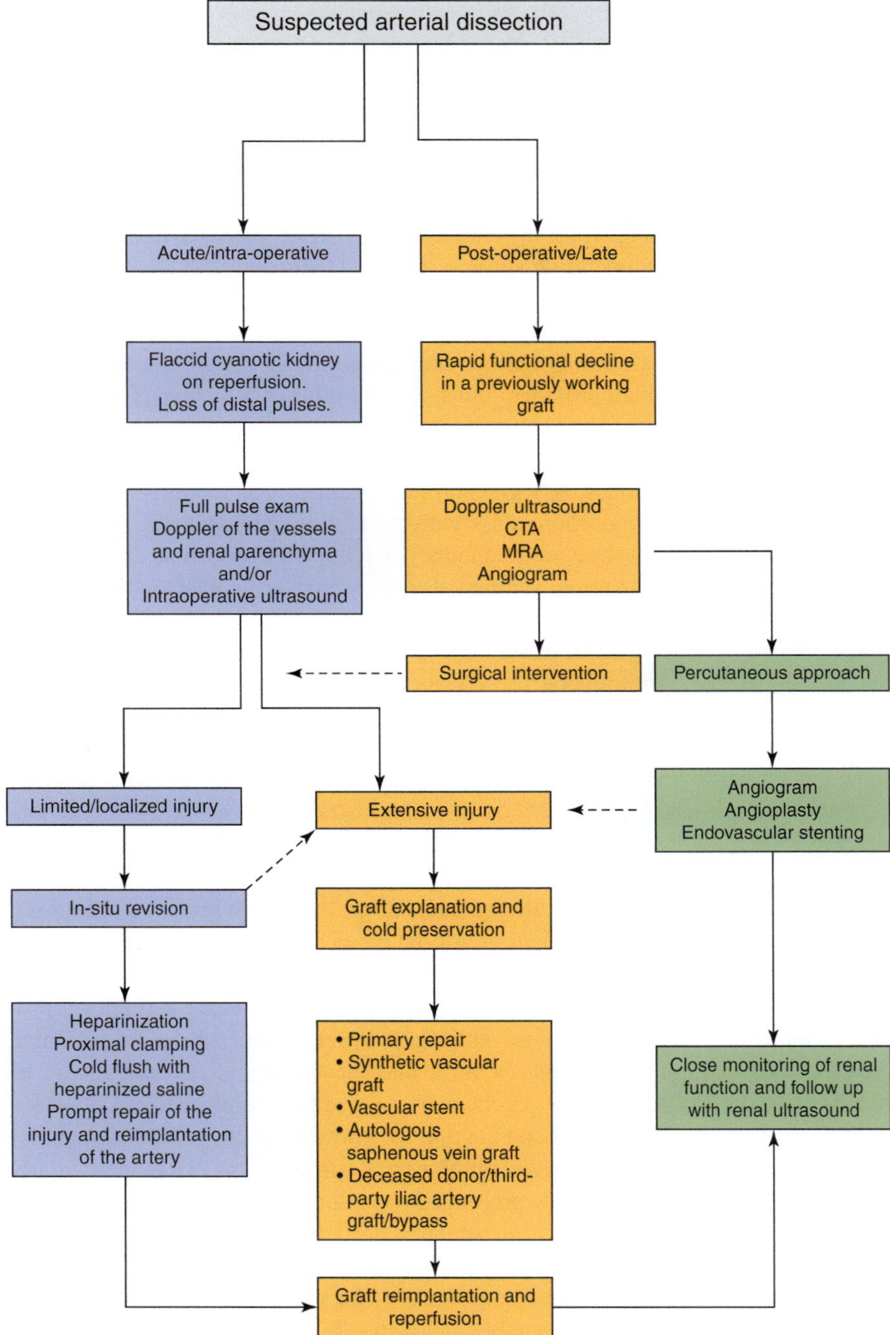

Fig. 12.1 Algorithm for diagnosis and management of arterial dissections after kidney transplantation. *CTA* computed tomography angiography, *MRA* magnetic resonance angiography

constructed using donor allograft, recipient saphenous vein, or synthetic materials. In a recent review of the literature by Lushina et al. the most common repair method described was the use of a synthetic vascular graft (52% of cases), followed by endovascular stent placement (17%), donor iliac artery graft (17%), saphenous vein graft (8%), and open endarterectomy with intimal tacking in approximately 1% of cases [2]. Unfortunately, most of the data on this subject is derived from case reports and institutional experience, but prospective long-term data on the outcomes of each repair method are lacking. Thus, the choice of appropriate approach and repair techniques still depends on operating surgeon ability, experience, and level of comfort with each of the described methods.

Arterial dissections diagnosed in the postoperative period require timely interventions to prevent graft loss but allow more flexibility in the choice of the initial approach. First, transplant providers must have a high index of suspicion for postoperative arterial thrombotic complications. Any patient exhibiting signs of acutely decreased graft function should undergo an immediate duplex ultrasound to evaluate blood flow to the kidney. A segmental infarct appears as a poorly marginated, hypoechoic area or a hypoechoic mass with a well-defined echogenic wall. In the case of complete flow obstruction, the kidney will appear hypoechoic and diffusely enlarged. On Doppler imaging, segmental infarcts appear as wedge-shaped areas without color flow. In total vascular obstruction, there is no perfusion to the transplanted kidney, and no arterial or venous blood flow is seen in the graft at an ultrasound. The authors recommend always starting with ultrasound due to its high accuracy, rapid and widespread availability, low cost, and safety profile. Computed tomography arteriography (CTA) is a great tool to detect perfusion deficits in the renal graft parenchyma, but it is generally avoided in renal transplant patients due to concern for nephrotoxic effects of contrast administration. If the ultrasound is non-diagnostic, magnetic resonance angiography (MRA) and digital subtraction angiography (DSA) can be performed and constitute reliable methods to evaluate diminished or absent flow to the allograft and abrupt changes in graft vascularity [4].

Once diagnosed, rapid treatment of arterial dissections is required for graft salvage. The first step is to determine whether a surgical or percutaneous intervention will be pursued. Surgical repair is definitive, rapid, and, as described above, provides a multitude of options for intervention. However, it does subject the patient to the physiologic stress of a second operation and anesthesia and may not always be indicated. Conversely, while a percutaneous procedure, typically percutaneous transluminal angioplasty (PTA) and stenting performed by interventional radiologists, avoids a second trip to the operating room, it carries its own risks, particularly to the graft. These hazards include prolonged procedure times, the use of high doses of nephrotoxic contrast agents, the potential need for postoperative antiplatelet agents or anti-coagulation, and concerns about the durability of repair. The authors tend to favor surgical repair of arterial dissections for these reasons, but several case reports have demonstrated acceptable outcomes from percutaneous procedural interventions [5]. In our institution, we have examined reconstruction of the transplant renal artery for specific indications, including anastomotic lesions, kinks, unsuccessful PTA, recurrent lesions, and bypass in association with definitive surgical treatment of recipient iliac artery aneurysms following renal transplant. Reported success rates for PTA are in the vicinity of 70–80% but with a recurrence rate of 20–40%. At our center, surgical reconstruction with cadaveric iliac artery graft was successful in 90% of cases, and no significant vascular or immune complications related to the use of these grafts [6].

While this discussion is focused primarily on the diagnosis and management of arterial dissection, prevention of these complications is the ideal strategy, especially considering that errors in surgical technique are a primary cause of these complications. Strategies to prevent arterial dissection include

- Careful arterial anastomoses incorporating intima with every bite of tissue, ensuring needle passage from in-to-out on the more diseased artery.
- Gentle vessel handling and cannulation during all stages of transplantation (procurement, back table graft preparation, and intraoperatively).
- Careful clamping technique.

Any instance of clamping has the potential to cause arterial dissection, so clamping should be performed as infrequently as possible. The surgeon must avoid clamping and re-clamping while consider not routinely clamping the donor artery, with only as much pressure as is required to occlude blood flow. Also, clamping calcified arterial segments should be discouraged, and if a clamp has to be applied over an area of arterial plaque, the surgeon must ensure that the clamp is oriented parallel and not perpendicular to the plaque to minimize the risk of fracture. Finally, careful setup of self-retaining retractor systems and gentle handling of the vessels during vascular exposure are required to minimize pressure or traction injuries to recipient arteries.

Arterial dissections are a rare but devastating post-transplant complication. A good surgical technique can limit, but not eliminate, postoperative dissections. Early recognition along with prompt treatment of arterial dissection is key to maximizing graft salvage.

References

1. Dimitroulis D, Bokos J, Zavos G, Nikiteas N, Karidis NP, Katsaronis P, et al. Vascular complications in renal transplantation: a single-center experience in 1367 renal transplantations and review of the literature. Transplant Proc. 2009;41(5):1609–14.
2. Lushina N, Lee A, Cuadra S, Whang M, Sun H. External iliac artery dissection during renal transplantation: a case report and literature review. Transplant Proc. 2019;51(2):538–40.
3. Hori S, Yoneda T, Tomizawa M, Ichikawa K, Morizawa Y, Nakai Y, et al. Unexpected presentation and surgical salvage of transplant renal artery dissection caused by vascular clamping: a case report. BMC Nephrol. 2020;21(1):1–6.
4. Sugi MD, Joshi G, Maddu KK, Dahiya N, Menias CO. Imaging of renal transplant complications throughout the life of the allograft: comprehensive multimodality review. Radiographics. 2019; https://doi.org/10.1148/rg.2019190096.
5. Takahashi M, Humke U, Girndt M, Kramann B, Uder M. Early posttransplantation renal allograft perfusion failure due to dissection: diagnosis and interventional treatment. AJR Am J Roentgenol. 2003;180(3):759–63.
6. Shames BD, Odorico JS, D'Alessandro AM, Pirsch JD, Sollinger HW. Surgical repair of transplant renal artery stenosis with preserved cadaveric iliac artery grafts. Ann Surg. 2003;237(1):116–22.

Chapter 13
Page Kidney After Kidney Biopsy

Michele Finotti and Eric J. Martinez

Introduction

Page kidney is a rare medical condition caused by kidney parenchymal compression that requires a high index of suspicion to diagnose. Most commonly resulting from blunt trauma with perinephric fluid accumulation and subsequently kidney compression, Page kidney can have nonspecific and variable clinical presentations. Though often asymptomatic, symptomatic manifestations typically include pain, acute kidney dysfunction, and hypertensive crisis. A prompt diagnosis and adequate treatment are mandatory, especially in kidney transplant recipients where the clinical presentation can be dramatic with a rapid worsening of the patient's condition given the inability of the contralateral kidney to compensate. Invasive procedures, such as kidney biopsies, are an important risk factor for Page kidney, especially in transplant recipients. Kidney ultrasound or computed tomography can be used to diagnose Page kidney, and the treatment options range from conservative to surgical intervention. We present in detail the case of a 56-year-old man with Page kidney after kidney transplant allograft biopsy. Diagnoses and management strategies of Page kidney are discussed, with particular attention to cases in the kidney transplant

M. Finotti
Annette C. and Harold C. Simmons Transplant Institute, Baylor University Medical Center, Dallas, TX, USA

4th Surgery Unit, Regional Hospital Treviso, University of Padua, Padua, Italy

E. J. Martinez (✉)
Annette C. and Harold C. Simmons Transplant Institute, Baylor University Medical Center, Dallas, TX, USA

Baylor Scott & White Transplant Services, Dallas, TX, USA
e-mail: Eric.Martinez1@BSWHealth.org

© The Author(s), under exclusive license to Springer Nature Switzerland AG 2022

F. Aziz, S. Parajuli (eds.), *Complications in Kidney Transplantation*,
https://doi.org/10.1007/978-3-031-13569-9_13

recipient where aggressive treatment is needed to reduce the risk of irreversible damage and graft loss.

Patient History

A 56-year-old man with a history of ESKD secondary to focal segmental glomerulosclerosis (FSGS) underwent an uncomplicated deceased donor left kidney transplant into the right iliac fossa. The recipient calculated panel reactive antibody (cPRA) was 0%, the flow crossmatch was T and B cell negative, and he received steroid induction. Maintenance immunosuppression consisted of tacrolimus (target level 8–10 ng/mL), mycophenolate mofetil, and prednisone. The early post-operative course was uneventful, and he was discharged home on a post-operative day (POD) 3 with adequate urine output, down-trending serum creatinine (sCr) 2.25 mg/dL (from 7.21 mg/dL), and a therapeutic tacrolimus level.

Increased sCr on POD-7 led to further investigation with a normal kidney doppler ultrasound and subsequent allograft biopsy with evidence of recurrent FSGS, granulomatous nephritis, and borderline rejection. He underwent various medical treatments, including plasmapheresis; however, sCr was maintained at 2.43 mg/dL, and a repeat allograft biopsy was performed on POD 68. On POD 70, the patient presented to the emergency department (ED) with progressively worsening right lower quadrant constant pain without radiation that had started a few hours after the biopsy. His vital signs in the ED were initially within normal limits other than the blood pressure of 160/93 mmHg and pain 7/10. Labs revealed hemoglobin of 10.1 g/dL (from 11.3 g/dL) and sCr of 3.78 mg/dL (from 2.43 mg/dL) relative to 2 days prior. A CT scan without contrast was performed by the ED (Fig. 13.1).

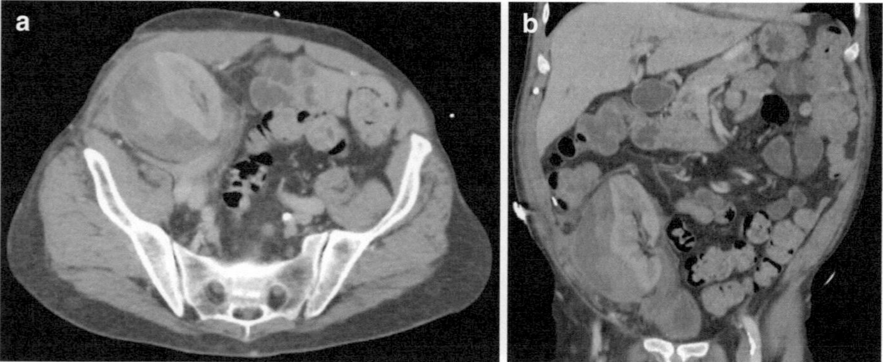

Fig. 13.1 CT abdominal scan without intravenous contrast demonstrating a heterogenous subcapsular kidney transplant fluid collection with allograft compression. (**a**) Axial and (**b**) Coronal view

Question 1

What is the most likely cause of this patient's symptoms and acute kidney dysfunction?

A. Acute rejection.
B. Renal vein thrombosis from lymphocele.
C. Hydronephrosis from urinoma.
D. Page kidney from subcapsular hematoma.
E. Sepsis from abscess formation.

The Correct Answer Is D.

Page kidney from subcapsular hematoma. Page kidney is a rare condition defined by the presence of kidney parenchymal compression with subsequent kidney dysfunction and hypertension. The low urine output is triggered by the compression on the kidney, leading to kidney hypoperfusion and ischemia. Figure 13.1 demonstrates a heterogenous subcapsular hematoma compressing the kidney parenchyma. Acute rejection may demonstrate parenchymal edema on CT with kidney dysfunction, usually requires a biopsy for definitive diagnosis, and does not cause kidney compression. Urine leaks (urinoma), lymphatic leaks (lymphoceles), and perinephric abscess can present as extracapsular perinephric fluid collections with variable degrees of kidney parenchymal compression, yet they appear as simple hypodense in the case of the first two, and complex rim-enhancing collections in the latter.

Hospital Course

The patient was initially managed in the ED with pain medication and control of vital parameters, and transplant services were consulted. Symptoms worsened promptly with pain increase to 9/10, worsening hypertension to 210/110 mmHg, and reduced urine output despite medical treatment.

Question 2

What is the next best step in the management of this patient?

A. Radiology-assisted percutaneous drainage.
B. Open surgical drainage.
C. Observation.
D. Increasing antihypertensive treatment.
E. Transplant nephrectomy.

The correct answer is B.

Open surgical drainage. Open surgical drainage for evacuation of the subcapsular hematoma is mandatory in cases with allograft compromise and uncontrolled hypertension despite pharmacotherapy as this is most often their only functioning kidney. Conservative treatment can be an attempt in the initial presentation of native kidneys, with angiotensin-converting enzyme inhibitors or aldosterone receptor antagonists but must be abandoned promptly if unsuccessful. Radiology-assisted percutaneous drainage can be an option, especially in the case of extracapsular fluid collections but may not adequately drain heterogenous fluid collections such as hematomas to appropriately relieve the compressive pressure. Transplant nephrectomy is performed in case of uncontrolled hypertensive crisis or when the extent of the compression has led to kidney hypoperfusion and graft loss [1].

Additional Clinical Course

The patient was taken to the operating room for exploration of the allograft through the previous incision. The subcapsular hematoma was identified and opened. Approximately 250 mL of hematoma was evacuated from the subcapsular space, with only small points of hemorrhage from the kidney parenchyma controlled with electrocautery. The kidney allograft appeared well perfused, and the surgical site was closed. Immediately after surgery, the blood pressure normalized, and the oliguric state resolved. The remainder of the hospital course was uneventful, and the patient was discharged 3 days post-op with a sCr of 2.16 mg/dL.

Discussion

Page kidney was first described by Irvine Page in 1939, and more than 100 cases have been described in the last decades [2, 3]. The kidney parenchyma is surrounded by two structures, the kidney capsule composed of fibrous and scarcely elastic tissue, and Gerota's fascia composed mainly of fat which allows it to expand. Kidney compression in the Page kidney can derive from either an extracapsular source though within Gerota's fascia, or from a source within the kidney capsule (subcapsular). A comprehensive list of causes of Page kidney can be found in Table 13.1 [4].

Kidney biopsy has been described as a possible mechanism of Page kidney due to subcapsular or intra-renal hematoma formation, especially in patients on therapeutic anticoagulation [5]. Considering the stiffness of the kidney capsule, even a small amount of subcapsular fluid can lead to a Page kidney. Kidney transplant allografts are usually placed in the extraperitoneal iliac fossa, a low compliance space after healing. Page kidney in transplant recipients can occur from fluid contained within the extraperitoneal space of the iliac fossa causing compression or from subcapsular fluid collections.

As in our patient, there are a few reports of Page kidney after biopsies in patients receiving plasmapheresis for AMR [6]. It is well known that plasmapheresis leads to a depletion of several coagulation factors that can lead to a prolonged prothrombin time and partial thromboplastin time [6].

Kidney parenchymal compression results in an inflammatory response and parenchymal microvascular occlusion and ischemia. In response to this vasoconstriction,

Table 13.1 Causes of Page kidney [4]

Etiology of Page kidney	
Traumatic bleeding	American football
	Other contact sports
	Motor vehicle accidents
Iatrogenic bleeding	Post-operative
	Kidney biopsy
	Extracorporeal shock wave lithotripsy
	Sympathetic nerve block
Spontaneous bleeding	Pancreatitis
	Warfarin therapy
	Polyarteritis nodosa
	Tumor
Nonbleeding causes	Pararenal lymphoceles
	Large simple cysts
	Retroperitoneal paraganglioma
	Urinoma
	Perirenal pseudocysts
	Peritransplant lymphocele

the renin—angiotensin—aldosterone system (RAAS) is activated, resulting in elevated plasma renin activity and hypertension. The Goldblatt model of renovascular hypertension can be comparable to the Page kidney, with the difference that the former is a result of compression on the major kidney vessels, while the latter results from microvascular ischemia and alteration of small-vessel hemodynamics [2].

Page kidney in the general population more commonly affects young men reflecting the demographics associated with the most common etiology of Page kidney, blunt trauma [2]. More recently, invasive procedures in an aging population have attributed to the incidence of Page kidney, with approximately 1% occurring after biopsy in a retrospective review of 518 transplants kidney biopsies [6].

The typical presentation of Page kidney is acute onset of flank pain and uncontrolled secondary hypertension. However, the clinical scenario can range from slow or nonspecific symptoms to a hypertensive crisis requiring emergent treatment. Furthermore, the kidney function is usually normal as the compression is rarely bilateral, and the contralateral kidney can compensate [7, 8]. Even when the contralateral kidney can compensate, due to the delay in diagnosis, chronic damage can occur to both kidneys. In the case of transplant patients, where the contralateral kidney cannot compensate, the clinical presentation and progression can be more rapid and severe, with hypertensive crisis and acute kidney failure. If not promptly treated in the transplant recipient, graft loss due to kidney compression can ensue.

The physical exam is usually negative, except in the case of recent trauma where a flank hematoma can be evident. A high clinical suspicion is usually required in diagnosing Page kidney as, except for a clear history of a causative factor, the onset may be slow with the interval from onset to presentation ranging from days to years at times.

Kidney ultrasound or contrast-enhanced computed tomography can be used to diagnose Page kidney. Kidney ultrasound with doppler, which usually demonstrates reduction or absence of diastolic flow and an elevated RI, can be a helpful initial tool [9]. CT scan is more accurately able to identify the location and extent of Page kidney and may better be able to guide subsequent therapeutic steps.

The goal of the treatment in Page kidney is to preserve the kidney parenchyma by removing the compression causing kidney ischemia. This allows resolution of the hypertensive state and kidney dysfunction. To date, there have been no randomized studies to address the best therapy for Page kidney. Most of the indications are derived from case series and retrospective studies [4, 6–8, 10]. In cases of slow-onset symptoms, the initial treatment is often pharmacological antihypertensive management targeting the renin–angiotensin–aldosterone system (angiotensin-converting enzyme inhibitors, angiotensin receptor blockers, or aldosterone receptor antagonists) [7, 11, 12].

Radiology-assisted percutaneous drainage is the preferred method of evacuation, especially in subcapsular fluid collections and/or hematomas of native kidneys. However, in the case of chronic Page kidney or organized hematoma, radiology-assisted percutaneous drainage is likely to fail [13]. A long-standing collection can result in fibrous pseudo capsules and chronic inflammation that can require more aggressive treatment and, in selected cases, laparoscopic or open surgery with the stripping of the fibrotic area from the kidney. In transplant recipients where Page kidney of the allograft is diagnosed, the evacuation of the causative compressive collection is imperative. This is usually achieved, as in the presented case, emergently with open surgery. Radical nephrectomy can be necessary if the kidney damage is irreversible as in case of a sub-acute presentation, with uncontrolled hypertensive crisis [10].

Lacking long-term studies, the real long-term effects of Page kidney are not well established. After removing the compressive agent from the affected kidney, a prompt normalization of the kidney function with adequate urine output and normalization of blood pressure is expected. In chronic Page kidney, even after nephrectomy of the affected kidney, a chronic state of hypertension may persist, requiring long-term hypertensive treatment. At least one-third of these patients may have had no prior history of hypertension [7]. As a result, close follow-up of blood pressure is recommended [7].

Page kidney is a clinical syndrome characterized by uncontrolled high blood pressure, kidney dysfunction, and pain. It is critical to correctly recognize and rapidly treat Page kidney to reverse the hypertensive state and prevent chronic kidney damage. Particular attention must be paid to kidney transplant recipients, where this can lead to acute clinical deterioration due to lack of compensation by a functioning contralateral kidney and damage or loss of their only functioning kidney.

Disclosures M. Finotti has no disclosures. E. Martinez reports employment with the Annette C. and Harold C. Simmons Transplant Institute at Baylor University Medical Center.

Funding None.

References

1. Kiczek M, Udayasankar U. Page Kidney. J Urol. 2015;194(4):1109–10. https://doi.org/10.1016/j.juro.2015.07.035.
2. Dopson SJ, Jayakumar S, Velez JCQ. Page kidney as a rare cause of hypertension: case report and review of the literature. Am J Kidney Dis. 2009;54(2):334–9. https://doi.org/10.1053/j.ajkd.2008.11.014.
3. Page IH. The production of persistent arterial hypertension by cellophane perinephritis. JAMA. 1939;113(23) https://doi.org/10.1001/jama.1939.02800480032008.
4. Butt FK, Seawright AH, Kokko KE, Hawxby AM. An unusual presentation of a page kidney 24 days after transplantation: case report. Transplant Proc. 2010;42(10):4291–4. https://doi.org/10.1016/j.transproceed.2010.09.042.
5. MAC O, Sharma V, Balogun O, Ghimire A. Page kidney complicating kidney biopsy after stopping apixaban: a physician's dilemma. Indian J Nephrol. 30(3):201–3. https://doi.org/10.4103/ijn.IJN_269_19.
6. Chung J, Caumartin Y, Warren J, Luke PPW. Acute page kidney following renal allograft biopsy: a complication requiring early recognition and treatment. Am J Transplant. 2008;8(6):1323–8. https://doi.org/10.1111/j.1600-6143.2008.02215.x.
7. Smyth A, Collins CS, Thorsteinsdottir B, et al. Page kidney: etiology, renal function outcomes and risk for future hypertension. J Clin Hypertens. 2012;14(4):216–21. https://doi.org/10.1111/j.1751-7176.2012.00601.x.
8. Kenis I, Werner M, Nacasch N, Korzets Z. Recurrent non-traumatic page kidney. IMAJ. 2012;14(7):452–3.
9. Heffernan E, Zwirewich C, Harris A, Nguan C. Page kidney after renal allograft biopsy: sonographic findings. J Clin Ultrasound. 2009;37(4):226–9. https://doi.org/10.1002/jcu.20465.
10. McCune TR, Stone WJ, Breyer JA. Page kidney: case report and review of the literature. Am J Kidney Dis. 1991;18(5):593–9. https://doi.org/10.1016/s0272-6386(12)80656-1.
11. Izekor BE, Odigwe C, Goraya N, Duran PA. Page kidney from a subcapsular urinoma following contralateral radical nephrectomy. Cureus. Published online June 14, 2021. https://doi.org/10.7759/cureus.15639.
12. Wahdat R, Schwartz C, Espinosa J, Lucerna A. Page kidney: taking a page from history. Am J Emerg Med. 2017;35(1):193.e1–193.e2. https://doi.org/10.1016/j.ajem.2016.06.095.
13. Kobel MC, Nielsen TK, Graumann O. Acute renal failure and arterial hypertension due to subcapsular haematoma: is percutaneous drainage a feasible treatment? BMJ Case Rep. 2016;2016 https://doi.org/10.1136/bcr-2015-212769.

Chapter 14
Prolonged Kidney Delayed Graft Function: Switching to Belatacept

Gillian Divard

Introduction

Kidney delayed graft function (DGF) remains a problem despite the many advances in kidney transplantation. This is mainly related to the increase in the use of marginal donor grafts. These organs with pre-existing vascular lesions are also more sensitive to the vascular effects of immunosuppressive treatments such as calcineurin inhibitors (CNI). This case illustrates a CNI sparing strategy with early conversion to a belatacept-based immunosuppressive regimen in prolonged DGF due to CNI toxicity after kidney transplantation.

Patient History

A 68-year-old man with a history of chronic kidney disease (CKD) stage 5 due to cholesterol embolization in the context of ischemic heart disease and hypertension underwent first kidney transplantation after 2 years of being on hemodialysis. The donor was a 73-year-old expanded criteria donor with a history of hypertension and death resulting from a stroke and terminal serum creatinine of 0.71 mg/dL without proteinuria. The donor was unstable during extraction and required norepinephrine up to 10 mg/h.

At the time of transplant, panel reactive antibody was 10%, no preformed donor-specific antibodies were found. Pre-implantation biopsy of the transplanted kidney

G. Divard (✉)
Université de Paris Cité, INSERM U970, PARCC, Paris Translational Research Centre for Organ Transplantation, Kidney transplant department, Saint-Louis hospital, Assistance Publique Hôpitaux de Paris, Paris, France
e-mail: gillian.divard@inserm.fr

© The Author(s), under exclusive license to Springer Nature Switzerland AG 2022
F. Aziz, S. Parajuli (eds.), *Complications in Kidney Transplantation*,
https://doi.org/10.1007/978-3-031-13569-9_14

demonstrated glomerulosclerosis in 2 out of 20 sampled glomeruli. Fibrosis and tubular atrophy affect up to 15% of the tubule interstitium (Banff score ci1 and ct1), mild arteriosclerosis (Banff score cv1), arteriolar hyalinosis (Banff score ah1), and large areas of acute tubular necrosis. The transplant surgery was uneventful, and the cold ischemia duration was 7 h in cold storage preservation. He received induction with basiliximab, and his maintenance immunosuppression included tacrolimus (target trough 6–8 ng/mL), mycophenolate sodium 720 mg twice a day, and steroids (10 mg/day). However, despite 1000 mg/day furosemide infusion, the patient stayed oligoanuric with a serum creatinine of over 4.8 mg/dL and needed four hemodialysis sessions for hyperkalemia and fluid overload during the first 10 days post-transplant. Four renal graft ultrasounds demonstrated normal echotexture of the transplanted kidney, and Doppler evaluation of the intraparenchymal vessels showed resistive indices ranging from 0.79 to 0.96. The urine culture test was negative, and no proteinuria was found. A biopsy of the transplanted kidney was performed on day 8 and found glomerulosclerosis in 4 out of 19 sampled glomeruli. Fibrosis and tubular atrophy affecting up to 20% of the tubule interstitium (Banff score ci1 and ct1), moderate arteriosclerosis (Banff score cv2), arteriolar hyalinosis (Banff score ah2), and large areas of acute tubular necrosis without any sign of rejection (Banff score g0ptc0i0t0). Polarized light was unremarkable.

Question 1
What is the most likely diagnosis?

A. Acute rejection.
B. Graft pyelonephritis.
C. Delayed Graft Function.
D. Calcineurin inhibitors toxicity.
E. Obstructive uropathy.

The correct answer is C.

The patient was at high risk for delayed graft function (DGF) based on the marginal donor (age, history of hypertension, stroke) and donor instability during extraction. DGF is an acute kidney failure post-transplantation and usually results from renal ischemia and reperfusion injuries based on risk factors from the procurement and the donor and the recipient [1]. Conversely, there is no sign of obstructive uropathy (normal graft ultrasound) or graft pyelonephritis (urine culture is negative) or acute rejection on the biopsy.

Hospital Course

Tacrolimus trough levels were at a range of 5–7 ng/mL. A second biopsy is performed on day 14 in the absence of functional improvement and found no additional lesions except cytoplasmic vacuolization of proximal tubular epithelial cells (Fig. 14.1). These findings have led to a conversion to belatacept-based

Fig. 14.1 Kidney graft biopsy performed at day 14 post-transplant, stained with trichrome, reveals cytoplasmic vacuolization of proximal tubular epithelial cells. (original magnification ×600). (*Courtesy* from Dr. Marion Rabant, Pathology department, Necker hospital, Assistance Publique-Hôpitaux de Paris, Paris, France)

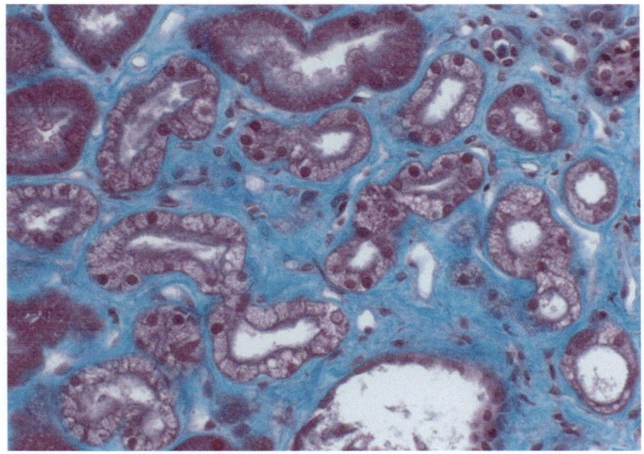

immunosuppression without calcineurin inhibitors (CNI) on day 16. Urine output started increasing at day 18 without diuretic support, and creatinine improved to 1.1 mg/dL in 10 days after CNI decreased.

Question 2

What are the most likely causes of the patient's prolonged delayed graft function?

A. Cold ischemia time.
B. Donor Age.
C. Calcineurin inhibitors toxicity.
D. Acute rejection.
E. Both B and C.

The correct answer is E.

In this case, we have multiple risk factors for DGF: donor age, donor history of hypertension, the instability of the donor reflected by the inotropic support, the cold storage preservation, the acute tubular necrosis, and the basiliximab induction [1, 2]. Additionally, there are signs of calcineurin inhibitors toxicity with the typic tubular cytoplasmic vacuolization on the figure and worsening of the arteriosclerosis and arteriolar hyalinosis on the biopsy compared to pre-implantation biopsy [3]. The rapid improvement of renal function after CNI reduction is also in favor of this diagnosis. Conversely, cold ischemia time is moderate here, and no signs of acute rejection were found on the biopsy in this low immunological risk patient.

Additional Clinical Course

With the new immunosuppressive regimen, including belatacept 5 mg/kg, mycophenolate sodium 720 mg twice a day, and steroids (10 mg/day), the patient stayed stable with an eGFR of 52 mL/min/1.73 m². At 1 year post-transplant, serum creatinine is 1.4 mg/dL and eGFR is 48.4 mL/min/1.73 m^2 without proteinuria. Circulating anti-HLA donor-specific antibodies were also tested and remained negative. A protocol biopsy was performed and found glomerulosclerosis in 5 out of 24 sampled glomeruli. Fibrosis and tubular atrophy affect up to 10% of the tubule interstitium (Banff score ci1 and ct1), mild arteriolar hyalinosis (Banff score ah1), and arteriosclerosis (Banff score cv1) without sign of rejection (Banff score g0ptc0i0t0). At 8 years after transplant, under a belatacept regimen, the eGFR remains stable at 45.3 mL/min/1.73 m^2 without proteinuria.

Discussion

Delayed graft function (DGF) has multiple definitions, but the most commonly used is clinical and is defined by the need for dialysis during the first week after kidney transplantation [2]. However, three main differential diagnoses must be considered: acute vascular complication, urological complication, and early allograft rejection. The incidence of DGF varies based on the various definitions; however, it is more prevalent in the donation after circulatory death donor at around 50% compared to the donation after brain death at around 20% [4]. This is an important post-transplant complication that impairs allograft survival and increases the incidence of early allograft rejection [1, 2]. Additionally, DGF duration seems to be an important factor. Prolonged DGF (longer than 15 days post-transplant) is associated with inferior renal function, patient, and graft survival at 1-year post-transplant [4]. Multiple DGF risk factors have been identified and can usually be divided into three categories: donor-related, recipient-related, and perioperative [1, 2]. Main donor-related risk factors are associated with marginal donors, including deceased donation, donor age, BMI. Regarding recipient-related risk factors, time on dialysis, previous kidney transplant, panel reactive antibody over 50%, ABO incompatibility, history of diabetes, BMI are the main risk factors, and perioperative risk factors are mainly driven by cold ischemia time duration. Several therapeutic approaches were tested to prevent or treat delayed graft function, but none demonstrates sufficient effect for clinical validation to be Food and Drug Administration-approved [5]. The only treatment that showed benefit in clinical settings and was routinely used is hypothermic machine perfusion [6].

Calcineurin inhibitors (CNIs) represented by cyclosporine and tacrolimus have remained the standard of care therapy for kidney transplantation for nearly 40 years [3]. CNIs prevent T-cell activation by inhibiting calcineurin, a cytoplasmic phosphatase required for the transcription of interleukin-2, which is upregulated when antigen is presented to the T cells. This treatment has transformed kidney transplantation by preventing graft rejection and improving graft survival [3]. However, CNIs are known to cause nephrotoxicity, hypertension, hyperlipidemia, diabetes, hirsutism, tremor, and may prolonged DGF, especially in the case of a marginal donor [3]. CNI nephrotoxicity is a non-specific clinical-histological diagnosis where the kidney graft biopsy is the cornerstone [7], Unfortunately, the serum levels of CNIs are not correlated well with the extent of graft injuries.

Two forms of CNI toxicity are described, acute and chronic. Histological features of acute CNI toxicity include early-stage hyalinization and vacuolization of myocytes in afferent arterioles and isometric vacuolization of proximal tubules [7]. Chronic CNI toxicity includes focal nodular hyalinosis, particularly adventitial, ultimately extending to the media of arterioles and arteries and striped interstitial fibrosis and tubular atrophy [7]. CNI toxicity can also cause thrombotic microangiopathy.

No specific treatment exists to prevent or avoid CNI toxicity [3]. Several immunosuppressive strategies were investigated for CNI toxicity, but currently, only two strategies are routinely used. The first is CNI sparing using low-dose CNI associated with mTOR inhibitors for de novo transplantation. In the TRANSFORM trial, this regimen was non-inferior to a standard of care regimen with the standard dose of CNI in terms of allograft function and graft survival at 2 years post-transplant [8]. However, mTOR inhibitor tolerability remains a real issue and limits the generalization of this practice. The other strategy is based on CNI avoidance using a belatacept-based immunosuppressive regimen.

Belatacept is a selective T-cell co-stimulation blocker approved by the FDA in 2011. Major studies evaluating belatacept showed that de novo kidney transplant patients treated with belatacept presented an improved renal function with a higher average estimated glomerular filtration rate (eGFR) compared to cyclosporine (CsA) regimen in patients with standard criteria donor (SCD) kidneys and extended criteria donor (ECD) kidneys, with a sustained effect at long follow-up [9]. Additionally, conversion to belatacept after transplant seems safe even in highly sensitized patients [10]. A meta-analysis of belatacept use as rescue therapy in case of CNI- toxicity, including 12 studies, showed that belatacept conversion improved eGFR. This effect was found significant, especially in the case of early conversion within 3 months post-transplant [10].

Due to the organ shortage in kidney transplantation, marginal donors are increasingly used and increase the risk of delayed graft function after kidney transplantation. The above patient and literature review suggest that multiple risk factors are associated with DGF, which impair long-term graft outcomes in kidney transplantation [1, 2]. The grafts with vascular lesions, for the most part, increase the risk of CNI toxicity and prolonged DGF. CNI avoidance seems to be the best option in this case. Early conversion to belatacept-based immunosuppression appears to be safe and improves kidney allograft function in observational studies [10]. Further studies are needed to determine long-term outcomes and safety profiles of early belatacept conversion in the case of DGF in kidney allograft recipients.

Disclosures G. Divard received grants from the French Foundation for Medical Research and the French-speaking Society of Nephrology, Dialysis, and Transplantation.

Funding None.

References

1. Ojo AO, Wolfe RA, Held PJ, Port FK, Schmouder RL. Delayed graft function: risk factors and implications for renal allograft survival. Transplantation. 1997;63(7):968–74.
2. Perico N, Cattaneo D, Sayegh MH, Remuzzi G. Delayed graft function in kidney transplantation. Lancet. 2004;364(9447):1814–27.
3. Liptak P, Ivanyi B. Primer: histopathology of calcineurin-inhibitor toxicity in renal allografts. Nat Clin Pract Nephrol. 2006;2(7):398–404. quiz following
4. Lim WH, Johnson DW, Teixeira-Pinto A, Wong G. Association between duration of delayed graft function, acute rejection, and allograft outcome after deceased donor kidney transplantation. Transplantation. 2019;103(2):412–9.
5. Nashan BA-FM, Citterio F. Prediction, prevention, and management of delayed graft function: where are we now? Clin Transpl. 2016;30:1198–208.
6. Moers C, Smits JM, Maathuis MH, Treckmann J, van Gelder F, Napieralski BP, et al. Machine perfusion or cold storage in deceased-donor kidney transplantation. N Engl J Med. 2009;360(1):7–19.
7. Lusco MA, Fogo AB, Najafian B, Alpers CE. AJKD atlas of renal pathology: Calcineurin inhibitor nephrotoxicity. Am J Kidney Dis. 2017;69(5):e21–e2.
8. Berger SP, Sommerer C, Witzke O, Tedesco H, Chadban S, Mulgaonkar S, et al. Two-year outcomes in de novo renal transplant recipients receiving everolimus-facilitated calcineurin inhibitor reduction regimen from the TRANSFORM study. Am J Transplant. 2019;19(11):3018–34.
9. Vincenti F, Rostaing L, Grinyo J, Rice K, Steinberg S, Gaite L, et al. Belatacept and long-term outcomes in kidney transplantation. N Engl J Med. 2016;374(4):333–43.
10. El Hennawy H, Safar O, Al Faifi AS, El Nazer W, Kamal A, Mahedy A, et al. Belatacept rescue therapy of CNI-induced nephrotoxicity, meta-analysis. Transplant Rev (Orlando). 2021;35(4):100653.

Chapter 15
A Case of De Novo Membranous Nephropathy in the Transplanted Kidney

Matthew Konz and Fahad Aziz

Introduction

Primary membranous nephropathy is one of the common causes of nephrotic syndrome [1]. The recurrence of primary membranous nephropathy after kidney transplantation is close to 10–45% [2, 3]. Usually, membranous nephropathy recurrence occurs 2–3 years after the transplant occurs [4]. Occasionally, de novo membranous nephropathy is identified on the kidney allograft biopsy. Here, we describe a case of de novo membranous nephropathy, focusing on management and outcomes.

Patient History

A 51-year-old African American male with end-stage kidney disease (ESKD) due to biopsy-proven focal segmental glomerular sclerosis (FSGS) (treated with a high dose of steroids) underwent a deceased donor kidney transplantation. At the time of transplant, his panel reactive antibody (PRA) was 15%, and he had no preformed donor-specific antibodies (DSA). He received induction with anti-thymocyte globulin. His maintenance immunosuppression included tacrolimus twice a day (target trough 6–8 ng/mL), mycophenolate sodium 720 mg twice a day, and prednisone

M. Konz (✉) · F. Aziz
Department of Medicine, University of Wisconsin–Madison School of Medicine and Public Health, University of Wisconsin Hospital and Clinics, Madison, WI, USA
e-mail: MKonz@uwhealth.org; faziz@wisc.edu

© The Author(s), under exclusive license to Springer Nature Switzerland AG 2022

F. Aziz, S. Parajuli (eds.), *Complications in Kidney Transplantation*,
https://doi.org/10.1007/978-3-031-13569-9_15

5 mg daily. He achieved a baseline creatinine of 1.2 mg/dL with eGFR of 60 mL/min/1.73 m^2. His post-transplant course was unremarkable. Three months after the transplant, he developed new proteinuria. His urine protein-creatinine ratio was more than 7 gm/gm. His creatinine worsened to 1.8 mg/dL. He presented for further management.

Question 1

What should be the next step in the management?

A. Start lisinopril.
B. Steroid pulse.
C. Transplant kidney biopsy.
D. Start spironolactone.

The correct answer is C.

There can be multiple reasons for proteinuria in kidney transplant recipients, including recurrence of glomerulonephritis, transplant glomerulopathy (TG), acute antibody-mediated rejection, and chronic antibody-mediated rejections. Though the addition of lisinopril and spironolactone can help reduce proteinuria, they would not treat the underlying disease process. The treatment should be focused on the histological diagnosis.

Further Course

The patient underwent a biopsy of the kidney allograft. His biopsy was negative for rejection (t0, g0, ptc0, cg0, c4d0). However, the electron microscopy showed numerous subepithelial electron-dense deposits and a few short basement membrane spikes (Fig. 15.1). There was severe foot process effacement. The glomerulus

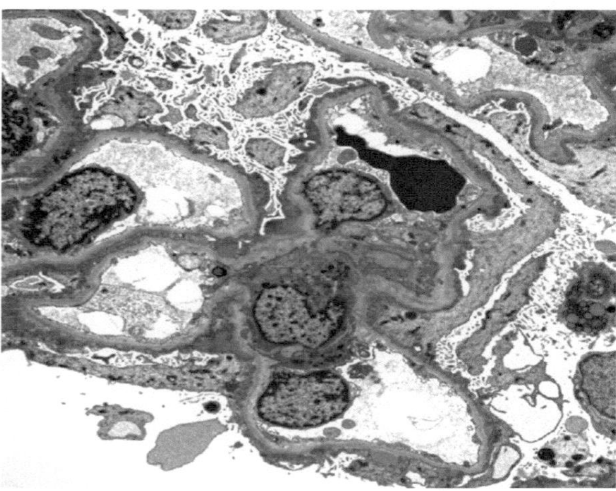

Fig. 15.1 Electron microscopy showing diffuse foot process effacement

showed normocellularity and no basement membrane double contours. The immunofluorescence showed no staining for IgG, IgM, IgA, C3, and C1q. These findings were suggestive of membranous nephropathy.

With the diagnosis of membranous nephropathy, he underwent an extensive workup to rule out secondary membranous nephropathy, including workup for malignancies. The workup was negative for monoclonal gammopathies, including serum protein electrophoresis (SPEP) and urine protein electrophoresis (UPEP). His serum anti-phospholipase A2 receptor antibodies (Anti-PLA2R antibodies) were elevated at 1:1280. With the negative workup and elevated anti-PLA2R receptor antibodies, it was labeled as de novo membranous nephropathy of the transplanted kidney.

Question 2
What will be the next step in managing the de novo membranous nephropathy in the transplanted kidney?

A. Observe.
B. Rituximab.
C. Lisinopril.
D. Belatacept.

The correct answer is B.
The optimal treatment of de novo or recurrent membranous nephropathy is not known. However, a few studies suggested that treating this condition with rituximab may improve graft outcomes [5], (option B). The recurrence of membranous nephropathy or de novo nephropathy is associated with significantly worse graft outcomes. Observation alone would not be a good option (option A). The addition of lisinopril can improve proteinuria, but it is not the primary treatment of membranous nephropathy (option C). An increase in immunosuppression by adding belatacept is not shown to improve the graft outcomes in patients with recurrence or de novo membranous nephropathy (option D).

Additional Clinical Course

After diagnosing idiopathic membranous nephropathy, the patient received two doses of rituximab 1 gm 2 weeks apart. An additional 1 gm of rituximab was given 1 month after the second dose. His baseline immunosuppression was also increased. The patient was also started on a combination of losartan and spironolactone. At 7-month post-transplant, anti-PLA2R antibodies titers dropped below 1:10, urine protein creatinine ratio dropped below 1 gm/gm, and serum creatinine improved to 1.3 mg/dL (Fig. 15.2).

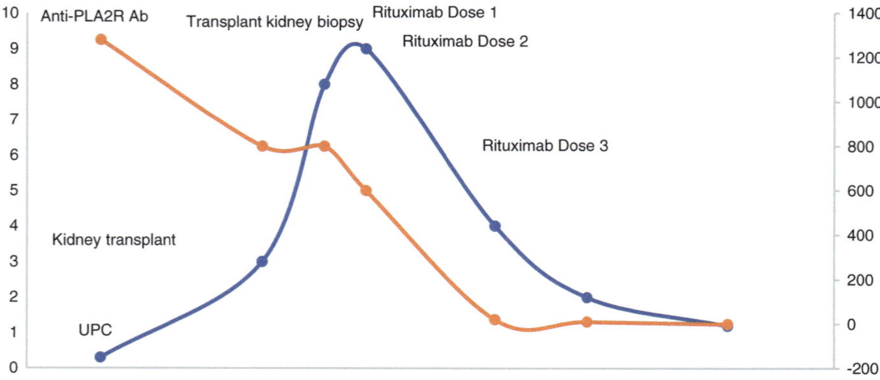

Fig. 15.2 Rituximab dosing and response to the treatment

Discussion

This case illustrates the successful treatment of de novo membranous nephropathy in the transplanted kidney. The incidence of de novo membranous nephropathy in the transplanted kidney is not known. Primary membranous nephropathy has been reported to recur in 10–45% of patients after kidney transplantation [3, 6–11]. Recurrent membranous nephropathy often occurs between the second and third-year post-transplantation, but earlier and later cases are also reported [12]. Briganti's study using the Australia and New Zealand Dialysis and Transplant Registry (ANZDATA) reported that renal allograft survival at 10-years was similar in patients with membranous nephropathy as their primary disease versus patients transplanted with other renal diseases [8]. Patients with membranous nephropathy have been reported to have a higher incidence of acute rejection after kidney transplantation. However, 10-years graft survival remained the same compared to the other GNs [13].

There are no known treatments to prevent and treat the recurrence of membranous nephropathy in kidney transplant recipients. The triple immunosuppression, including steroids, calcineurin inhibitors, and antiproliferative agents, does not have a role in preventing membranous nephropathy recurrence [5]. On the other hand, their role in treating membranous nephropathy recurrence is not well established. Rituximab can significantly reduce the phospholipase A2 receptor (PLA2R) antibodies and is an important therapeutic option for patients with primary membranous nephropathy [5, 14]. Rituximab is shown to be an effective therapeutic option for recurrence or de novo membranous nephropathy [15]. Prophylactic use of rituximab for the prevention of membranous nephropathy is not known. No high-quality studies are looking at the treatment response in patients with recurrence or de novo membranous nephropathy. A response is usually assessed by decreasing anti-PLA2R antibodies and urine protein creatinine ratio [16].

Post-transplant de novo membranous nephropathy is a significant cause of kidney allograft dysfunction. Aggressive treatment of the de novo membranous nephropathy in the transplanted kidney with rituximab and appropriate up-titration in the immunosuppression can improve graft outcomes. Further, studies are needed to determine the risk factors, diagnosis, management, and long-term outcomes in kidney allograft recipients with idiopathic membranous nephropathy.

References

1. Cattran DC. Idiopathic membranous glomerulonephritis. Kidney Int. 2001;59(5):1983–94.
2. Taylor DM, Cameron PA, Eddey D. Recurrent overdose: patient characteristics, habits, and outcomes. J Accid Emerg Med. 1998;15(4):257–61.
3. Ponticelli C, Passerini P. Can prognostic factors assist therapeutic decisions in idiopathic membranous nephropathy? J Nephrol. 2010;23(2):156–63.
4. Ponticelli C, Passerini P. Management of idiopathic membranous nephropathy. Expert Opin Pharmacother. 2010;11(13):2163–75.
5. Dahan K, Debiec H, Plaisier E, Cachanado M, Rousseau A, Wakselman L, et al. Rituximab for severe membranous nephropathy: a 6-month trial with extended follow-up. J Am Soc Nephrol. 2017;28(1):348–58.
6. Cameron JS. Recurrent renal disease after renal transplantation. Curr Opin Nephrol Hypertens. 1994;3(6):602–7.
7. Moroni G, Gallelli B, Quaglini S, Leoni A, Banfi G, Passerini P, et al. Long-term outcome of renal transplantation in patients with idiopathic membranous glomerulonephritis (MN). Nephrol Dial Transplant. 2010;25(10):3408–15.
8. Briganti EM, Russ GR, McNeil JJ, Atkins RC, Chadban SJ. Risk of renal allograft loss from recurrent glomerulonephritis. N Engl J Med. 2002;347(2):103–9.
9. Dabade TS, Grande JP, Norby SM, Fervenza FC, Cosio FG. Recurrent idiopathic membranous nephropathy after kidney transplantation: a surveillance biopsy study. Am J Transplant. 2008;8(6):1318–22.
10. El-Zoghby ZM, Grande JP, Fraile MG, Norby SM, Fervenza FC, Cosio FG. Recurrent idiopathic membranous nephropathy: early diagnosis by protocol biopsies and treatment with anti-CD20 monoclonal antibodies. Am J Transplant. 2009;9(12):2800–7.
11. Hogan SL, Muller KE, Jennette JC, Falk RJ. A review of therapeutic studies of idiopathic membranous glomerulopathy. Am J Kidney Dis. 1995;25(6):862–75.
12. Ponticelli C, Glassock RJ. Posttransplant recurrence of primary glomerulonephritis. Clin J Am Soc Nephrol. 2010;5(12):2363–72.
13. Singh T, Astor B, Zhong W, Mandelbrot D, Djamali A, Panzer S. Kidney transplant recipients with primary membranous glomerulonephritis have a higher risk of acute rejection compared with other primary Glomerulonephritides. Transplant Direct. 2017;3(11):e223.
14. Fervenza FC, Abraham RS, Erickson SB, Irazabal MV, Eirin A, Specks U, et al. Rituximab therapy in idiopathic membranous nephropathy: a 2-year study. Clin J Am Soc Nephrol. 2010;5(12):2188–98.
15. Passerini P, Malvica S, Tripodi F, Cerutti R, Messa P. Membranous nephropathy (MN) recurrence after renal transplantation. Front Immunol. 2019;10:1326.
16. Francis J BL. Kidney transplantation in adults: membranous nephropathy and kidney transplantation. 2021

Chapter 16
Postoperative Complications Urine Leak

Ashlee M. Griffin and Praise Matemavi

Introduction

Kidney disease is a highly morbid condition that results in significant impairment in the quality of life for affected individuals. Treatment options are limited and include hemodialysis, peritoneal dialysis, and kidney transplantation, with the latter being the superior treatment modality. While kidney transplantation is preferred, complications can arise in the postoperative period requiring additional interventions. These complications include urine leak, ureteral strictures, obstruction, renal artery stenosis, and rejection. Urine leak is the most common complication with management ranging from conservative with external urinary drainage, minimally invasive with ureteral stents, or invasive with surgical intervention. We present a case of a urine leak after a kidney transplant requiring additional procedural interventions and re-operation for definitive repair.

Patient History

A 48-year-old female with a history of ESKD secondary to diabetic nephropathy on hemodialysis for 8 years and anuric underwent routine deceased circulatory death donor kidney transplant. The kidney donor profile index (KDPI) was 10%, with a cold ischemia time of 22 h and 46 min and a warm ischemia time of 28 min. Her

A. M. Griffin · P. Matemavi (✉)
Division of Transplant and Hepatobiliary Surgery, Department of Surgery, University of Mississippi Medical Center, Jackson, MS, USA
e-mail: amgriffin@umc.edu; pmatemavi@umc.edu

© The Author(s), under exclusive license to Springer Nature Switzerland AG 2022
F. Aziz, S. Parajuli (eds.), *Complications in Kidney Transplantation*,
https://doi.org/10.1007/978-3-031-13569-9_16

Fig. 16.1 CT scan after removal of the stent

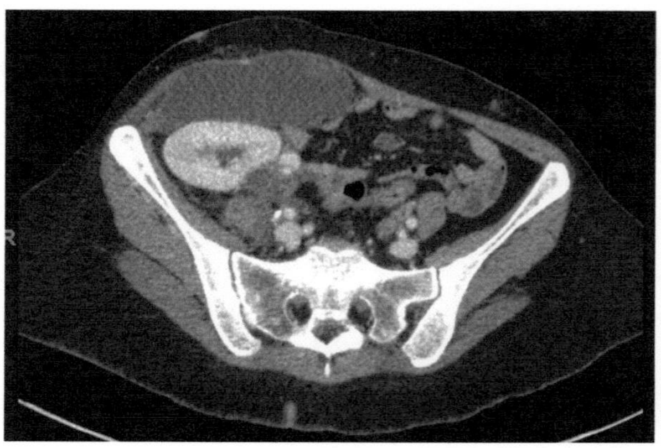

initial postoperative course was uneventful, and she was discharged on postoperative day 3 with excellent allograft function. Approximately 2 weeks postoperatively, her ureteral stent was removed, which she initially tolerated well. 2 days after stent removal, she began experiencing right lower quadrant pain, nausea, and anorexia. Her pain progressively worsened, resulting in her presentation to the emergency department for evaluation. She was afebrile and hemodynamically stable. On exam, she was tender to palpation over her incision, but there was no evidence of wound dehiscence, erythema, or drainage. Pertinent laboratory results showed WBC 14.2 K/uL, potassium 6.9 mmol/L, BUN 34 mg/dL, and Cr 1.95 mg/dL. Ultrasound of the transplanted kidney showed a non-specific fluid collection, hydroureteronephrosis with normal resistive indices. CT imaging was obtained and shown below (Fig. 16.1).

Question 1

Given the patient's presentation and imaging, what is the most likely cause of the patient's symptoms?

A. Acute rejection.
B. Renal artery stenosis.
C. Wound infection.
D. Urine leak.

The correct answer is D.

Given the patient's acute onset of abdominal pain and fluid collection after removing her ureteral stent, a urine leak is the most likely explanation. While she does have leukocytosis and a subcutaneous fluid collection under her incision on imaging, the acute onset, lack of drainage, and erythema make wound infection less likely. Resistive indices on ultrasound were within normal limits ruling out renal artery stenosis. Although acute rejection could be a consideration given her elevated lab values, this would not explain her clinical presentation and imaging findings.

Clinical Course

The patient was admitted to the hospital, and interventional radiology was consulted for drain placement. Urine creatinine confirmed urinoma. A percutaneous nephrostomy tube was placed, and imaging demonstrated a focal leak at the mid to distal ureter. Conservative management was attempted for a month, but unfortunately, she developed a long segment mid-ureteral stricture. She then underwent an antegrade placement of a nephroureteral stent after balloon dilation of the stricture. She required multiple upsizing and stent exchanges without success. Her serum creatinine nadir was 0.7 mg/dL.

Question 2

What is the next best treatment option for her ureteral stricture after failed conservative management?

A. Upsize stent and nephrostomy tube placement.
B. Return to the operating room for definitive repair.
C. Balloon dilation of the ureteral stricture with stent replacement.
D. Laser endoureterotomy.

The correct answer is B.

This patient has failed conservative management with nephroureteral stent with upsizing and stent exchanges. While balloon dilation may help with a short segment stricture, it is less successful in long segment strictures. Surgical management with a return to the operating room for definitive repair is the best option as it is likely to have a long-term solution, especially in this young patient with normal allograft function.

Additional Clinical Course

The patient underwent surgical repair of ureteral stricture. In this case, because it was a right donor kidney in the right iliac fossa with the blood vessels anterior to the renal pelvis, it was challenging to perform a pyelo-ureterostomy. Nephrogram of the transplanted kidney and the collecting system showed a patent proximal ureter for a length of 4 cm from the renal pelvis. The right native ureter was anastomosed to the proximal transplant ureter without tension. The surgery went well without complications, and the patient was discharged home on postoperative day 2. She continues to do well 24 months postoperative with a creatinine of 0.7–0.9 mg/dL.

Discussion

Kidney transplantation is the preferred management for ESKD in appropriate candidates. The overall 5-year survival rate for a kidney transplant is more than double that of dialysis, with the added benefit of the decreased overall cost. While transplant remains the preferred treatment option, surgical intervention is not without the inherent risk of peri-operative complications [1]. Urologic complications are the most common surgical complications encountered in the postoperative period and include urine leak, ureteral stenosis/stricture, and obstruction. Urine leak after kidney transplantation is the most common early surgical complication encountered postoperatively. Several studies report that the estimated incidence of postoperative urine leak ranges from 1.5 to 6% [2].

Clinical presentations may vary amongst patients based on whether the urine leak occurs early or late in the postoperative period. Early urine leaks generally occur within the first 48 h postoperatively and are likely a result of technical failure. Presentations may include excess drainage of clear yellow fluid from the incision or surgical drain (if one is present), oliguria, and increased pain or pressure near the surgical site [3]. Late urine leaks are seen around postoperative days 5–14 and typically result from ischemic necrosis of the distal ureter secondary to the compromised blood supply [1–3]. Presentation is similar to early urine leak with increased abdominal pain or swelling, oliguria, drainage of yellow fluid from the surgical incision with impaired wound healing, and/or signs of infection.

If a urine leak is suspected, workup should include routine labs and imaging studies with a transplant kidney ultrasound and/or CT. Lab values may show a leukocytosis if there is an infected fluid collection or elevated serum creatinine. CT imaging will likely demonstrate a simple fluid collection near the transplanted kidney, with or without hydronephrosis. Ultrasound findings suspicious for urine leak include a well-defined, anechoic fluid collection without septations with or without the presence of hydronephrosis [4]. Additionally, a contrasting study to evaluate the urologic system is a useful adjunct in reaching the diagnosis.

Management of a urine leak is generally conservative. Maximal decompression of the urologic system via percutaneous nephrostomy (PCN) tube, foley catheter, and ureteral stent is preferred when a small volume leak is suspected. Additionally, drainage of any notable fluid collections can provide further confirmation of urine leak by evaluating the fluid creatinine, which will be much more elevated than serum creatinine. A PCN and stent should remain for approximately 6–8 weeks to allow for optimal ureteral healing. If a persistent leak occurs or an initial large volume, uncontrolled leak, then surgical intervention should be pursued [1–5].

Disclosures P. Matemavi reports employment with the University of Mississippi Medical Center and has received research funding through the American Society of Transplant Surgeons – Natera Socio Economic and Racial Disparity grant. A. Griffin reports employment with the University of Mississippi Medical Center.

Funding None.

References

1. Sarier M, Yayar O, Yavuz A, Turgut H, Kukul E. Update on the management of urological problems following kidney transplantation. Urol Int. 2021;105:541–7. https://doi.org/10.1159/000512885.
2. Buttigieg J, Agius-Anastasi A, Sharma A, Halawa A. Early urological complications after kidney transplantation: an overview. World J Transplant. 2018;8(5):142–9. https://doi.org/10.5500/wjt.v8.i5.142.
3. Gunawansa N, Sharma A, Halawa A. Post-transplant urinary leak; the perennial 'Achilles heel' in renal transplant surgery. Trends Transplant. 2018; https://doi.org/10.15761/TiT.1000246.
4. Veeratterapillay R, Sharma A, Halawa A. Management of urine leak following renal transplantation: an evidence-based approach. J Urol Nephrol Open Access. 2018;4(1):1–5. https://doi.org/10.15226/2473-6430/4/1/00141.
5. Akbar S, Jafri S, Amendola M., Madrazo B, Salem R, Bis K. Complications of renal transplantation. 2005 [online] Available at: https://doi.org/10.1148/rg.255045133. Accessed 14 Dec 2021.

Chapter 17
Post-Kidney Transplant Lymphocele

Matthew Rosenzweig and Eric J. Martinez

Introduction

Lymphoceles are lymph-containing fluid collections covered by a fibrous capsule and are a well-described complication of renal transplant. They are often the result of extensive vascular dissection of the lymphatic tissue overlying the iliac vessels. Through the study of renal transplant, several contributing factors have been associated with postoperative lymphoceles, including immunosuppression, obesity, delayed graft function, and rejection. With advances in modern imaging, lymphoceles have been identified in up to 50% of renal transplant recipients, most asymptomatic and self-resolving. However, 5–10% of symptomatic lymphoceles require intervention. It is imperative for teams managing renal transplant recipients to be vigilant for and familiarize themselves with this complication to optimize the postoperative care of the patient and the allograft. We present a case of a 54-year-old male who received a deceased donor renal transplant and developed a postoperative lymphocele. We discuss several physical exam findings aiding in the early identification of post-renal transplant lymphoceles. Additionally, we provide a stepwise approach to diagnosis and outline a management algorithm to address this postoperative complication.

M. Rosenzweig
Annette C. and Harold C. Simmons Transplant Institute, Baylor University Medical Center, Dallas, TX, USA
e-mail: Matthew.Rosenzweig@BSWHealth.org

E. J. Martinez (✉)
Annette C. and Harold C. Simmons Transplant Institute, Baylor University Medical Center, Dallas, TX, USA

Baylor Scott & White Transplant Services, Dallas, TX, USA
e-mail: Eric.Martinez1@BSWHealth.org

© The Author(s), under exclusive license to Springer Nature Switzerland AG 2022

F. Aziz, S. Parajuli (eds.), *Complications in Kidney Transplantation*,
https://doi.org/10.1007/978-3-031-13569-9_17

Patient History

A 54-year-old man with a history of heart transplant secondary to cardiomyopathy, and bilateral native nephrectomy secondary to polycystic kidney disease, underwent a brain-dead donor kidney transplant into the left iliac fossa. The patient had a kidney ultrasound on a postoperative day (POD) 1 due to oliguria which revealed mild hydronephrosis and no surrounding fluid collections (Fig. 17.1). On POD 14, despite adequate urine output and down-trending serum creatinine (sCr) of 1.68 mg/dL down from 5.38 mg/dL, the patient presented with generalized fatigue and a new leukocytosis of 21.8 K/uL. The patient's hemoglobin was stable at 9.5 g/dL compared to his preoperative levels. A CT (Fig. 17.2a, b) was ordered of his chest, abdomen, and pelvis, revealing a left perinephric fluid collection.

Question 1

What is the most likely diagnosis of the patient's presentation?

A. Urinoma.
B. Lymphocele.
C. Hematoma.
D. Abscess.

The correct answer is B.

Lymphoceles form from leakage of lymph from the recipient iliac or donor renal lymphatic channels. On imaging, they may appear homogeneous and hypoechoic, usually inferior and medial to the allograft. Lymphoceles can result in pain, ipsilateral lower extremity edema, and renal allograft dysfunction via the mass effect on the surrounding recipient or renal vasculature, ureter, or bladder [1]. Urine leaks, usually diagnosed in the early postoperative period and presenting with elevated sCr or wound leaking with elevated fluid creatinine, may occur from injury during the

Fig. 17.1 Ultrasound of renal allograft on POD 1

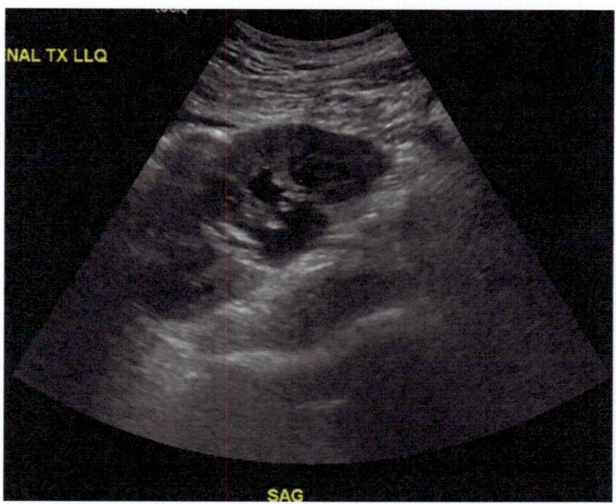

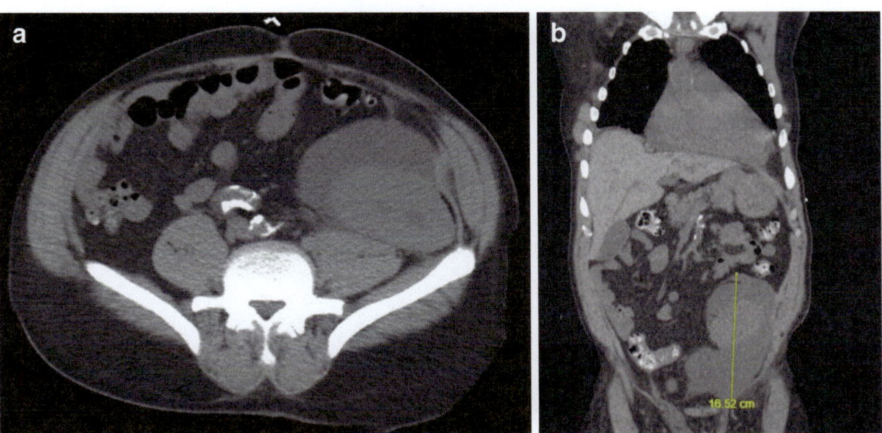

Fig. 17.2 Computed tomography (CT) scan of the abdomen and pelvis demonstrating a left perinephric fluid collection. (**a**) Axial. (**b**) Coronal

procurement, technical error during implantation, or from ischemic necrosis of the distal transplanted ureter. Hematomas, though common and often asymptomatic, appear heterogenous on imaging and can cause graft dysfunction, hemodynamic instability, or wound complications. Surgical site infections have been documented to occur in 7.5% of renal transplants. While a WBC of 21.8 K/uL is concerning for an abscess, no additional symptoms or objective findings in the physical exam, lab work, or imaging suggested an abscess, making lymphocele more likely.

Hospital Course

Under ultrasound guidance, interventional radiology aspirated 300 mL of serous perinephric fluid and sent it for analysis (Fig.17.3). Fluid creatinine was 1.61 mg/dL, and sCr was 1.66 mg/dL. The culture of the fluid was negative for growth. Lymphocytes accounted for 93% of the leukocytes within the aspirated fluid. The fluid collection reaccumulated 14 days later, and the patient was symptomatic with left lower quadrant bulging, left lower extremity edema, and pain with ambulation. He remained afebrile and had a leukocyte count of 9.9 K/uL.

Question 2
What is the most definitive treatment?

A. Repeat aspiration with percutaneous drain placement.
B. Percutaneous aspiration of fluid collection.
C. Laparoscopic marsupialization or peritoneal window.
D. Open marsupialization or peritoneal window.

   The correct answer is C.

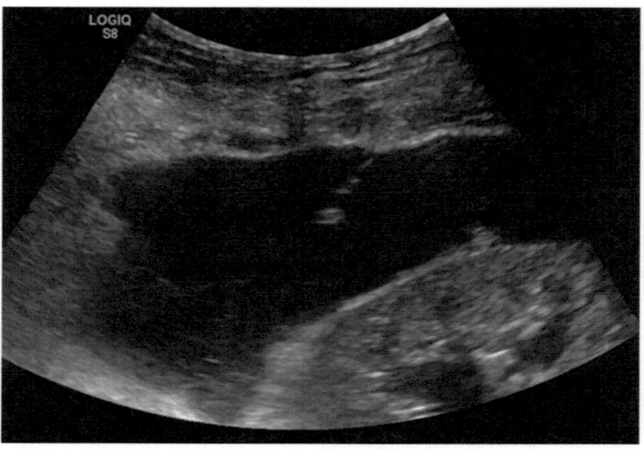

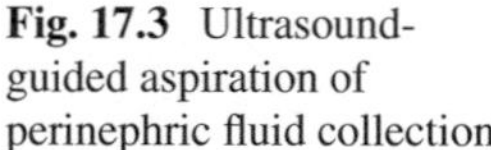

Fig. 17.3 Ultrasound-guided aspiration of perinephric fluid collection

Laparoscopic marsupialization of lymphoceles status post-kidney transplant is the most definitive treatment. The laparoscopic approach and open approaches have recurrence rates of 8% and 16%, respectively [2]. Percutaneous aspiration and drain placement of perinephric lymphoceles are effective at relieving symptoms and aid in the diagnosis; however, the recurrence rates are 60% and 50%, respectively, for these approaches and introduce the possibility of contaminating the collection.

Additional Clinical Course

The patient underwent laparoscopic marsupialization of the lymphocele 1 month after his renal transplant. In the operating room, 600 mL of clear, serous fluid was aspirated. A 2 × 2 cm area of the peritoneal wall overlying the lymphocele was excised to ensure continued drainage. Upon follow-up, his only lingering symptom was edema to his left lower extremity, which subsequently resolved. He reported normal urine output, and his sCr trended down to 1.24 mg/dL at the 6-month mark.

Discussion

General Information

Lymphoceles are lymph-containing fluid collections covered by a fibrous capsule localized around the renal allograft. Lymphoceles in kidney transplant patients have been noted since the 1970s as a complication of extensive vascular dissection of the lymphatic tissue overlying the iliac vessels. Over time, other contributing factors that have been associated with lymphoceles in the post-kidney transplant recipient include immunosuppression, obesity, delayed graft function, and rejection [3].

Incidence/Frequency/Timing

The diagnosis of lymphoceles typically occurs between the second week and 6-month postoperative mark, with a peak incidence at 6 weeks [4]. With the routine use of postoperative renal ultrasound, the incidence of lymphoceles has increased, and collections may be demonstrated in up to 50% of scans [5]. The incidence of symptomatic lymphoceles, however, has been documented at 6%, requiring treatment in 5–10% of diagnosed cases [4, 5].

Common Clinical Presentation

Most cases of lymphocele are asymptomatic. Symptomatic lymphoceles are usually found anterior to the iliac vessels between the allograft and bladder. Lymphatic vessels injured during recipient iliac vascular dissection or during the donor renal hilum backbench preparation that are not ligated can leak lymphatic fluid into the retroperitoneum [6]. When large enough (>300 cc), clinical symptoms are often secondary to mass effect as the peritoneum keeps the fluid contained. Presenting features include wound or ipsilateral lower extremity swelling, ureteral obstruction, graft dysfunction, and pain [7]. In some instances, the mass effect of the lymphocele on the external iliac vein can be severe enough to cause deep vein thrombosis [8]. Other subjective findings may include urinary urgency and frequency [9]. Additionally, infected lymphoceles may present as an abscess with fevers, chills, and signs of sepsis, an important consideration in the workup.

Evaluation

Though many lymphoceles are incidentally identified on imaging, symptomatic lymphoceles are typically detected after a workup for allograft dysfunction with ultrasound, or less commonly, CT scans. Lymphoceles on ultrasound are anechoic and may contain septations. On CT, lymphoceles usually demonstrate water-attenuation levels, differentiating them from hematomas and abscesses. Though rarely clinically indicated, MRI or nuclear scintigraphy may be performed to exclude the presence of blood or urine, respectively. The diagnosis is typically confirmed after biochemical analysis of percutaneous needle aspirate, effectively ruling out a urine leak (or urinoma) with a fluid creatinine similar to the sCr [3].

Management (Evidence-Based)

Most small lymphoceles containing <100 mL of lymph are asymptomatic and resolve spontaneously with time [4, 9]. For those that require treatment, there are several treatment modalities available. Aspiration is a logical first step that serves both a diagnostic and therapeutic role. Unfortunately, the rate of recurrence ranges between 10 and 95% [2]. The addition of leaving a drain yields similar if not worse results with a recurrence rate of 50%. Sclerotherapy is another minimally invasive option with an overall recurrence rate of 31% [2, 10]. Different sclerotic agents have included povidone-iodine, human fibrinogen, human thrombin, calcium chloride, gentamycin, ethanol, tetracycline, and streptomycin with varying degrees of success. The mainstay of treatment is surgical marsupialization. This allows continued leaking lymphatic fluid to drain into the peritoneal cavity and get absorbed by the peritoneum, effectively relieving the symptoms of the mass effect and managing the fluid. The recurrence rate of laparoscopic marsupialization has been documented at 8%, better than that for the open approach at 16% [2]. For this reason, the standard algorithm for management of symptomatic lymphoceles has become an aspiration for diagnostic and therapeutic purposes, followed by laparoscopic marsupialization of the lymphocele if there is a recurrence.

Clinical Meaning

While most post-renal transplant lymphoceles are asymptomatic, symptomatic lymphoceles pose a clinical challenge due to a high recurrence rate. To minimize the morbidity of the transplant recipient and maximize allograft function, the transplant physician must develop an understanding of significant risk factors that may predispose recipients to lymphocele formation, an algorithm for working through the differential diagnosis of peri-allograft fluid collections and familiarize themselves with the goals and effectiveness of various treatment options. A stepwise approach from minimally invasive diagnostic to more invasive treatment options is recommended to manage post-transplant lymphoceles.

Disclosures M. Rosenzweig has no disclosures. E. Martinez reports employment with the Annette C. and Harold C. Simmons Transplant Institute at Baylor University Medical Center.

Funding None.

References

1. Moreno CC, Mittal PK, Ghonge NP, et al. Imaging complications of renal transplantation. Radiol Clin N Am. 2016;54:235–49. https://doi.org/10.1016/j.rcl.2015.09.007.
2. Lucewicz A, Germaine W, Lam VW, et al. Management of primary symptomatic lymphocele after kidney transplantation: a systematic review. Transplantation. 2011;92:663–73.
3. Ranghino A, Segolomo G, Lasaponara F, et al. Lymphatic disorders after renal transplantation: new insights for an old complication. Clin Kidney J. 2015;8(5):615–22.
4. Bzoma B, Kostro J, Debska-Slizien A, et al. Treatment of the lymphocele after kidney transplantation: a single-center experience. Transplant Proceedings. 2016;48:1637–40.
5. Barlow A, Nicholson M. Kidney transplantation surgery. Comprehensive. Clin Nephrol. 2018;103:1174–1185. e1.
6. Hakim N, Haberal M, Maluf D. Surgical complications after kidney transplant. Transplantation Surgery. 2021;10:802–48.
7. El-Hennawy H, Morrill C, Orlando G, et al. Vascular complications in renal transplantation, kidney transplantation, bioengineering and regeneration. 2017;27:373–402. 34:491–502
8. Knight S, Allen R. Vascular and lymphatic complications after kidney transplantation. In: Kidney Transplantation-Principles and Practice, vol. 28. 8th ed; 2019. p. 458–86.
9. Ghavamian R, Chalouhy C. Complications of urologic surgery. Campbell-Walsh-Wein. Urology. 2021;17:260–281.e3.
10. Gipson M. Percutaneous management of lymphocele after renal transplantation. Semin Intervent Radiol. 2013;30:215–8.

Chapter 18
Transplant Renal Artery Stenosis

Ashlee M. Griffin and Praise Matemavi

Introduction

Transplant renal artery stenosis (TRAS) is a known cause of post-transplant arterial hypertension, graft dysfunction, and loss. An ultrasound, though non-discriminating, is a safe and non-invasive first step in evaluation. For those with creatinine levels less than 2 mg/dL, a contrasted CT scan accurately delineates arterial anatomy, while in patients with elevated creatinine, a magnetic resonance imaging angiography is preferred. When kidney function is stable, and hypertension is well controlled, no specific indication is required. In uncontrolled hypertension on pharmacologic agents and or worsening renal function, percutaneous transluminal renal angioplasty and stent placement are the first-choice therapy. A surgical approach is necessary in cases that are not amenable to angioplasty.

Patient History

A 62-year-old male with a history of ESKD secondary to hypertension presents to the emergency department 14 weeks after a deceased donor kidney transplant. The donor was a 40-year-old brain-dead donor who died from a drug overdose. The donor kidney anatomy was notable for two arteries: a main artery and a much smaller inferior pole artery. The two arteries were 15 mm apart on a common aortic patch; however, due to their distance apart, the smaller artery was anastomosed to the main artery. A single arterial anastomosis was performed end-to-side to the

A. M. Griffin · P. Matemavi (✉)
Division of Transplant and Hepatobiliary Surgery, Department of Surgery, University of Mississippi Medical Center, Jackson, MS, USA
e-mail: amgriffin@umc.edu; pmatemavi@umc.edu

© The Author(s), under exclusive license to Springer Nature Switzerland AG 2022

F. Aziz, S. Parajuli (eds.), *Complications in Kidney Transplantation*,
https://doi.org/10.1007/978-3-031-13569-9_18

external iliac artery. Reperfusion of the kidney was normal; the kidney made very little urine in the operating room. The patient had delayed graft function requiring two sessions of hemodialysis post-operatively. Induction immunosuppression was steroids and anti-thymocyte globulin, and he was on maintenance tacrolimus, mycophenolate mofetil, and corticosteroids. Blood pressure (BP) after transplant ranged between 130/80 and 160/90. At the time of transplant discharge from the hospital, the patient was on nifedipine 60 mg twice daily and metoprolol 50 mg twice daily.

On presentation to the emergency department, the patient complained of being unwell over the last week. BP was 225/115, HR 89. He reported headaches, new-onset dyspnea, and oliguria. Over the last 3 weeks before presentation, his transplant nephrologist had titrated up his antihypertensives, and he was now on nifedipine 90 mg twice daily, metoprolol 100 mg twice daily, and clonidine 0.1 mg three times a day. There was no evidence of medication noncompliance. On examination, he was in moderate respiratory distress had rales in bilateral lungs on auscultation. His abdominal exam was significant for a bruit to auscultation in the right lower abdomen. Laboratory studies were notable for serum creatinine that had increased from a baseline of 1.3–4.6 mg/dL. Chest X-ray showed pulmonary edema. An echocardiogram showed a normal ejection fraction. Duplex sonography of allograft revealed high peak systolic velocity of the donor renal artery at the anastomosis of 485 cm/s with spectral analysis showing a "tardus-parvus" waveform. A nicardipine drip was started in the emergency department with no improvement in his blood pressure. The patient was admitted to the intensive care unit with plans to go for an angiogram the following day.

Question 1

What additional workup or studies would be helpful at this time in reaching a diagnosis in this patient?

A. CT angiography of the abdomen and pelvis (CTA).
B. Digital subtraction angiography.
C. Contrast-enhanced magnetic resonance angiography (MRA).
D. No need for additional studies; duplex sonography is enough.

The correct answer is B.

Digital subtraction angiography has been shown to correlate highly with conventional angiography and uses a smaller amount of contrast material, making it a more suitable choice for evaluating transplant renal artery stenosis (TRAS) [1, 2]. CTA is a great non-invasive study because it provides three-dimensional images of the vascular anatomy and uses less iodinated contrast. In this case, however, the clinical picture, laboratory, and imaging studies point to a diagnosis of TRAS; therefore, it is imperative to do an angiogram with the intervention plan. MRA is also a great alternative with a high degree of diagnostic accuracy but also lacks the therapeutic option. A duplex sonogram is a typical first test of choice but is not definitive.

Clinical Course

The patient was taken to the interventional radiology suite, and an angiogram was performed, which demonstrated stenosis at the anastomosis (Fig. 18.1).

Question 2
Given the patient's transplant renal artery stenosis on angiography, what is the next best step in managing this patient's complication?

A. No intervention indicated at this time; continue medical therapy
B. Surgical bypass of the stenotic segment of the renal artery using the internal iliac artery as a conduit
C. Percutaneous transluminal angioplasty with stent placement
D. Surgical endarterectomy with excision and reimplantation of the renal artery to the common iliac artery

The correct answer is C.

Percutaneous transluminal angioplasty with stent placement is currently the first-line therapy to manage TRAS. Complications associated with this therapy are renal artery dissection, stent restenosis, thromboembolism, hematoma, and pseudoaneurysm at the puncture site. Open surgical revision is reserved for cases of unsuccessful angioplasty and stent [3]. Surgical options include bypassing the stenotic segment, excision and revision of anastomosis, and local endarterectomy with reimplantation [4].

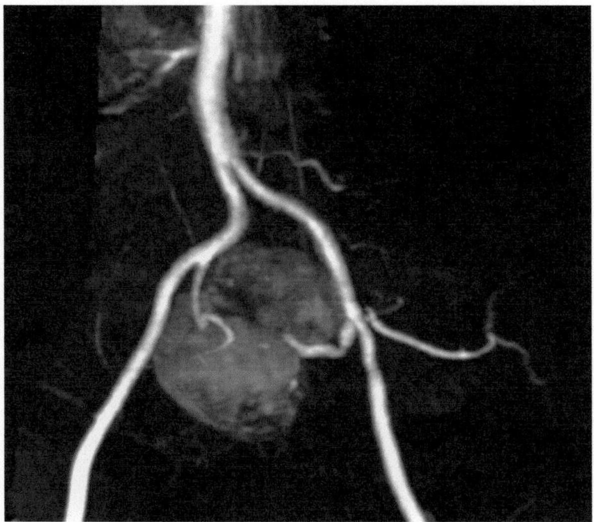

Fig. 18.1 MRA-transplant renal artery stenosis

Additional Clinical Course

The patient underwent percutaneous transluminal angioplasty with stent placement (Fig. 18.2). He tolerated the procedure well. Throughout his hospitalization, his clinical course improved, and he was discharged home on hospital day eight on nifedipine 90 mg twice a day and metoprolol 50 mg twice a day. Serum creatinine was down to 2.3 mg/dL.

Discussion

Transplant renal artery stenosis (TRAS) is a known complication after kidney transplant accounting for 1–5% of cases of post-transplant hypertension and at least 75% of all post-transplant vascular complications. Generally becoming apparent between 3 months and 24 months [5, 6]. Renal artery stenosis has been reported in up to 10% of recipients [7]. It is simply narrowing of the renal artery that causes hemodynamic significance in the renal allograft. The hypoperfusion, in turn, results in activation of the renin—angiotensin—aldosterone system causing refractory hypertension, fluid retention, and overload, as well as dysfunction in the allograft. Early diagnosis and treatment are crucial in preserving allograft function.

Risk factors for developing TRAS are atherosclerotic disease in the donor's vessel, cytomegalovirus infection (CMV), delayed graft function, transplantation of pediatric kidney in an adult recipient, and kinking or twisting of the renal artery at the time of wound closure [8]. The stenosis is usually situated near the anastomosis of the renal artery to an iliac artery and can be short, diffuse, or multiple sites and

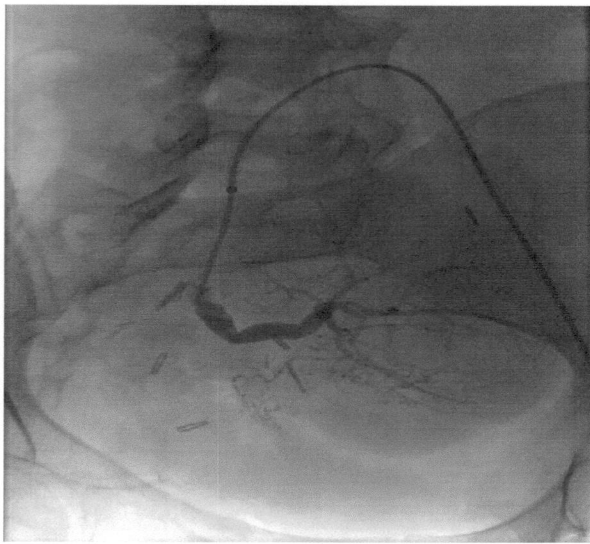

Fig. 18.2 Percutaneous transluminal angioplasty

can also occur at different times. In about half of all TRAS cases, the stenosis involves the anastomotic site, and it is iatrogenic. Most commonly caused by scarring related to poor procurement technique, clamping of the vessels, or other trauma to the donor and recipient arteries during cold ischemia, as well as suture technical failure [8]. The long and more diffuse stenosis tends to occur later and has been attributed to immune-mediated endothelial injury with progressive intimal proliferation [9].

Angiography is the gold standard for diagnosis of TRAS because of the quality of the images and ability to measure pressure gradients across the stenosis; it is especially valued because of the ability to intervene at the time of angiography. Doppler ultrasonography is the first-choice test and a great tool in the differential diagnosis of allograft dysfunction. A peak systolic velocity greater than 250 cm/s and a "tardus-parvus" arterial waveform are both highly suspicious for TRAS [7].

Conservative treatment has a role in managing TRAS in asymptomatic patients without renal allograft dysfunction or those who have easily treated hypertension. Serial ultrasonography is prudent in these cases to observe for worsening stenosis. It is believed that conservative management of the stenosis is acceptable for TRAS in the order of less than 70%. For patients with greater than 70% stenosis, even though asymptomatic without allograft dysfunction, there is concern that this degree of stenosis is more susceptible to occlusion in the presence of periods of dehydration or cardiovascular instability, and intervention should be highly considered [9].

Percutaneous transluminal angioplasty (PTA) is the initial treatment of choice and has been reported to be most successful in lesions that are short, linear, and distal from the anastomosis [5].

Surgical correction is considered a rescue effort or last resort in cases unsuitable to PTA or after failed PTA. Challenges to open surgery are safe access to the renal artery, availability of arterial conduit and inflow, and the resultant warm ischemia time that is required to do the anastomosis. Excision of the stenotic segment with direct anastomosis to the adjacent iliac artery, as well as interposition graft using a saphenous vein or recipient internal iliac artery and autotransplantation have been described by Morris and Knechtle [9]. The risk of surgery has to be carefully weighed against the potential benefit of improving blood flow to the kidney. Morris and colleagues recommend a biopsy to evaluate the renal parenchyma.

TRAS is a potentially treatable problem associated with allograft loss and high morbidity and mortality; therefore, it is imperative to have a high index of suspicion when a post-kidney transplant patient presents with uncontrollable hypertension, fluid retention, and allograft dysfunction.

Disclosures P. Matemavi reports employment with the University of Mississippi Medical Center and has received research funding through the American Society of Transplant Surgeons – Natera Socio-Economic and Racial Disparity grant. A. Griffin reports employment with the University of Mississippi Medical Center.

Funding None.

References

1. Rath M, Castro L, Schuler M, et al. Digital subtraction angiography in the diagnosis of arterial complications after renal transplantation. Eur J Radiol. 1984;4:34–7.
2. Cavalcanti A, Durao M, Santos B, Tonato E, Doher M, Guimaraes-Souza N, Moreira VL, Affonso B, Nasser F, Pacheco-Silva A. Endovascular management of transplant renal artery stenosis: a safe and effective treatment. Am J Transplant. 2017;17(Suppl. 3)
3. Seratnahaei A, Shah A, Bodiwala K, et al. Management of transplant renal artery stenosis. Angiology. 2011;62:219–24.
4. Shames BD, Odarico JS, D'Alessandro AM, et al. Surgical repair of transplant renal artery stenosis with preserved cadaveric iliac artery grafts. Ann Surg. 2003;237:116–22.
5. Chen W, Liise K, Martin Z, et al. Transplant renal artery stenosis: clinical manifestations, diagnosis and therapy. Clin Kidney J. 2015;8:71–8.
6. Roberts JP, Ascher NL, Fryd DS, Hunter DW, Dunn DL, Payne WD, Sutherland DE, Castaneda-Zuniga W, Najarian JS. Transplant renal artery stenosis. Transplantation. 1989;48:580–3.
7. Danovitch, G. Handbook of kidney transplantation. 6th Edition. Wolters Kluwer. Chapter 9. p. 250.
8. Weir MR, Salzberg DJ. Management of hypertension in the transplant patient. J Am Soc Hypertens. 2011;5:425–32.
9. Morris PJ, Knechtle SJ. Kidney transplantation: principles and practice, vol. 28. 7th ed. Elsevier. 452, 456, 458

Chapter 19
Hydronephrosis

Ashlee M. Griffin and Praise Matemavi

Introduction

Kidney transplantation is the preferred treatment modality for end-stage kidney disease in appropriate candidates. Overall graft survival has improved over the years due to advancements in immunosuppressive medication regimens leading to an increase in the number of transplants. Surgical intervention, however, is not without complications. Urologic complications occur most frequently, including urine leak, ureteral stricture/stenosis, and obstruction. Hydronephrosis of the transplanted kidney can occur as a result of ureteral strictures or any obstruction along the urinary tract. Conservative management with decompression remains the first-line treatment for hydronephrosis. We present a case of hydronephrosis secondary to ureteral stenosis successfully treated with minimally invasive interventions.

Patient History

A 52-year-old female with a history of ESKD secondary to polycystic kidney disease underwent a deceased donor kidney transplant. Her immediate postoperative course was complicated by delayed graft function, requiring one hemodialysis session. Her allograft function improved, and she was discharged on postoperative day 6. Approximately 1 week after scheduled ureteral stent removal, she presented for routine clinic follow-up and was subsequently admitted to the hospital for further

A. M. Griffin (✉) · P. Matemavi
Division of Transplant and Hepatobiliary Surgery, Department of Surgery, University of Mississippi Medical Center, Jackson, MS, USA
e-mail: amgriffin@umc.edu; pmatemavi@umc.edu

© The Author(s), under exclusive license to Springer Nature Switzerland AG 2022
F. Aziz, S. Parajuli (eds.), *Complications in Kidney Transplantation*,
https://doi.org/10.1007/978-3-031-13569-9_19

workup for acute weight gain, bilateral pitting edema, and elevated serum creatinine. Pertinent labs include WBC of 6.2×10^9/L, BUN 53 mg/dl, and Cr 6.51 mg/dL, which was increased from 2.3 mg/dL the week prior. CT imaging demonstrated hydroureteronephrosis of the transplanted kidney. The transplant kidney US indicated Grade 2 hydronephrosis and an 8.6×4.5 cm fluid collection.

Question 1

What additional workup or studies would be helpful at this time in reaching a diagnosis in this patient?

A. Biopsy of the transplanted kidney.
B. Contrasted Imaging Study.
C. MRI.
D. Echocardiogram.

The correct answer is B.

The best next step in the workup of this patient would be to obtain a contrasted imaging study of the urologic system. This study would allow a more detailed view of the collecting system to further assess for leak, obstruction, or stricture. While there is an acute elevation in the serum creatinine, biopsy for graft rejection is not indicated. An echocardiogram may ultimately be necessary if the patient's pedal edema and weight gain persist after resolving the acute renal process. MRI would likely not give us any additional information.

Additional Clinical Course

Interventional radiology was consulted for antegrade pyelogram (Fig. 19.1) to evaluate the collecting system further. Results of the study demonstrated stenosis of the distal ureter, causing hydronephrosis of the transplanted kidney.

Question 2

Given the patient's ureteral stricture seen on a contrasted imaging study (Fig. 19.1), what is the next best step in managing this patient's complication?

A. No intervention indicated at this time.
B. Return to the operating room for immediate repair.
C. Medical management with calcium channel blocker or alpha-blocker.
D. Decompression of the collecting system with percutaneous nephrostomy tube, balloon ureteroplasty, and ureteral stent placement.

The correct answer is D.

The best treatment option of those listed above is placing a percutaneous nephrostomy (PCN) tube and balloon dilation with a ureteral stent to decompress the urinary tract. Offloading the pressure through the PCN and placing a stent across the stricture following dilation allow the ureter time to heal and remodel. Surgical intervention may be warranted if this method fails to relieve the stricture. Medical

Fig. 19.1 Pyelogram of the transplanted kidney

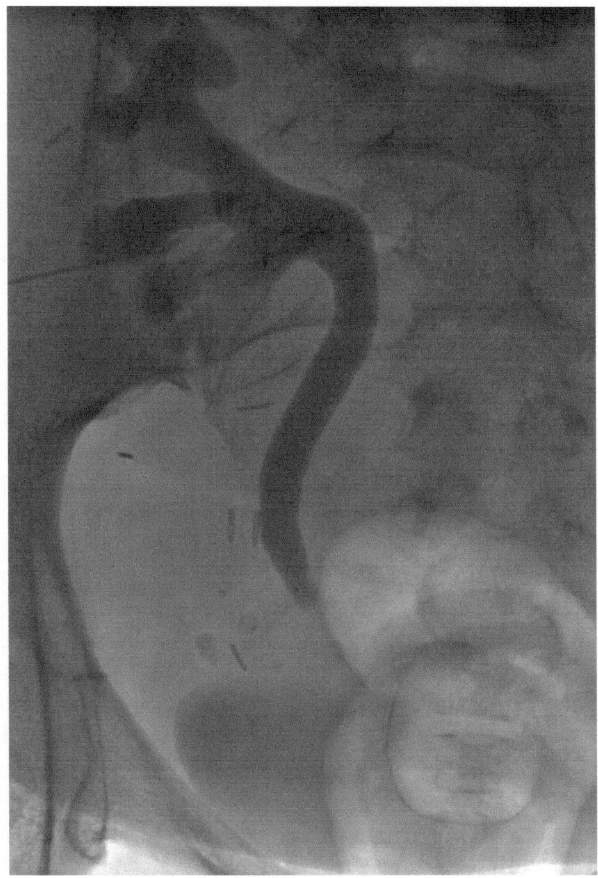

management with calcium channel blockers or alpha-blockers may help relieve ureteral spasms in patients with nephrolithiasis to facilitate stone passage; however, this would be of no use in urethral stricture.

Clinical Course Continued

The patient underwent placement of percutaneous nephrostomy tube (PCN) by our interventional radiologist, and our urologist colleagues placed a retrograde ureteral stent. The patient tolerated the procedures well. She was discharged home on hospital day 2. Four weeks later, her PCN was capped and removed without problems when she demonstrated that she could void without difficulty. Her ureteral stent was removed 6 weeks later. Repeat ultrasound did not show any evidence of fluid collections, obstruction, or hydronephrosis. She is doing well with normal allograft function 3 years post-transplant.

Discussion

According to the United States Renal Data System Annual Report, end-stage kidney disease (ESKD) remains a prevalent and highly morbid disease affecting over 780,000 people in the US [1]. Kidney transplantation is the preferred treatment method for ESRD, with approximately 22,817 transplants performed in 2020 [2]. Continued advancements in the management of kidney transplants have led to an overall improvement in allograft survival since its onset as an accepted treatment modality. However, a wide array of surgical complications can occur post-operatively, ultimately affecting graft survival. Surgical complications are generally grouped into vascular or urologic. Vascular complications include renal artery stenosis, infarction, pseudoaneurysm, arteriovenous fistula, and renal vein thrombosis. Urologic complications occur more frequently, including urine leaks and urinary obstruction resulting in hydronephrosis [3].

Hydronephrosis is typically caused by outlet obstruction at some point along the urinary tract. In kidney transplant patients, urinary obstruction can occur at any location along the urinary tract; however, it most commonly occurs distally at the ureterovesical junction [3]. This is thought to result from ischemic necrosis leading to ureteral stricture or stenosis. Other causes include kinking of the ureter, extrinsic compression, or technical error. Hydronephrosis can also result from kinking or clogging of the foley catheter, impairing urine drainage, nephrolithiasis, or in patients with BPH history.

Clinical presentations may vary in patients with hydronephrosis; however, they commonly manifest as decreased urine output and elevation in serum creatinine. Workup for kidney transplant patients with oliguria and lab abnormalities generally includes an ultrasound of the transplanted kidney as this test is non-invasive and helps differentiate vascular from urologic complications. If hydronephrosis is noted on the ultrasound, CT imaging may be a valuable adjunct for further evaluation of the etiology. The presence of a large fluid collection on imaging causing extrinsic compression may be percutaneously drained and result in resolution of the hydronephrosis. Fluid analysis with creatinine levels should be obtained to evaluate for urine leak as a further intervention may be necessary.

Additionally, a contrasted imaging study of the urinary system should be pursued as it will allow for a more detailed view of the collecting system. Decompression of the urinary system is the standard approach for initial management of hydronephrosis, including placement of a foley catheter and percutaneous nephrostomy tube [3, 4]. If the ureteral stricture is noted on imaging, balloon dilation with stent placement has a success rate of up to 60–80% [5]. Ureteral stents should remain for approximately 6–8 weeks to maximize healing and can usually be removed in an outpatient setting. Surgical intervention is typically reserved for complete obstruction unable to be repaired percutaneously or failure of conservative management.

Disclosures P. Matemavi reports employment with the University of Mississippi Medical Center and has received research funding through the American Society of Transplant Surgeons – Natera Socio-Economic and Racial Disparity grant.

A. Griffin reports employment with the University of Mississippi Medical Center.

Funding None.

References

1. United States Renal Data System. 2020 USRDS annual data report: epidemiology of kidney disease in the United States. Bethesda, MD: National Institutes of Health, National Institute of Diabetes and Digestive and Kidney Diseases; 2020.
2. Organ Procurement and Transplantation Network. National data—OPTN. [online] Available at 2021. https://optn.transplant.hrsa.gov/data/view-data-reports/national-data/. Accessed 15 Dec 2021.
3. Akbar SA, Jafri SZ, Amendola MA, Madrazo BL, Salem R, Bis KG. Complications of renal transplantation. [online] RadioGraphics 2021. https://doi.org/10.1148/rg.255045133. Accessed 15 Dec 2021.
4. Sarier M, Yayar O, Yavuz A, Turgut H, Kukul E. Update on the management of urological problems following kidney transplantation. Urol Int. 2021;105:541–7. https://doi.org/10.1159/000512885.
5. Mor E, Mehjibovsky V, Eizner S, Gurevich M, Ginea R, Tennak V, Nesher E, Kniznik M. Long-term results of percutaneous balloon dilatation of ureteral stricture after kidney transplantation. Transplantation. 2018;102:S640. https://doi.org/10.1097/01.tp.0000543557.68087.1d.

Chapter 20
Management of Post-Kidney Transplantation Ureteral Stricture

Oren Shaked and Robert Redfield

Introduction

Ureteral complications following kidney transplants are among the most common surgical complications affecting patients in the short and long term. Ureteral obstruction occurs in 2–10% of kidney transplant recipients, and the vast majority of these are from ischemic stricturing of the ureter [1]. Other types of ureteral obstruction that need to be differentiated from stricture following transplant include intrinsic factors, such as thrombus, caliculi, tumor, and edema, or extrinsic factors, such as kinking of the ureter, pelviureteric junction obstruction, or a misplaced ureteral anastomosis [2]. Risk factors associated with the development of ureteral strictures post-transplant include recipients aged greater than 65, the presence of more than two donor arteries, a prolonged cold ischemic time, and not using a stent for the ureteral anastomosis. Often, stricturing presents after the first few weeks of transplant, if not within the first year.

Patient History

A 61-year-old male with a history of coronary artery disease status post percutaneous coronary stent placement with drug-eluting stents, insulin-dependent type-2 diabetes, obstructive sleep apnea, and end-stage renal disease secondary to diabetes, previously on peritoneal dialysis, with 0% panel reactive antibodies, underwent a living unrelated kidney transplant. Cytomegalovirus (CMV) antibody IgG was positive in the donor and negative in the recipient. Cold ischemic time was 67 min. Warm ischemic time was 46 min. There was a single renal artery, renal vein, and ureter. An extravesical ureteroneocystostomy was performed by direct anastomosis of the transplant ureter to the mucosa of the bladder. Prior to the closure of the

O. Shaked (✉) · R. Redfield
Division of Transplant Surgery, Department of Surgery, Hospital of the University of Pennsylvania, Philadelphia, PA, USA
e-mail: oren.shaked@pennmedicine.upenn.edu; robert.redfield@pennmedicine.upenn.edu

© The Author(s), under exclusive license to Springer Nature Switzerland AG 2022

F. Aziz, S. Parajuli (eds.), *Complications in Kidney Transplantation*,
https://doi.org/10.1007/978-3-031-13569-9_20

ureteroneocystostomy, a double J nephroureteral stent was positioned across the anastomosis. An anti-reflux tunnel was created over the distal ureter by approximation of the detrusor muscle using interrupted suture.

In the immediate post-transplant period, the patient's course was notable for a slow recovery of the transplanted kidney compared to what might be expected from a living donor operation, with low urine output and slow clearance of creatinine until postoperative day 3. Renal ultrasounds of the transplanted kidney demonstrated appropriate flow through the renal artery and vein, and no evidence of hydronephrosis. The patient was discharged on postoperative day 4 with signs of ongoing recovery. His discharge immunosuppressive regimen included tacrolimus, mycophenolate mofetil, and a prednisone taper, and prophylactically he was maintained on a 6-month course of sulfamethoxazole-trimethoprim and a 3-month course of valacyclovir. His creatinine nadired at 1.67 mg/dL. 3 months after transplant, the patient got a booster dose of the Moderna SARS-CoV-2 vaccine. Two weeks after the booster, routine labs demonstrated leukopenia and an acute kidney injury, with creatinine elevation to 2.64 mg/dL. The patient was readmitted for expedited workup. Despite a bolus of intravenous fluid administration, the patient's creatinine continued to rise. Mycophenolate mofetil was held in the setting of his leukopenia. Infection studies, including a chest X-ray, urine analysis and culture, blood cultures, and assays for cytomegalovirus, Epstein–Barr virus, and BK virus were negative. Donor-specific antibodies were checked and were negative. An ultrasound of the transplanted kidney showed appropriate flow in the renal artery and vein and new moderate hydronephrosis.

Question 1

What is the most probable cause of the patient's presentation?

A. Medication side effect.
B. Infection.
C. Dehydration.
D. Ureteral obstruction.
E. Rejection.

The correct answer is D.

Discussion of Question 1

The patient's acute kidney injury (AKI) was most likely secondary to ureteral obstruction. His creatinine did not improve with intravenous fluid administration, making dehydration an unlikely diagnosis. It is unclear whether the SARS-CoV-2 booster vaccine that was administered was directly or temporally linked to the development of leukopenia. Other common causes of leukopenia include viral infections, for which this patient was at higher risk given the CMV mismatch status of his transplant and medication side effects. A complete infectious workup was negative, making infection less likely. His medications were adjusted to decreased doses but did not significantly impact his leukopenia, which persisted for an additional month. While antibody-mediated rejection seemed less likely in the setting of negative DSAs, in the absence of a biopsy of the transplanted kidney, this potential cause of his AKI was not entirely ruled out at this time.

Hospital Course

Given the moderate hydronephrosis seen on ultrasound, the patient was sent for a nephrostogram with interventional radiology (IR), which showed multiple filling defects within the collecting system as well as a distal ureteral stricture. A percutaneous nephrostomy tube (PCN) was placed, which initially drained 900 mL of bloody output, and was associated with a rising creatinine. The patient was taken back to IR for a repeat nephrostogram wherein they noted that the previously identified filling defects within the ureter were, in fact, a duplicated collecting system. They again saw the distal ureteral stricture, as well as new contrast extravasation into the retroperitoneum. The tube was removed and exchanged for a larger caliber multipurpose drain. The patient's creatinine remained elevated after confirming that the new PCN was in an appropriate position. A kidney biopsy showed no evidence of acute cellular or antibody-mediated rejection. A nuclear medicine MAG3 study showed appropriate perfusion to the kidney, no focal perfusion defects, and concentration of tracer in the renal cortex consistent with a diagnosis of acute tubular necrosis. The patient was managed with ongoing supportive care, and ultimately his creatinine began to normalize.

Question 2
Once diagnosed, what are the next steps in the management of ureteral strictures?

A. Open ureteric reimplantation.
B. Ureteric dilation.
C. Open ureteroureterostomy.
D. Endoureological endoureterotomy.
E. Endourological laser ablation.

The correct answer is B.

Discussion of Question 2
There are no standardized pathways for the management of post-transplant ureteral stricture. Decisions about when and how to intervene are institution-specific and depend on provider experience, center-specific outcomes, and patient condition. Choosing the best intervention option involves consideration of the patient, comorbidities, anatomy, nutritional status, and time from surgery. In general, endourological approaches have the advantages of being less morbid, with faster recovery times, and lower costs. Open operations have a higher overall success rate, as discussed below. Often a tiered approach starting with less invasive treatment options followed by more invasive treatments for refractory cases is needed.

Additional Clinical Course

The patient was discharged home with a percutaneous nephrostomy tube in place. He represented a week later with pseudomonas urosepsis, which was treated with a course of antibiotics. His percutaneous nephrostomy tube was converted to a

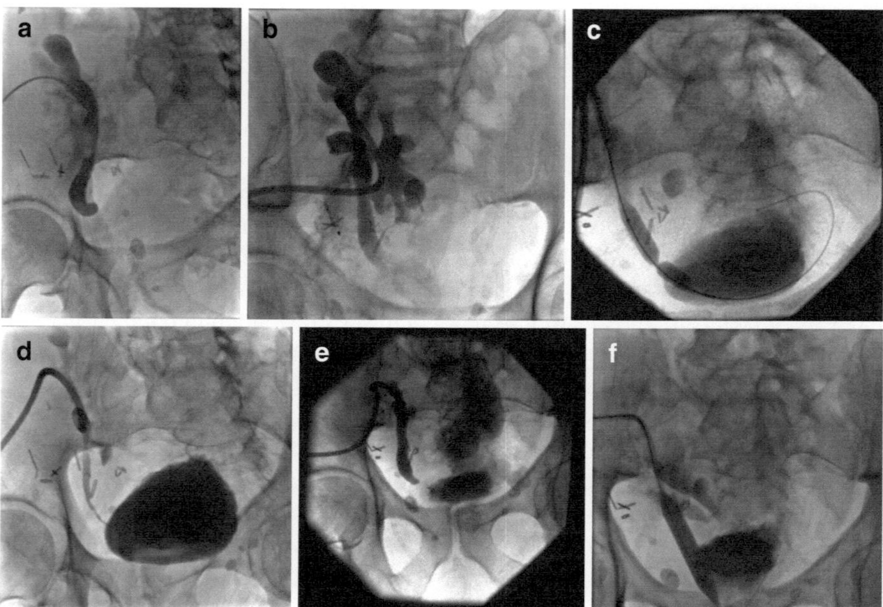

Fig. 20.1 Images from top to bottom, left to right: (**a**) initial antegrade nephrostogram demonstrating possible filling defects. (**b**) Repeat antegrade nephrostogram demonstrating duplicated collecting system. (**c**) Identification of distal ureteral stricture and stricturoplasty. (**d**) PCNU to PCN conversion for capping trial. (**e**) Persistent distal ureteral narrowing. (**f**) Second stricturoplasty and conversion back to PCNU

percutaneous nephroureteral tube (PCNU), and a ureteroplasty was performed 1 month after the initial diagnosis. Nephrostograms with tube exchanges occurred every 2–4 weeks, showing persistent distal ureteral narrowing. A second attempt at ureteroplasty was performed, after which the patient developed fever and malaise and was directly admitted for monitoring and antibiotics. At that time, the patient expressed a desire to undergo surgical intervention to attempt to treat the persistent stricture.

He was taken to the operating room approximately 6 months after his kidney transplant for open revision of the ureter. A ureteral stent was placed in the native right ureter pre-incision to facilitate identification of the native right ureter intraoperatively. The transplant ureteral anastomosis was identified taken down, and the edges of the transplant ureter were cut back and freshened up to healthy tissue. The transplanted ureter was, in fact, able to reach the patient's bladder under no tension, and so a new ureteroneocystostomy was performed, this time with a full-thickness anastomosis. In addition to repositioning the PCNU across the new anastomosis, an internal double J ureteral stent was positioned across the anastomosis in anticipation of future removal of the PCNU (Fig. 20.1).

Two weeks after the open operation, a nephrostogram through the PCNU showed a patent anastomosis with a brisk flow of contrast into the bladder. The PCNU was converted to a PCN. After 2 days, the PCN was capped with no complications, which the patient tolerated well. With no evidence of complications after the PCN was capped for 2 weeks, the double J stent was retrieved by interventional radiology. After an additional 2 weeks of tolerating the PCN capped, the PCN was removed, which the patient tolerated without issue.

Discussion

Traditionally, ureteric strictures in transplant patients were treated with an open surgical approach. While the overall success rate of open approaches is reportedly higher, the decreased morbidity, decreased cost, and faster recovery times associated with minimally invasive treatment modalities have made these an increasingly popular first step in the management algorithm of these challenging cases. Open approaches to repair have a success rate in the range of 80–90%, while minimally invasive treatments are successful in approximately 60–70% of cases [3, 4]. There are definite advantages of minimally invasive therapeutic options in patients who are poor surgical candidates, have multiple comorbidities, or in patients who already demonstrate signs of significant graft dysfunction and would have marginal benefits from intervention or formal revision of a ureteric stricture. But there is also data to suggest that long-term graft survival is improved with upfront surgical approaches to ureteral stricture post transplant [5].

Many patients benefit from a stepwise approach to the management of ureteral strictures following kidney transplant, as was the management strategy described in the presented case. The first step in managing a ureteral stricture is to decompress the collecting system before permanent damage to the allograft can occur. A percutaneously placed nephrostomy tube is an excellent minimally invasive option allowing for early decompression, which affords time for the physician to categorize the nature of the ureteral stricture and develop a management plan. Of note, as described in the case, even minimally invasive procedures are associated with challenges and complications. Early identification of potential issues and a low threshold to repeat minimally invasive procedures can help prevent a rush back to the operating room and an open operating in a patient who is potentially poorly optimized from surgery with a heavy inflammatory burden.

Once the collecting system is decompressed, the physician can categorize a ureteral stricture as early or late, proximal or distal, and the underlying etiology. There is also time to classify the patient's candidacy for open operative intervention, optimize comorbidities, ensure appropriate nutritional status, and critically, to allow for decompression and reduce the inflammatory burden of the stressed renal allograft collecting system. After a period of decompression, converting a PCN to a PCNU establishes access to the bladder for urine collection and good bladder habits for transplanted patients and also provides access for several minimally invasive treatments, including balloon dilation, stent placement, dilation with electrocautery, and cold-knife incision [6, 7].

Once access has been established across a stricture, it is up to the patient and surgeon to determine how many attempts and minimally invasive stricturoplasty and via which approach is appropriate. If the patient tolerates intervention, there are no established guidelines on how many interventions or over what timeframe minimally invasive techniques can be employed. It is reasonable to try at least several times at minimally invasive management of a ureteral stricture given the overall high success rate, as well as the significantly reduced morbidity from these procedures. In the case presented, the ureteral stricture was associated with recurrent episodes of urosepsis necessitating inpatient hospitalization and risk to the patient.

Open intervention is the next best step in patients who are not tolerating a more conservative approach. Open interventions include ureteral reimplantation, pyeloureterostomy, ureteroureterostomy, and ileal interposition conduit. There is no standard accepted open approach, and treatment choices often depend heavily on patient anatomy and surgeon experience. Having a targeted preoperative plan is crucial, but the surgeon must be nimble and flexible in the operating room and ready to make changes to their surgical approach depending on how much healthy ureter they are able to identify, the distance of the healthy ureter to the bladder, the presence of an ipsilateral native ureter, or access to the bowel. It is critical that healthy ureteral tissue be identified and used for a revised anastomosis and that the repair be performed without tension. Outcomes after open intervention are generally favorable, and long-term graft survival is improved with aggressive open surgical management in those patients able to tolerate a second invasive operation. Given the heterogeneity of approaches in management for post-kidney transplant ureteral strictures, further studies are needed before a definitive management algorithm can be established. A randomized trial of minimally invasive versus open surgical approach to treatment would be reasonable, given the relative frequency of ureteral complications post-kidney transplant.

References

1. Dinckan A, Tekin A, Turkyilmaz S, Kocak H, Gurkan A, Erdogan O, Tuncer M, Demirbas A. Early and late urological complications corrected surgically following renal transplantation. Transpl Int. 2007;20(8):707–2.
2. Kumar S, Ameli-Renani S, Hakim A, Jeon JH, Shrivastava S, Patel U. Ureteral obstruction following renal transplantation: causes, diagnosis, and management. Br J Radiol. 2014;87(1044):20140169.
3. Doehn C, Böse N, Meyer AJ, Jocham D. Results of secondary ureteral implantation after kidney transplantation. Int Urol Nephrol. 2011;43(3):669–74.
4. Kwong J, Schiefer D, Aboalsamh G, Archambault J, Luke PP, Sener A. Optimal management of distal ureteric strictures following renal transplantation: a systematic review. Transpl Int. 2016;29(5):579–88.
5. Arpali E, Al-Qaoud T, Martinez E, Redfield RR III, Leverson GE, Kaufman DB, Odorico JS, Sollinger HW. Impact of ureteral stricture and treatment choice on long-term graft survival in kidney transplantation. Am J Transplant. 2018;18(8):1977–85.

6. Collado A, Caparros J, Guirado L, Rosales A, Martí J, Solà R, Vicente J. Balloon dilatation in the treatment of ureteral stenosis in kidney transplant recipients. Eur Urol. 1998;34(5):399–403.

7. Juaneda B, Alcaraz A, Bujons A, Guirado L, Diaz JM, Marti J, De La Torre P, Sabaté S, Villavicencio H. Endourological management is better in early-onset ureteral stenosis in kidney transplantation. Transplant Proc. 2005;37(9):3825–7.

Chapter 21
Mycotic Pseudoaneurysms

Melissa Chen and Robert Redfield III

Introduction

Mycotic pseudoaneurysms are a rare complication following kidney transplantation, occurring in fewer than 1% of all recipients [1]. Presentation varies widely, ranging from asymptomatic to life-threatening hemorrhage. Due to the possibility of graft loss and patient death, it is essential to diagnose and treat mycotic pseudoaneurysms in a prompt fashion.

Patient History

A 70-year-old man with end-stage renal disease secondary to AL-amyloid with both liver and kidney involvement underwent deceased-donor kidney transplant. The donor had no signs of infection, and standard microbiological tests were negative. At the time of transplant, the recipient had no donor-specific antibodies and his panel reactive antibody was 0%. He received standard perioperative cefazolin for surgical prophylaxis. He developed delayed graft function (DGF) requiring dialysis within the first week of transplantation but was ultimately discharged home with a functioning graft. His creatinine (Cr) nadired at 1.3. Three months after transplant he was found to have acute kidney injury on routine labs with a Cr 1.9. Workup included urinalysis and urine culture, as well as a duplex ultrasound of his renal allograft, which demonstrated a new 5.7 cm pseudoaneurysm arising at the

M. Chen (✉) · R. Redfield III
Division of Transplant Surgery, Department of Surgery, Hospital of the University of Pennsylvania, Philadelphia, PA, USA
e-mail: Melissa.Chen@pennmedicine.upenn.edu; robert.redfield@pennmedicine.upenn.edu

© The Author(s), under exclusive license to Springer Nature Switzerland AG 2022
F. Aziz, S. Parajuli (eds.), *Complications in Kidney Transplantation*, https://doi.org/10.1007/978-3-031-13569-9_21

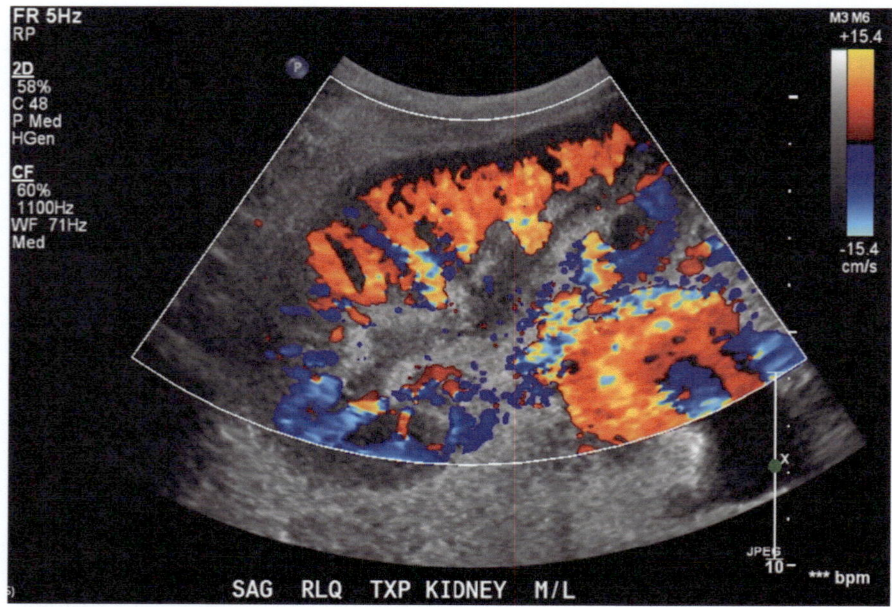

Fig. 21.1 Duplex ultrasound of renal allograft

anastomosis between the renal artery and the recipient external iliac artery (Fig. 21.1). He was admitted for further studies and management.

Question 1

What is the most likely cause of the pseudoaneurysm?

A. Technical complication.
B. Donor or recipient arteriosclerosis.
C. Bacterial infection.
D. Fungal infection.

The correct answer is A.

Technical complications (typically related to donor or recipient atherosclerosis) are the most likely to lead to an anastomotic pseudoaneurysm. Mycotic aneurysms (including both bacterial and fungal etiologies) are infrequent (<1%) but given the potential for life-threatening complications including suture line disruption and rupture, early recognition and intervention are key.

Clinical Course

At time of his hospital admission, he was afebrile with normal vital signs. He had no complaints of pain or tenderness over his renal allograft. Blood and urine cultures were obtained, and he was treated with empiric antibiotic and antifungal

Fig. 21.2 Iliac angiogram demonstrating pseudoaneurysm arising from proximal aspect of the renal artery anastomosis

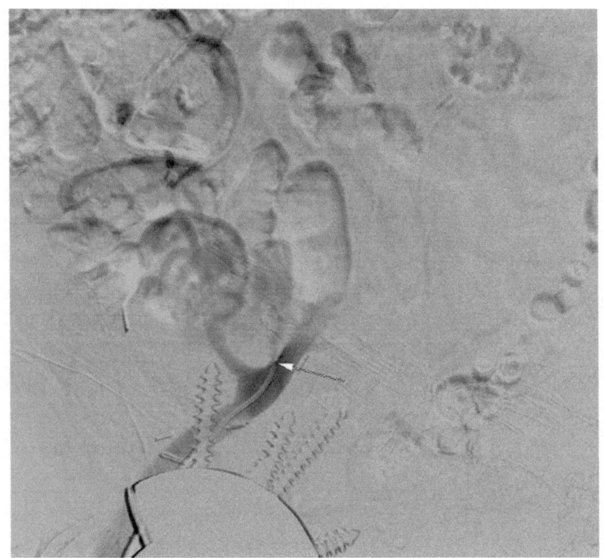

agents. In spite of serially negative blood cultures, there was a high index of suspicion for mycotic aneurysm (likely fungal or an indolent pathogen). He was recommended to undergo exploration with aneurysmectomy and reconstruction of the renal artery with the potential need for nephrectomy, but ultimately refused an operation. He was treated with a covered stent graft to exclude both the renal allograft and the pseudoaneurysm (Fig. 21.2). He recovered from the procedure without immediate complications.

Question 2

What are the treatment options for a mycotic pseudoaneurysm?

A. Long-term suppressive antibiotics and antifungals.
B. Angiographic embolization and thrombin injection.
C. Surgical excision of mycotic pseudoaneurysm.
D. Surgical debridement with vascular reconstruction and possible graft nephrectomy.

The correct answer is D.

Historically, surgical excision and/or wide debridement were the only definitive options for mycotic pseudoaneurysms. This often necessitates graft nephrectomy as direct reconstruction of the transplant renal artery in a contaminated and scarred field was prohibitive. There have been case reports published more recently documenting less invasive and at times nonsurgical approaches. These must be considered with caution, as any treatment option that does not remove the infected artery wall puts patients at risk for significant hemorrhage.

Continued Clinical Course

Multi-disciplinary discussions were held between transplant surgery, transplant nephrology, interventional radiology, and transplant infectious disease. The patient discussed in this case had no evidence of active infection (no fevers, no leukocytosis, no positive blood or urine cultures). Consideration was given to tagged white blood cell scan, but ultimately he was recommended to undergo exploration with aneurysmectomy and reconstruction of the renal artery with the potential need for nephrectomy. After extensive counseling, he declined an operation. He was treated with a covered stent graft to exclude both the renal allograft and the pseudoaneurysm. He recovered from the procedure without immediate complications. He was gradually taken off of immunosuppression as an outpatient.

Discussion

Mycotic pseudoaneurysms are an exceedingly rare complication of kidney transplantation, occurring in fewer than 1% of recipients [1]. Pseudoaneurysms develop as with the patient presented in this case, many are found on imaging studies performed for other indications. Symptomatic patients may present with non-specific complaints of malaise, fever, abdominal pain, or peri-graft tenderness. Others may present with thromboembolic complications including acute kidney injury, claudication, or with mass effect on the renal vein or ureter. Regardless of symptoms, patients found to have a mycotic aneurysm should be treated urgently. There is significant associated morbidity and mortality from suture line disruption and subsequent hemorrhage, similar to graft infections in general vascular surgery. Fungal sources remain more common than bacterial. Absence of documented microbial systemic infection does not preclude the presence of a mycotic aneurysm.

Historic recommendations have been for aneurysmectomy, arterial reconstruction, possible allograft nephrectomy depending on degree of damage identified in the operating room [2]. Graft loss was expectedly inevitable when surgeries were performed emergently for life-threatening hemorrhage. This highlights the importance of rapid diagnosis to strategize treatment options.

There is an emerging role for endovascular treatment options in conjunction with culture-directed antimicrobial therapy as a less invasive alterative to open repair [3]. This is an attractive option in frail patients, but there remains a risk of prosthetic stent infection and rupture. Many of these studies have been conducted in immunocompetent participants. There are fewer available reports of endovascular therapy in the transplant population [4]. While some authors have reported durable success, placement of endoprosthetic material in an infected field in an immunocompromised patient should be approached with caution. The role for endovascular interventions is likely strongest as temporizing or bridging therapy to avoid hemorrhagic complications while patients are being treated with long-term antibiotic and/or antifungal therapy with plans for definitive repair.

References

1. Leonardou P, Gioldasi S, Zavos G, Pappas P. Mycotic pseudoaneurysms complicating renal transplantation: a case series and review of the literature. J Med Case Reports. 2012;6:59.
2. Bracale UM, Santangelo M, Carbone F, et al. Anastomotic pseudoaneurysm complicating renal transplantation: treatment options. Eur J Vasc Endovasc Surg. 2010;39(5):565–8.
3. Luo CM, Chan CY, Chen YS, Wang SS, Chi NH, Wu IH. Long-term outcome of endovascular treatment for mycotic aortic aneurysm. Eur J Vasc Endovasc Surg. 2017;54:464–71.
4. Yao J, Vicaretti M, Lee T, Amaratunga R, et al. Endovascular management of mycotic pseudoaneurysm after pancreas transplant: case report and literature review. Transplant Proc. 2020;52(2):660–6.

Chapter 22
COVID-19 and Kidney Transplantation: An Approach to Acute Rejection in a Kidney Transplant Recipient with SARS-CoV-2 Infection

Vidya A. Fleetwood and Fadee Abualrub

Case Report

A 29-year-old kidney transplant recipient presented to the outpatient clinic with complaints of 5 days of fatigue, anorexia, and anosmia. His medical history was significant for end-stage kidney disease due to IgA nephropathy, and he had undergone living unrelated kidney transplantation 1 year prior. He had received a 4-antigen mismatch kidney with a negative flow crossmatch and had received anti-thymocyte globulin for induction. His postoperative course had been unremarkable, and his creatinine had reached a nadir of 0.8 mg/dL. He was maintained on tacrolimus with trough levels of 6–8 mg/mL, mycophenolic acid 360 mg BID, and 5 mg of prednisone daily.

Upon presentation, his physical exam was significant for poor skin turgor and dry mucous membranes. His breathing was nonlabored, with an oxygen saturation of 97% on room air. His vital signs and physical exam were otherwise unremarkable. Laboratory testing revealed a normal electrolyte panel and a normal hematology panel; however, his kidney function panel was significant for a creatinine level of 1.2 mg/dL from a nadir of 0.8 mg/dL and a blood urea nitrogen of 31 mg/dL. A chest X-ray was significant for mild ground-glass opacification with no infiltrates or consolidation. He was admitted for hydration and administered an anti-SARS-CoV-2 spike protein monoclonal antibody solution.

V. A. Fleetwood (✉) · F. Abualrub
Center for Abdominal Transplantation, Saint Louis University, St. Louis, MO, USA
e-mail: Vidyaratna.fleetwood@health.slu.edu; Fadee.Abualrub@health.slu.edu

© The Author(s), under exclusive license to Springer Nature Switzerland AG 2022
F. Aziz, S. Parajuli (eds.), *Complications in Kidney Transplantation*,
https://doi.org/10.1007/978-3-031-13569-9_22

Question 1

How should his maintenance immunosuppression be handled, inpatient?

A. Continue all home immunosuppressive medications at current doses.
B. Discontinue calcineurin inhibitor (CNI) and continue other therapies.
C. Discontinue mycophenolic acid (MPA) and continue other therapies.
D. Discontinue prednisone and continue other therapies.
E. Discontinue all immunosuppressive medications and start stress dose steroids.

The correct answer is C.

In the setting of acute SARS-CoV-2 infection, the immunosuppressive regimen must be tailored to the patient's acuity of illness and risk factors for worsening the disease. Completely asymptomatic disease in a low-risk patient may be approached by continuing all current immunosuppressives (a) and monitoring for clinical decompensation. In this patient with the mild symptomatic disease on triple therapy, the antimetabolite should be discontinued (c), and the calcineurin inhibitor and prednisone continued. In hypoxia, the CNI may be dose reduced or discontinued and the prednisone replaced with dexamethasone for the preservation of lung function [1].

Treatment Course

Antimetabolites were discontinued, and tacrolimus dose was lowered to target a trough of 2–4 mg/mL. The patient's physical exam improved with hydration, and his creatinine normalized although his anosmia persisted. He was able to hydrate sufficiently to be discharged home. He remained without dyspnea and on room air. Five days after discharge, he presented with mild graft tenderness and was found to have a creatinine level of 2.3 mg/dL despite being well-appearing and clinically euvolemic. Urinalysis was negative for infection, and tacrolimus level was 4 mg/mL. Doppler ultrasound of the kidney allograft is unremarkable.

Question 2

What is the next step in diagnosis and treatment?

A. Restart mycophenolic acid.
B. Repeat monoclonal antibody treatment.
C. Obtain percutaneous kidney allograft biopsy.
D. Start empiric treatment for allograft rejection.

The correct answer is C.

Once hypovolemia, infection, and vascular abnormalities have been excluded, the acute rejection must be considered, particularly in patients who have recently had their immunosuppression lowered. Increasing immunosuppression (a) would likely be ineffective without pulse dose steroids (d); however, neither can be done until rejection has been demonstrated with an allograft biopsy (c). Although SARS-CoV-2 infection can lead to various pathologic changes in the transplanted kidney [2], monoclonal antibody treatments will be ineffective outside of the acute phase of the disease [1].

Additional Clinical Course

An allograft biopsy was significant for grade II T cell-mediated rejection (TCMR). The patient was admitted and treated with 3 days of pulse dose steroids and an extended prednisone taper. The creatinine trended down and returned to a nadir of 1.1 mg/dL 2 weeks after treatment.

Discussion

The coronavirus disease 2019 (COVID-19) pandemic significantly impacted kidney transplant activity: within the first week of the pandemic declaration in March 2020, 80% of United States kidney transplant programs placed restrictions or complete holds on transplantation due to concerns for donor transmitted disease, recipient safety, and hospital system overload [3]. Over the following year, these concerns were seen to be warranted, with studies demonstrating COVID-19 mortality of 13–30% in kidney transplant recipients (KTRs) [4]. Initial review suggested that this high mortality may be due to the comorbid conditions—obesity, diabetes, and cardiovascular disease—frequently present in the KTR population; however, matched cohort study has demonstrated similar rates of severe disease, but higher COVID-19 associated mortality, in kidney transplant patients [5].

Treatment of SARS-CoV-2 infection in KTRs consists primarily of supportive care and appropriate immunosuppression management. The data remains limited and mixed on other agents. Monoclonal antibody treatment has shown some effectiveness at preventing severe disease. Remdesivir, an antiviral with preliminary data against other coronaviruses, exhibited some decrease in length of stay but was inconsistent across trials. Tocilizumab has been widely used but is off-label and still under investigation. Dexamethasone may reduce mortality in patients with hypoxia [1]. At this time, our approach was to start monoclonal antibody when outpatient and administer remdesivir if admitted, as well as dexamethasone if hypoxic.

No formal guidelines exist regarding managing immunosuppression in kidney transplant recipients who develop SARS-CoV-2 infection. Before the COVID-19 pandemic, KDIGO guidelines recommended temporary lowering or discontinuation of immunosuppression in the presence of other viral infections [6]. Although no consensus COVID-19 guidelines have been released, the European Renal Association (ERA-EDTA-DESCARTES) has published an expert opinion regarding immunosuppression in SARS-CoV-2 infected renal transplant recipients (Table 22.1) [1] the crux of which is a wait-and-see approach in low-risk asymptomatic patients and discontinuation of antimetabolites and mTOR inhibitors in high-risk asymptomatic or any symptomatic patients. CNIs are generally maintained at current doses unless more severe infection develops. Worldwide, clinical practice has closely aligned with these recommendations on systematic review [7].

Table 22.1 Expert opinion statement regarding immunosuppression management in the setting of acute SARS-CoV-2 infection. Any of the following defines the high-risk patient: age $\geq$ 70, diabetes, cardiac disease, pulmonary disease including tobacco abuse, BMI >30 kg/m^2, eGFR <30 mL/min/1.73 m^2, recent lymphocyte depletion within 3–6 months

Clinical status	Expert opinion [1]
Asymptomatic	
Low-risk patient	No change in immunosuppression
High-risk patient	Consider stopping AZA/MPA/mTORi if on triple therapy
Mild disease	
Without pulmonary involvement	Triple therapy:
Afebrile	Stop AZA/MPA/mTORi
O$_2$ saturation > 95%	Continue CNI
Respiratory rate < 25/min	
No evidence of pneumonia	Dual therapy (with steroids):
	Continue dual therapy
	Dual therapy (no steroids):
	Continue CNI[a]
	Replace AZA/MPA/mTORi with low-dose steroids
With pulmonary involvement	
Low-risk patient	As above
	Reduce tacrolimus level to 3 ± 1 ng/mL
High-risk patient	Stop AZA/MPA/mTORi
	Stop CNI
	Increase steroids 15–25 mg/day
Severe disease	
Febrile	Discontinue all immunosuppressive drugs
O$_2$ saturation <94%	Increase steroids 15–25 mg/day
Respiratory rate >30/min	
Clinical decompensation	

[a]Consider reducing tacrolimus if there is no improvement in 3–5 days

Lowering immunosuppression to prevent severe disease carries an inherent risk of graft rejection. In a systematic review of 554 KTRs with SARS-CoV-2 infection [7], 10.3% of patients developed worsening renal function or graft loss; however, a review of almost 1400 KTRs failed to demonstrate increased 90-day rejection rates following infection [8]. Nevertheless, the differential diagnosis of AKI after SARS-CoV-2 infection must include rejection. A biopsy is mandatory to confirm the diagnosis, both because COVID-19 has been associated with a variety of pathologic findings in the kidney—including acute tubular necrosis, glomerular damage, and podocytopathy [2]—and because empiric treatment of rejection in the setting of active SARS-CoV-2 infection is prohibitively risky.

Biopsy-proven rejection poses a unique clinical challenge. Generally, rejection is treated in a graded approach, with low-grade acute cellular rejections (ACR) treated with pulse steroids and higher-grade ACR or AMR treated additionally with lymphodepleting agents. However, reports of kidney transplant rejection in COVID-19 patients are scarce, and the treatment details are even more limited. A recent case report has demonstrated the efficacy of using pulse dose steroids alone in a patient with grade II ACR [9]. The use of anti-thymocyte globulin for treatment of acute rejection in two patients with active, although asymptomatic, SARS-CoV-2 infection has been described; both of these patients did well with no worsening of the disease [10]. However, the timeframe from initial infection and the presence or absence of neutralizing antibodies in these patients is unclear, leading to the limited applicability of these cases to clinical decision-making. In our case, we elected to treat only with pulse dose steroids, with good resolution of clinical rejection. Until further data has been presented, cautious use of steroid-only regimens appears to be the safest course of action in this clinical scenario.

The progression of the pandemic will no doubt lead to further reports of COVID-19 associated kidney allograft rejection. A systematic review will be necessary to elucidate better the safety of using lymphodepletion in refractory cases of rejection and the ideal candidates for such an approach. Until the data has been clarified, providers must approach rejection primarily by prevention, both by encouraging appropriate COVID-19 precautions and identifying pandemic-related gaps in access to post-transplant care.

References

1. Maggiore U, Abramowicz D, Crespo M, et al. How should I manage immunosuppression in a kidney transplant patient with COVID-19? An ERA-EDTA DESCARTES expert opinion. Nephrol Dial Transplant. 2020;35(6):899–904.
2. de Oliveira P, Cunha K, Neves P, et al. Renal morphology in coronavirus disease: a literature review. Medicina (Kaunas). 2021;57(3)
3. Lentine KL, Mannon RB, Josephson MA. Practicing with uncertainty: kidney transplantation during the COVID-19 pandemic. Am J Kidney Dis. 2021;77(5):777–85.
4. Azzi Y, Bartash R, Scalea J, Loarte-Campos P, Akalin E. COVID-19 and solid organ transplantation: a review article. Transplantation. 2021;105(1):37–55.
5. Caillard S, Chavarot N, Francois H, et al. Is COVID-19 infection more severe in kidney transplant recipients? Am J Transplant. 2021;21(3):1295–303.
6. Kasiske BL, Zeier MG, Chapman JR, et al. KDIGO clinical practice guideline for the care of kidney transplant recipients: a summary. Kidney Int. 2010;77(4):299–311.
7. Angelico R, Blasi F, Manzia TM, Toti L, Tisone G, Cacciola R. The management of immunosuppression in kidney transplant recipients with COVID-19 disease: an update and systematic review of the literature. Medicina (Kaunas). 2021;57(5)
8. Vinson AJ, Agarwal G, Dai R, et al. COVID-19 in solid organ transplantation: results of the national COVID cohort collaborative. Transplant Direct. 2021;7(11):e775.
9. Mohamed M, Smith J, Parajuli S, et al. Successful management of T-cell mediated rejection in a recent kidney transplant recipient with COVID-19 associated severe acute respiratory syndrome. Transpl Infect Dis. 2021;23(4):e13598.
10. Kolonko A, Więcek A. Safety of antithymocyte globulin use in kidney graft recipients during the COVID-19 pandemic. Ann Transplant. 2021;26:e933001.

Chapter 23
Disseminated Histoplasmosis After Kidney Transplantation

Alissar El Chediak and Beatrice P. Concepcion

Introduction

Kidney transplant recipients are at increased risk for developing infections, including opportunistic infections, due to their immunocompromised state. Histoplasmosis is a common endemic mycosis that can go unnoticed in immunocompetent individuals but can be disseminated and cause severe disease in immunocompromised patients. Here, we review the clinical presentation, diagnosis, and management of disseminated histoplasmosis in a kidney transplant recipient.

Clinical History

A 36-year-old man with a past medical history of end-stage kidney disease secondary to autosomal dominant polycystic kidney disease underwent a deceased donor kidney transplant. He received alemtuzumab and steroid induction and was maintained on tacrolimus, mycophenolate mofetil, and prednisone. The patient completed cytomegalovirus (CMV) prophylaxis with valganciclovir and *Pneumocystis* prophylaxis with trimethoprim-sulfamethoxazole. He had immediate graft function with a baseline serum creatinine (SCr) of 1.6–1.8 mg/dL. He was doing well, without any history of acute rejection or infections up until 6 years after his transplant,

A. El Chediak · B. P. Concepcion (✉)
Division of Nephrology and Hypertension, Vanderbilt University Medical Center, Nashville, TN, USA
e-mail: Alissar.el.chediak@vumc.org; Beatrice.p.concepcion@vumc.org

© The Author(s), under exclusive license to Springer Nature Switzerland AG 2022
F. Aziz, S. Parajuli (eds.), *Complications in Kidney Transplantation*,
https://doi.org/10.1007/978-3-031-13569-9_23

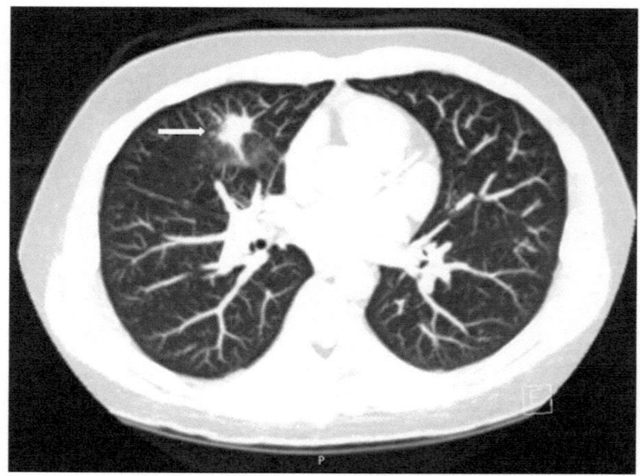

Fig. 23.1 Irregular nodule in the inferior right upper lobe with surrounding micronodules

when he presented with 2 weeks of non-productive cough and high-grade fever. This was associated with headaches, malaise, and loss of appetite. On presentation, he had a temperature of 101 °F, blood pressure 101/64, heart rate 122/min, respiratory rate 16/min. He was ill-appearing but was not in distress. He had no palpable lymphadenopathy. Lungs were clear. He was tachycardic but had no audible murmurs. The abdomen was soft, and the allograft was non-tender. Initial workup was notable for a SCr of 2.6 mg/dL, white blood cell count 3100 mcL, platelet count 132,000 mcL, aspartate aminotransferase 214 units/L, alanine aminotransferase 96 units/L. A chest X-ray was normal. Computed tomography (CT) of the chest showed a new irregular nodule in the inferior right upper lobe with surrounding micronodules and mildly enlarged left hilar lymph node (Fig. 23.1).

Question 1

What is the most likely diagnosis?

A. CMV disease.
B. Disseminated Histoplasmosis (DH).
C. Nocardiosis.
D. *Pneumocystis jirovecii* pneumonia.

The correct answer is B.

Although all of the above choices are possible, the patient's clinical presentation of fever, cough, headache, leukopenia, transaminitis, and the radiologic findings of pulmonary nodules and perihilar lymphadenopathy are most consistent with DH [1]. A study of 152 patients with post-transplant histoplasmosis reported that 81% of post-transplant histoplasmosis had evidence of dissemination, and the lungs were the most commonly involved (81%), followed by bone marrow (26%) and liver (18%). Less commonly involved organs were the spleen, gastrointestinal tract, central nervous system, and cutaneous sites [2].

Hospital Course

Urine Histoplasma antigen was positive. CMV was not detected by the polymerase chain reaction (PCR) test. Fungal blood cultures were negative. The patient was admitted for further management. Intravenous liposomal amphotericin B (5 mg/kg) was started for 3 days, after which he received itraconazole. Itraconazole was given orally at 200 mg three times daily for 3 days as a loading dose, then 200 mg twice daily as a maintenance dose. The patient started to improve clinically on day 3 of hospital admission with the resolution of fever. SCr trended down to baseline with intravenous fluids.

Question 2

Which drug levels should be monitored in this patient?

A. Tacrolimus.
B. Mycophenolate mofetil.
C. Itraconazole.
D. A and C.

The correct answer is D.

Both the calcineurin inhibitor and the itraconazole drug levels must be monitored. Azole antifungals increase the level of calcineurin inhibitors by inhibiting the drug-metabolizing enzyme cytochrome (CYP) P450. A significant reduction in tacrolimus dosage can be expected after the initiation of itraconazole. Blood levels of itraconazole should be measured after a steady state has been reached to ensure adequate drug exposure [3]. It is recommended that an itraconazole level be obtained approximately 2 weeks into therapy. Dose adjustments need to be made if the random serum level is lower than 1 mg/mL [3].

Additional Clinical Course

The patient's mycophenolate was held in the setting of DH. Prednisone was increased from 5 mg to 10 mg daily. Tacrolimus levels and itraconazole levels were monitored closely. The patient required a 75% reduction in the dose of his tacrolimus to maintain therapeutic levels. The itraconazole level was therapeutic at the prescribed dose of 200 mg twice a day. On outpatient follow-up at 1 month after his initial presentation, the patient's symptoms had resolved, and blood counts had normalized. Thus, mycophenolate was resumed, and prednisone was reduced back to 5 mg daily. Urine Histoplasma antigen was undetectable at 3 months after initiation of therapy. Antifungal therapy with itraconazole was continued for 1 year. Tacrolimus dosage was re-adjusted to his original dose prior to itraconazole.

Discussion

Histoplasmosis is caused by the dimorphic fungus *Histoplasma capsulatum* and is the most prevalent endemic mycosis in the United States [4]. Despite histoplasmosis being rare in kidney transplant patients, it can be severe and disseminated. The incidence of post-transplant histoplasmosis is reported to be 1 per 1000 person years per a retrospective study, which included 3436 solid organ transplant patients [5]. Einollahi et al. reported similar results with only one patient out of 2410 patients developing histoplasmosis [6].

There are three mechanisms of infection with Histoplasma: primary infection via inhalation, activation of latent infection, and direct spread from the donor allograft [7]. Neutrophils, macrophages, lymphocytes, and natural killer cells are involved in response to the infection [8]. In addition, T-cell mediated immunity plays a role in further activating macrophages to kill the organism. Therefore, patients on immunosuppressive therapy are unable to mount an adequate response and are at risk for DH. Similarly, being a solid organ transplant recipient is a risk factor for developing DH. Most Histoplasma infections occur within 1–2 years post-transplant [7]. However, a case series in India reported a median duration for presentation to be 5 years after transplant [9].

DH in a kidney transplant recipient can present in an unspecific manner. As mentioned above, organ systems involved in DH include pulmonary (most common), bone marrow, liver, central nervous system, and skin [6]. Fever, cough, malaise, weight loss, and cutaneous lesions are all symptoms that have been reported. The most common clinical sign of DH in immunocompromised patients is fever, with a frequency of 54–66% [9]. This makes it challenging to make a timely diagnosis of DH since symptoms coincide with other opportunistic infections like CMV. Several abnormal laboratory values are described in DH, most commonly elevated liver function tests (aspartate aminotransferase, alanine aminotransferase) [10].

Diagnosis of DH requires a high level of suspicion. Diagnosis can be made by combining different modalities. These include blood and urine antigen tests, radiology, and appropriate biopsies for culture and histology [2]. Tuberculated conidia detected in tissue cultures are characteristic of the infection [10]. Urine antigen tests are more than 95% sensitive to detect DH [3]. Histoplasma antigen can also be detected in bronchoalveolar lavage fluid in patients undergoing bronchoscopy to evaluate pulmonary infiltrates. Thus, body fluids and tissue should always be submitted for fungal cultures and stains when DH is suspected. A peripheral blood smear can show intracellular yeast organisms leading to the diagnosis of DH [3]. Serologic tests may be negative in acute infections, especially in immunocompromised patients [9].

Nonetheless, they may complement the results of antigen testing, especially in patients whose diagnosis is still uncertain. CT can identify pulmonary involvement in DH. Chest CT shows focal consolidation or nodules, with or without pleural effusions [3]. Mediastinal adenopathy can also be seen.

The mainstay treatment of DH is antifungals. As per the Infectious Disease Association of America (IDSA), treatment of histoplasmosis depends on the location and extent of the infection. For pulmonary involvement or significant disseminated infection, liposomal amphotericin B or lipid-associated amphotericin B is recommended until the patient is symptomatically improved (usually for 1–2 weeks) [10]. Once the clinical response is established, the patient can be switched to oral itraconazole (200 mg three times daily for 3 days and then 200 mg twice daily) for at least 12 months in the immunocompromised patient [11]. The levels of both immunosuppressive agents, particularly calcineurin inhibitors and itraconazole, must be monitored due to the CYP P450 interaction with the azole antifungals. A balance between infection treatment and organ rejection prevention must be maintained while managing DH. With appropriate therapy, the prognosis of histoplasmosis is good in transplant patients, highlighting the importance of its timely diagnosis and proper treatment.

Disclosures None.

Funding None.

References

1. Gajurel K, Dhakal R, Deresinski S. Histoplasmosis in transplant recipients. Clin Transpl. 2017;31:e13087.
2. Assi M, Martin S, Wheat LJ, et al. Histoplasmosis after solid organ transplant. Clin Infect Dis. 2013;57:1542–9.
3. Freifeld AG, Wheat LJ, Kaul DR. Histoplasmosis in solid organ transplant recipients: early diagnosis and treatment. Curr Opin Organ Transplant. 2009;14(6):601–5.
4. Chu JH, Feudtner C, Heydon K, Walsh TJ, Zaoutis TE. Hospitalizations for endemic mycoses: a population-based national study. Clin Infect Dis. 2006;42(6):822–5.
5. Cuellar-Rodriguez J, Avery RK, Lard M, Budev M, Gordon SM, Shrestha NK, et al. Histoplasmosis in solid organ transplant recipients: 10 years of experience at a large transplant center in an endemic area. Clin Infect Dis. 2009;49(5):710–6.
6. Einollahi B, Lessan-Pezeshki M, Pourfarziani V, Nemati E, Nafar M, Pour-Reza-Gholi F, et al. Invasive fungal infections following renal transplantation: a review of 2410 recipients. Ann Transplant. 2008;13(4):55–8.
7. Miller R, Assi M, Practice ASTIDCo. Endemic fungal infections in solid organ transplant recipients-guidelines from the American society of transplantation infectious diseases Community of Practice. Clin Transpl. 2019;33(9):e13553.
8. Horwath MC, Fecher RA, Deepe GS Jr. Histoplasma capsulatum, lung infection, and immunity. Future Microbiol. 2015;10(6):967–75.
9. Rana A, Kotton CN, Mahapatra A, Nandwani A, Sethi S, Bansal SB. Post kidney transplant histoplasmosis: an under-recognized diagnosis in India. Transpl Infect Dis. 2021;23(3):e13523.
10. Johnston RB Jr, Thareja S, Shenefelt PD. Disseminated histoplasmosis in a renal transplant patient. Cutis. 2013;91(6):295–9.
11. Wheat LJ, Freifeld AG, Kleiman MB, Baddley JW, McKinsey DS, Loyd JE, et al. Clinical practice guidelines for managing patients with histoplasmosis: 2007 update by the Infectious Diseases Society of America. Clin Infect Dis. 2007;45(7):807–25.

Chapter 24
Post-Transplant Progressive Multifocal Leukoencephalopathy Secondary to JC Polyomavirus

Arpita Basu

Introduction

JC polyomavirus is a human polyomavirus that causes progressive multifocal leukoencephalopathy (PML), a rare, often fatal, demyelinating disease particularly in immunocompromised hosts such as solid organ transplant recipients (SOTRs). The literature evidence of PML in SOTRs is limited. Through this case vignette, the authors discuss this rare disease entity, review the disease prevalence, clinical spectrum, and overall disease prognosis while highlighting the need for a timely diagnosis which is crucial for good outcomes.

Patient History

A 42-year-old female underwent preemptive living-related kidney transplantation for stage V Chronic Kidney Disease (CKD) secondary to biopsy-proven Focal Segmental Glomerular Sclerosis (FSGS). Her past medical history was significant for depression, well-controlled on sertraline, and migraine headaches. Pre-transplant she had failed several immunosuppressive therapies to manage FSGS spanning over 20 years. Her panel reactive antibody was 0%, and she had no preformed donor-specific antibodies. Cytomegalovirus (CMV) serology was donor positive and recipient negative (CMV High Risk). She received basiliximab induction and was on a maintenance immunosuppression regimen of tacrolimus (target trough 8–12 ng/mL in the first 6 months post-transplant), mycophenolate mofetil (MMF)1000 mg

A. Basu (✉)
Division of Nephrology and Hypertension, Department of Medicine, Emory School of Medicine, Atlanta, GA, USA
e-mail: arpita.basu@emory.edu

© The Author(s), under exclusive license to Springer Nature Switzerland AG 2022

F. Aziz, S. Parajuli (eds.), *Complications in Kidney Transplantation*,
https://doi.org/10.1007/978-3-031-13569-9_24

twice a day, and prednisone 5 mg daily. She was also on valganciclovir and sulfamethoxazole-trimethoprim prophylaxis for 6 months. The immediate post-transplant course was unremarkable, with creatinine stabilizing between 1.3 and 1.5 mg/dL. Five months post-transplant, the patient presented to an outside facility with headache, altered mentation, and aphasia following a subacute gastrointestinal illness with nausea and diarrhea. The family reported an increase in the patient's baseline migraines a few weeks prior to hospitalization and an unintentional 20-pound weight loss for which she had not pursued any medical assistance. At the outside facility, as part of her workup, she underwent a Computerized Tomography (CT) head, Magnetic Resonance Imaging (MRI) brain, and Electroencephalogram (EEG), all of which were normal. She had symptomatic improvement following administration of a migraine cocktail and was subsequently discharged a day later with the diagnosis of migraine with an aura. The following day the patient presented to our hospital with nonsensical speech, increased somnolence, and motor difficulty. Physical exam on presentation was unremarkable except for several pertinent neurological findings, including euthymic affect, attention difficulty, incoherent speech, and upper extremity tremor. There were no strength or sensory deficits observed. Vital signs were stable with no evidence of fever. She was admitted for further evaluation and management of her symptoms.

Question 1

What is the most likely cause of her abnormal neurologic findings?

A. Infectious process.
B. Calcineurin Inhibitor (CNI) toxicity.
C. Malignancy
D. Cerebrovascular event.
E. Any of the above.

The correct answer is E.

The differential diagnosis for abnormal neurological findings in an immunosuppressed patient is extensive, including several infectious and non-infectious disease possibilities. Infectious evaluation including, but not limited to, COVID-19 encephalopathy, Herpes Simplex Virus (HSV) Encephalitis, HIV encephalopathy, CMV encephalitis, Epstein Barr Virus (EBV) associated lymphoproliferative disorder, Progressive Multifocal Leukoencephalopathy (PML), toxoplasmosis, cryptococcus encephalitis should be considered. Primary and metastatic central nervous system (CNS) malignancies can present similarly and need to be assessed, particularly in a patient presenting with unintentional weight loss. Immunosuppressive agents including CNIs such as tacrolimus or cyclosporine, purine synthesis inhibitors, such as MMF or azathioprine, and glucocorticoids have direct neurotoxic effects. They can be responsible for neurological abnormalities, particularly early post-transplant, when the drug levels are maintained at a higher range to minimize the likelihood of allograft rejection [1]. Also, solid organ transplant recipients (SOTRs) are at a higher risk of cerebrovascular events than the general population, with a reported incidence of 5% in the first year post-transplant [1].

Hospital Course

Following hospitalization, the patient had another MRI brain which was normal, and a repeat EEG that showed generalized slowing without seizures or epileptiform activity. Blood and urine toxicology screen and cultures were negative. Lumbar puncture was done, and the cerebrospinal fluid (CSF) was without pleocytosis, with normal glucose and mildly elevated protein. Laboratory results were all normal except for supratherapeutic tacrolimus trough levels, thus tacrolimus was held. Other medications likely to cause CNS depression, like sertraline, were discontinued. The patient was given nutritional supplements and started on para-enteral nutrition. Over the next 2 days, extensive Infectious and non-infectious workup remained negative, and the patient had some improvement in her neurological status with the above-mentioned interventions. On hospitalization day 4, she again developed worsening mentation, with dystonia and hyperreflexia. This coincided with the re-introduction of sertraline and concern for possible serotonin syndrome. All serotonergic medications were discontinued.

To minimize immunosuppression associated neurotoxicity, tacrolimus was discontinued, sirolimus was initiated (target trough 5–8 ng/mL), MMF was reduced to 500 mg daily, and prednisone 5 mg daily was continued. On hospitalization day 8, the patient had status epilepticus warranting ICU transfer due to the need for intubation for airway protection and sedation. MRI brain was repeated and now showed hyperintensity in bilateral thalamus and fluid-attenuated inversion recovery (FLAIR) signal non-suppression in the sulci suggestive of the meningo-encephalitic process of unclear etiology. Repeat lumbar puncture done on hospitalization day 9 showed markedly elevated protein with mild pleocytosis. Repeat EEG done following seizures was consistent with toxic metabolic encephalopathy. She was empirically started on broad-spectrum antibiotics and acyclovir for possible bacterial or viral meningitis, which was discontinued when blood, urine, and CSF biofire were negative. As the hospitalization progressed, the patient remained critically ill with no specific etiology identified for her illness despite another exhaustive infectious workup. Entertaining the possibility of truly uncommon infections, CSF was sent for metagenomic deep sequencing to an outside lab. Unfortunately, on hospitalization day 16, the patient had significant changes in her neurologic status. Brain imaging showed severe edema and brain herniation. She then went into pulseless electrical activity arrest and ultimately expired. Posthumous, the CSF metagenomic deep sequencing was positive for JC virus.

Question 2

JCPyV belongs to which family of viruses?

A. Human herpes virus.
B. Human polyoma virus.
C. Human T-lymphotropic virus (HTLV-I).
D. Japanese encephalitis virus.
E. Enteroviruses.

The correct answer is B.

Table 24.1 The clinical manifestations observed in JCPyV, BKPyV, and MCPyV

	BK polyomavirus (BKPyV)	JC human polyomavirus(JCPyV)	Merkel cell polyomavirus (MCPyV)
Genotypes	4	1	5
Seroprevalence %	90	86	79
During latent period found in	Kidney, bone marrow, brain	Kidney	Skin
Clinical presentation	• Nephropathy • Ureteral stenosis • Hemorrhagic cystitis • Extra-renal manifestations(rare)	• Classic progressive multifocal Leukoencephalopathy • Progressive multifocal leukoencephalopathy—Immune reconstitution inflammatory syndrome • JC virus granule cell neuronopathy • Meningitis • Encephalitis	• Invasive Merkel cell carcinoma

JCPyV is a human polyomaviruses (HPyVs) of the DNA virus genus in the Polyomaviridae family [2]. A total of 14 HPyV species have been identified to date with literature evidence primarily on JCPyV, BK polyomavirus (BKPyV), and Merkel cell polyomavirus (MCPyV) [2]. HPyVs are ubiquitous worldwide with high sero-prevalence (50–90%) that is known to increase with advancing age [2]. The majority of primary infections are either asymptomatic or result in a nonspecific viral syndrome. Following the primary infection, HPyVs remain latent in varied organs such as the kidney until it is reactivated when immunocompromised or with a greater burden of viral replication. The clinical manifestations observed in JCPyV, BKPyV, and MCPyV are described in Table 24.1.

Final Diagnosis: Progressive multifocal leukoencephalopathy secondary to JC virus (JCPyV).

Discussion

Progressive multifocal leukoencephalopathy (PML) is a rare, often fatal, demyelinating disease resulting from lytic infection of the glial cells in the brain by JCPyV. First described as a complication in patients with primary B cell lymphoproliferative disorder, it has since been reported in several other immunocompromised populations such as patients with acquired immunodeficiency syndrome (AIDS), SOTRs, bone marrow transplantation (BMT) recipients, and patients who received humanized, monoclonal antibody, natalizumab [3].

JCPyV infects approximately 70–85% of the human population [2, 4]. The pathological transformation of JCPyV is poorly understood; however, a strong correlation between the duration of immunosuppression and PML incidence has been documented in the literature [5]. Our patient, who was immunosuppressed for more than 20 years in the pre-transplant era, was at a heightened risk of PML given prolonged immunosuppression exposure. The literature evidence of PML in SOTRs is scant in risk factors and clinical spectrum, and incidence in this cohort is uncertain. In one review of 427 heart or lung transplant recipients, the calculated incidence rate of PML was reported as 1.2 cases per 1000 post-transplantation years [6]. PML does not uniformly occur in all immunocompromised patient populations. Studies suggest several risk-modifying factors at play; for example, JCPyV reactivation is most common in those with a cluster of differentiation 4(CD4+) T cells deficiencies or host genetic risk factors such as the human leukocyte antigen (HLA)-DRB1*0401 allele increasing susceptibility to PML [7].

Clinically, PML commonly presents with hemiparesis, cognitive disturbances, or visual field deficits. Behavioral and cognitive changes are the most prevalent symptoms in SOTRs [3, 8]. The mean time from the introduction of immunosuppressive agents to the development of first symptoms in SOTRs is reported to be 34.9 months [8]. The disease course of PML is progressive, and the disease fatality is high due to a lack of effective treatment, as discussed later. Mateen et al. estimated an 84% case fatality and a 56% 1-year survival in SOTRs with PML [6].

Neuroimaging, including CT and MRI, are a useful diagnostic tool. Demyelinating white matter lesions appearing as subcortical hypodensities, particularly in frontal and parietal lobes, are typically seen, though lesions in the corpus callosum, thalamus, and basal ganglia, though rare, have also been reported. In a study, thalamic involvement similar to that observed in our patient was reported in only 12% of SOTRs with PML [8]. Imaging coupled with the identification of JCPyV in the CSF is adequate to diagnose PML. Our patient had multiple imaging studies showing no abnormalities before the thalamic hypodensities were observed, and her CSF never showed evidence of JCPyV, thus making it a challenge to identify the etiology of her presentation. Brain biopsy, along with detection of JCPyV DNA by in situ hybridization or immunohistochemistry, remains the most reliable method of diagnosing PML [1]. Demyelination, bizarre astrocytes, and enlarged oligodendrocyte nuclei are the typical triad seen on histopathology that establishes diagnosis and should be pursued if able [1].

Currently, there is no effective treatment for PML. Antiviral medications like cidofovir, cytarabine, and mefloquine, tested in randomized trials or prospective studies, have shown no significant clinical benefits [9]. In SOTRs, discontinuation or reduction in immunosuppression has been recommended, but no proven changes in fatality outcomes have been observed with the same [9]. Studies exploring the benefits of boosting the adaptive immune response with dendritic cell vaccines or using virus-specific cytotoxic T cells generated from the patient (autologous) or allogenic third-party donors are still in the investigational phase [2, 9].

In conclusion, this case showcases the challenges of diagnosing rare opportunistic infections in SOTRs particularly as the differential diagnosis is very broad. In our patient, given the lack of any effective therapy, a timely diagnosis may not have changed the outcome. However, in other situations, timely diagnosis remains crucial for good outcomes. Patients and families must be educated continuously of the risks associated with an immunocompromised state and the need to alert their medical providers in the event of any new, abnormal, or significant worsening of an existing symptom.

References

1. Faravelli I, Velardo D, Podestà MA, et al. Immunosuppression-related neurological disorders in kidney transplantation. J Nephrol. 2021;34:539–55. https://doi.org/10.1007/s40620-020-00956-1.
2. Imlay H, Limaye A. Overview of JC polyomavirus, BK polyomavirus, and other polyomavirus infections. 2021. Uptodate.com. https://www.uptodate.com/contents/overview-of-jc-polyomavirus-bk-polyomavirus-and-other-polyomavirus-infections?search=jc%20virus&source=search_result&selectedTitle=1~91&usage_type=default&display_rank=1#H1143005128. Accessed 3 Jan 2022.
3. Waggoner J, Martinu T, Palmer SM. Progressive multifocal leukoencephalopathy following heightened immunosuppression after lung transplant. J Heart Lung Transplant. 2009;28(4):395–8. https://doi.org/10.1016/j.healun.2008.12.010.
4. Harypursat V, Zhou Y, Tang S, Chen Y. JC Polyomavirus, progressive multifocal leukoencephalopathy and immune reconstitution inflammatory syndrome: a review. AIDS Res Ther. 2020;17(1):37. Accessed 6 July 2020. https://doi.org/10.1186/s12981-020-00293-0.
5. Pavlovic D, Patera AC, Nyberg F, Gerber M, Liu M. Progressive multifocal Leukoencephalopathy consortium. Progressive multifocal leukoencephalopathy: current treatment options and future perspectives. Ther Adv Neurol Disord. 2015;8(6):255–73. https://doi.org/10.1177/1756285615602832.
6. Mateen FJ, Muralidharan R, Carone M, van de Beek D, Harrison DM, Aksamit AJ, Gould MS, Clifford DB, Nath A. Progressive multifocal leukoencephalopathy in transplant recipients. Ann Neurol. 2011 Aug;70(2):305–22. https://doi.org/10.1002/ana.22408.
7. Cortese I, Reich DS, Nath A. Progressive multifocal leukoencephalopathy and the spectrum of JC virus-related disease. Nat Rev Neurol. 2021;17(1):37–51. https://doi.org/10.1038/s41582-020-00427-y.
8. Maas RP, Muller-Hansma AH, Esselink RA, Murk JL, Warnke C, Killestein J, Wattjes MP. Drug-associated progressive multifocal leukoencephalopathy: a clinical, radiological, and cerebrospinal fluid analysis of 326 cases. J Neurol. 2016;263(10):2004–21. https://doi.org/10.1007/s00415-016-8217-x.
9. Saji AM, Gupta V. Progressive multifocal leukoencephalopathy. StatPearls [Internet]. Treasure Island (FL): StatPearls Publishing; 2021.

Chapter 25
Central Nervous System Aspergillosis in a Kidney Transplant Recipient

Emily Joachim and Judy Hindi

Introduction

Infectious complications are a significant cause of morbidity and mortality in kidney transplant recipients and remain the second leading cause of mortality in kidney transplant recipients.

Clinicians must have a high suspicion for atypical and fungal infections, given that typical manifestations of infections are not always present in this immunocompromised patient population. While less common than bacterial infections, fungal infections comprise up to 10% of infections in kidney transplant patients, with candida and aspergillus species being the most frequent infections [1–3]. Mortality with invasive fungal infections may approach 100%, thus prompt recognition and treatment with the most effective agents are necessary. In this chapter, we present a case of invasive aspergillosis in a post-kidney transplant recipient and discuss the diagnostic and treatment modalities available and the complications that may arise from these treatments.

Patient History

A 73-year-old male with end-stage kidney disease (ESKD) secondary to diabetes and hypertension underwent a 3/6 HLA-matched living unrelated kidney transplant. He was on dialysis for 10 months pre-transplant. Pre-transplant cytomegalovirus (CMV) status was donor negative, recipient positive, and Epstein–Barr virus (EBV)

E. Joachim (✉) · J. Hindi
Division of Nephrology, Department of Medicine, Medical College of Wisconsin, Milwaukee, WI, USA
e-mail: ejoachim@mcw.edu; jhindi@mcw.edu

© The Author(s), under exclusive license to Springer Nature Switzerland AG 2022

F. Aziz, S. Parajuli (eds.), *Complications in Kidney Transplantation*,
https://doi.org/10.1007/978-3-031-13569-9_25

status was donor and recipient positive. Pre-transplant panel reactive antibody was 0% for both classes I and II. For induction, he received anti-thymocyte globulin and was maintained on tacrolimus (goal trough 6–10 ng/mL), mycophenolate mofetil 1000 mg twice daily, and prednisone 5 mg daily. The patient received valganciclovir for 6 months post-transplant and trimethoprim/sulfamethoxazole 400 mg/80 mg daily indefinitely for infection prophylaxis.

Four months post-transplant, he developed acute rhinosinusitis treated with amoxicillin/clavinulate 875/125 BID for 10 days. Subsequently, he developed recurrent sinusitis 2 and 3 months after the initial episode, treated again with amoxicillin/clavinulate for 10 days and then cefdinir 300 mg BID for 10 days. At this time, he was referred to otolaryngology, and a CT sinus demonstrated pan-sinusitis. A sinus culture was obtained and grew 1+ staphylococcus pseudointermedius, sensitive only to vancomycin, and one colony of aspergillus fumigatus. He was treated with a short burst of steroids but no further antimicrobials.

Two weeks later, he underwent sinus surgery, and the operative report noted that thick mucopus was debrided from bilateral sphenoid sinuses and the right ethmoid sinus. The right sinus contents demonstrated a mycetoma with no definitive tissue invasion. Surgery was felt curative, and thus no antibiotics or antifungals were started. Six weeks postoperatively, he presented to the emergency department with altered mental status and right-sided weakness. MRI showed a 1.4 cm left inferior frontal lobe lesion with thin peripheral rim enhancement. (Fig. 25.1).

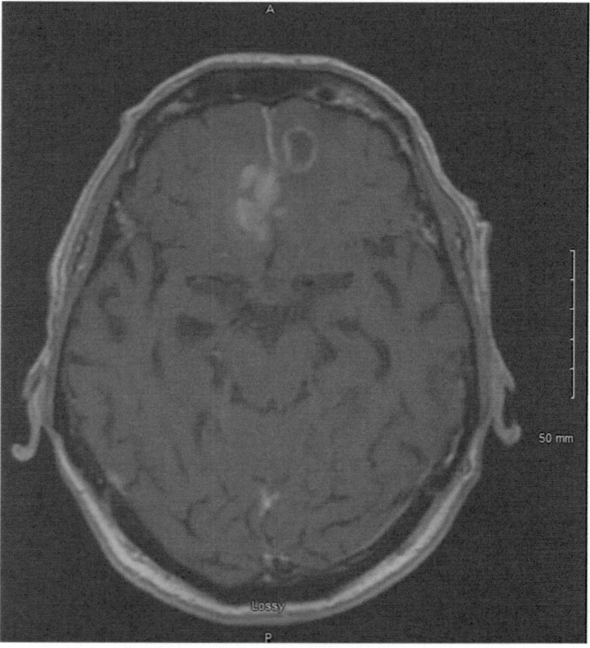

Fig. 25.1 MRI showed a 1.4 cm left inferior frontal lobe lesion with thin peripheral rim enhancement

Question 1

What is the most likely cause of his ring-enhancing lesion?

A. Bacterial abscess.
B. Fungal abscess.
C. Post-transplant lymphoproliferative disorder (PTLD).
D. CNS vasculitis.

The correct answer is B.

Given a ring-enhancing lesion in the setting of known sinusitis with recent instrumentation, the main differential would be bacterial versus fungal abscess. He was previously treated for bacterial infection, and sinus surgery demonstrated mycetoma, thus increasing the possibility of fungal abscess, especially in previous cultures showing Aspergillus fumigatus. While post-transplant lymphoproliferative disorder (PTLD) does peak within the first year post-transplant, his history of sinus instrumentation points towards an infectious etiology.

Hospital Course

The patient underwent craniotomy and evacuation of the frontal lobe lesion. Intraoperatively, he was found to have a small epidural abscess and pachymeningitis with adjacent intraparenchymal hemorrhage. He additionally was noted to have osteomyelitis of his skull based on intraoperative bone biopsy. Cultures returned positive for 1+ aspergillus fumigatus, with no aerobic or anerobic growth of bacteria.

He was treated with 7 days of IV liposomal amphotericin and started on hyperbaric oxygen therapy. His mycophenolate mofetil was reduced to 500 mg BID, and he was continued on tacrolimus, but the goal level was reduced to 2–5 ng/mL. He developed acute kidney injury (Cr peak 1.62 mg/dL), and hyperkalemia with amphotericin despite IV hydration, which resolved with the transition to oral voriconazole. He had a repeat sinus endoscopic evaluation with no concern for active fungal sinusitis and was subsequently discharged on voriconazole with a plan for at least 6 months of therapy.

Question 2

What risk factors does this patient have for an invasive fungal infection?

A. Advanced age.
B. Induction immunosuppression with anti-thymocyte globulin.
C. Surgical disruption of sinuses.
D. Use of systemic antibiotics.
E. All of the above.

The correct answer is E.

Risk factors for invasive fungal infections are the level of immunosuppression, including both induction and maintenance therapy, multiple transplants, chronic allograft rejection (necessitating an increase in immunosuppression), broad-spectrum antibiotics, indwelling catheters, disruption of mucosal membranes, infection with cytomegalovirus, chronic liver disease, advanced age, diabetes/hyperglycemia, prolonged pre-transplant dialysis, and abnormal kidney function post-transplant including the need for dialysis post-transplant [1].

Additional Clinical Course

Two months into therapy with voriconazole, his alkaline phosphatase rose to 1190 U/L, AST to 87 U/L, and ALT to 92 U/L, which was attributed to voriconazole, and he was transitioned to IV micafungin as an outpatient with normalization of his liver function tests. He was hospitalized 1 week later with worsening headaches, and repeat CT demonstrated increasing air-fluid level in the left frontal lobe. He underwent repeat surgical decompression; the fluid culture was sterile, and he was discharged on isavuconazole. He was maintained on this for 5 months with therapeutic plasma levels and then readmitted with worsening left-sided headache, new blurry vision, and MRI was concerning for progressive aspergillosis. Given concern for isavuconazole failure and intolerance of other therapies, he underwent placement of a central nervous system (CNS) reservoir and began intrathecal amphotericin initially three times weekly, tapered to once weekly over 8 months. He had severe headaches that lasted 1–2 days post-therapy, and after 8 months, he was transitioned to oral posaconazole as maintenance therapy.

Discussion

Overall, fungal infections make up around 5% of post-transplant infections [1], with studies reporting the incidence of invasive fungal infections between 1.4 and 9.4% in kidney transplant recipients [2, 3]. Invasive aspergillosis has been reported to be the second leading cause of invasive infections after candida species, with an incidence of 0.5–2.2% [4, 5]; a more recent study found that aspergillus was the most frequent invasive fungal infection in solid-organ transplant recipients [6]. Pulmonary aspergillosis is the most frequent presentation, although cutaneous or cerebral aspergillosis can occur, and autopsy studies have demonstrated that CNS involvement is present in 20% of patients with invasive aspergillosis [7]. Unfortunately, the prognosis associated with invasive aspergillosis is poor; the mortality rate ranges between 88 and 100% depending on the infection site, with mortality reaching 100% in CNS infection [5, 8].

CNS aspergillosis usually results in brain abscess formation, but it can rarely present as cerebral infarction with or without hemorrhage or meningitis [8]. MRI brain will typically show ring-enhancing lesions with possible infarction and vascular infiltration. In cases of aspergillus meningitis, cerebral spinal fluid galactomannan will be positive in up to 90% of patients and thus can aid in the diagnosis, as only around 30% of fungal cultures will be positive [9].

The therapy of choice for CNS aspergillosis is voriconazole, given its superior clinical activity and CNS penetration compared to IV amphotericin, even liposomal preparations [10]. A retrospective case series of patients with CNS aspergillosis treated with voriconazole either as initial or salvage therapy had a 31% survival rate with a median observation time of 390 days [11]. The most common voriconazole-related adverse events in this study were elevated liver function tests, visual changes, and rash [11]. There is limited data on the efficacy of echinocandins, and given their poor CNS penetration, are not recommended as initial therapy. While there are no clear recommendations on neurosurgical interventions in CNS aspergillosis, several studies have demonstrated that patients who underwent neurosurgical procedures had significantly improved survival, regardless of the type of procedure performed (stereotactic drainage, intracavitary catheters or craniotomy with evacuation) [11, 12].

References

1. Pérez-Sáez MJ, Mir M, Montero MM, Crespo M, Montero N, Gómez J, Horcajada JP, Pascual J. Invasive aspergillosis in kidney transplant recipients: a cohort study. Exp Clin Transplant. 2014;12(2):101–5.
2. Nampoory MR, Khan ZU, Johny KV, et al. Invasive fungal infections in renal transplant recipients. J Infect. 1996;33(2):95–101.
3. Badiee P, Kordbacheh P, Alborzi A, Zeini F, Mirhendy H, Mahmoody M. Fungal infections in solid organ recipients. Exp Clin Transplant. 2005;3(2):385–9.
4. Alangaden GJ, Thyagarajan R, Gruber SA, et al. Infectious complications after kidney transplantation: current epidemiology and associated risk factors. Clin Transpl. 2006;20(4):401–9.
5. Morgan J, Wannemuehler KA, Marr KA, et al. Incidence of invasive aspergillosis following hematopoietic stem cell and solid organ transplantation: interim results of a prospective multicenter surveillance program. Med Mycol. 2005;43(Suppl. 1):S49–58.
6. Bodro M, Sabé N, Gomila A, et al. Risk factors, clinical characteristics, and outcomes of invasive fungal infections in solid organ transplant recipients. Transplant Proc. 2012;44(9):2682–5.
7. Bodey G, Bueltmann B, Duguid W, Gibbs D, Hanak H, Hotchi M, Mall G, Martino P, Meunier F, Milliken S, Naoe S, Okudaira M, Scevola D, van't Wout J. Fungal infections in cancer patients: an international autopsy survey. Eur J Clin Microbiol Infect Dis. 1992;11:99–109.
8. Lin SJ, Schranz J, Teutsch SM. Aspergillosis case-fatality rate: systematic review of the literature. Clin Infect Dis. 2001;32(3):358–66.
9. Sonneville R, Magalhaes E, Meyfroidt G. Central nervous system infections in immunocompromised patients. Curr Opin Crit Care. 2017 Apr;23(2):128–33.
10. Schwartz S, Thiel E. Update on the treatment of cerebral aspergillosis. Ann Hematol. 2004;83(Suppl. 1):S42–4.
11. Schwartz S, Ruhnke M, Ribaud P, Corey L, Driscoll T, Cornely OA, Schuler U, Lutsar I, Troke P, Thiel E. Improved outcome in central nervous system aspergillosis, using voriconazole treatment. Blood. 2005;106(8):2641–5.
12. Coleman JM, Hogg GG, Rosenfeld JV, Waters KD. Invasive central nervous system aspergillosis: cure with liposomal amphotericin B, itraconazole, and radical surgery–case report and review of the literature. Neurosurgery. 1995;36:858–63.

Chapter 26
A Case of West Nile Virus Infection in a Kidney Transplant Recipient

Quarshie Glover and Fahad Aziz

Introduction

Viral encephalitis has a distinct course of illness and is even more of a medical challenge in the immunosuppressed individual. West Nile virus is the most common cause of viral encephalitis in the United States, with historical outbreaks in several parts of the country over the last few decades. Kidney Transplant Recipients (KTR) are a large cohort of solid organ transplant recipients who are at risk of severe infections.

This chapter discusses the clinical approach to managing kidney transplant recipients presenting with fever and altered mental state. We highlight WNV encephalitis as a possible differential that should be considered. A high index of suspicion, followed by a robust workup, is needed to develop this diagnosis, as clinical presentation widely varies.

Patient History

A 40-year-old male with a history of chronic kidney disease stage 5, due to diabetes, underwent a simultaneous kidney and pancreas transplantation. At the time of transplant, his panel reactive antibody (PRA) was 0%, and he had no preformed donor-specific antibodies (DSA). He received induction with anti-thymocyte globulin. His maintenance immunosuppression included tacrolimus (target trough 6–8 ng/mL), mycophenolate sodium 720 mg twice a day, and prednisone 5 mg daily. He achieved

Q. Glover (✉) · F. Aziz
Department of Medicine, University of Wisconsin–Madison School of Medicine and Public Health, University of Wisconsin Hospital and Clinics, Madison, WI, USA
e-mail: QGlover@uwhealth.org; faziz@wisc.edu

© The Author(s), under exclusive license to Springer Nature Switzerland AG 2022

F. Aziz, S. Parajuli (eds.), *Complications in Kidney Transplantation*,
https://doi.org/10.1007/978-3-031-13569-9_26

a baseline creatinine of 1 mg/dL with eGFR of 80 mL/min/1.73 m^2. His post-transplant course was unremarkable. Eight months after the transplant, he presented to the hospital with fever and altered mental status. His initial infectious workup was normal, including urine analysis, blood cultures, and chest X-ray. A CT scan of the head was also unremarkable.

Question 1

What should be the next step in the management?

A. Observation.
B. Lumbar puncture.
C. Stop anti-rejection medications.

The correct answer is B.

A lumbar puncture should be performed in the immunocompromised transplant patients with altered mental status and fever. Observation alone would not be a good choice for an immunocompromised patient with altered mental status. Stopping immunosuppression altogether would not be a good option either. In the transplant recipient, immunosuppression can be reduced in the setting of acute infection; however, stopping anti-rejection medications can put the kidney and pancreas allografts at the risk of acute rejection.

Further Course

The patient was started on broad-spectrum antibiotics. He underwent a lumbar puncture. The cerebrospinal fluid (CSF) analysis showed pleocytosis with lymphocyte predominance. Serological testing of CSF detected immunoglobulin M (IgM) to West Nile virus (WNV). On MRI of the brain, a new focus T2 flair signal abnormality was identified within the midbrain. Subsequently, he felt worsening generalized weakness and difficulty in swallowing. He had decreased power in lower extremities 4/5, tremors were noted bilaterally in lower extremities. He also had an ataxic gait pattern decrease in coordination, balance, and functional mobility. MRI of the spine showed epidural lipomatosis extending from T3–7, with no evidence of space-occupying lesions. The electromyography (EMG) showed diffuse demyelinating disease and polyneuropathy, likely from WNV encephalitis.

Question 2

What will be the next best step in managing WNV encephalitis in solid organ transplant recipients?

A. Intravenous immunoglobulins.
B. Observation and immunosuppression adjustment.
C. Broad-spectrum antibiotics.
D. Anti-viral medications.

The correct answer is B.

There is currently no known treatment for WNV encephalitis. The transplant recipients are managed conservatively with appropriate modification in the immunosuppression (option A). Currently, there is no evidence that the addition of IVIG helps in patients with this severe neurological deficit; however, the use of IVIG is approved by The US Food and Drug Administration (FDA) for neurologic conditions such as Guillain-Barré syndrome (GBS) and chronic inflammatory demyelinating polyneuropathy (CIDP) [1]. With the neurological manifestation of WNV infection, adding IVIG, with a gradual reduction in immunosuppression, is reasonable. It is possible that IVIG could have the additional benefit of immunomodulation against alloreactivity in the setting of aggressive immunosuppression reduction. There is no role in using antibiotics or anti-viral medication in patients with WNV encephalitis (option C & D).

Further Course

With the diagnosis of WNV encephalitis, he was taken off mycophenolate. His tacrolimus goals were adjusted to 4–6 ng/mL, and prednisone was kept at 5 mg daily. He received IVIG 500 mg/kg weekly for 4 weeks.

He underwent aggressive physical therapy. With the supportive care and adjustments in immunosuppression, he had marked improvement in his weakness over 1 month. He was successfully discharged home. At his last follow-up, both kidney and pancreas allografts were functional.

Discussion

West Nile virus (WNV) is the most common cause of viral encephalitis in the United States [2, 3]. Most of the infections from WNV are asymptomatic; however, it can cause severe neurological diseases in humans, especially in the immunosuppressed population. Several case reports and small case series have described WNV disease in solid organ transplant recipients [4–6]. However, the data on kidney transplant recipients is limited. Although the native kidney involvement in WNV is described in the literature [7–12], the effect of WNV infection on the transplanted kidney has not been explained well in the literature.

Aziz et al. described the largest series of WNV infections in the KTRs. During the 24-year study period, 11 cases of WNV infection were reported. Most of the patients in this series presented with altered mental status, followed by fever and headaches. Nine patients recovered with no residual deficiency; however, two patients suffered permanent neurological damage. WNV infection was associated with relatively small reductions in eGFR at 1 year. Three patients suffered acute rejection within 1 year after the infection episode, likely attributable to aggressive immunosuppressive reduction. Most of the patients in this series recovered fully with supportive care and immunosuppression adjustment [13].

In another series, Kleinschmidt-DeMasters et al. published the series of WNV infections in solid organ transplants. This series also had 11 patients, although mixed allograft subtype (four KTRs, two stem cell recipients, two liver recipients, one lung, and two SPK recipients). 10 of 11 patients presented with severe meningoencephalitis. 9 of 11 patients survived the infection, but 3 had significant residual deficits, and one patient died 17 days after diagnosis. They concluded that WNV encephalitis in transplant recipients involved neurological damage at the severe end of the spectrum compared to immunocompetent patients [14] (Table 26.1).

In 2014, Yango et al. described three KTRs with WNV infection. All three patients had a rapid decline in their mental status. All three patients received IVIG 400 mg/kg weekly, 2–3 doses, reducing baseline immunosuppression. Survival was only 67% in this series, suggesting severe disease [4] (Table 26.1). Ravindra et al. also described three cases of WNV infection in KTRs. Two of these patients presented with altered mental status, and one presented with fevers. All these patients were managed by the reduction of immunosuppression and supportive care. None

Table 26.1 Studies in WNV infection in solid organ transplant recipients

Studies	Number of patients	Type of transplant	Most common presentation	Number of patients with permanent neurological deficit	Number of patients died within 1 year of diagnosis	Treatment
Aziz et al. [13]	11	7 KTR 4 SPK	Altered mental status	3	0	Immunosuppression reduction 2 patients received IVIG
Kleinschmidt-DeMasters et al. [14]	11	4 KTR 2 stem cell recipients 2 liver recipients 1 lung transplant 2 SPK recipients	Altered mental status	3	1	Immunosuppression reduction
Yango et al. [4]	3	2 KTR 1 SPK	Altered mental status	1	1	Immunosuppression reduction All patients received IVIG
Ravindra et al. [15]	3	1 KTR 1 PTA 1 SPK	Altered mental status	0	0	Immunosuppression reduction

KTR kidney transplant recipients, *SPK* simultaneous pancreas and kidney transplants, *PTA* pancreas transplant alone

of these patients received IVIG. All of these patients completely recovered [15] (Table 26.1).

The treatment of WNV infection is primarily supportive with careful modification in immunosuppression. In the setting of neurologic manifestations in a patient with a WNV infection that encompasses polyneuropathy, it is reasonable to pursue the use of IVIG at doses recommended for that neurologic manifestation. The American Society of Transplantation—Infectious disease community of practice (ID COP) guidance does not take a firm stance on IVIG, agreeing that further study is necessary [16].

Although not well described in the literature, post-transplant WNV encephalitis is a significant cause of morbidity in kidney transplant recipients. Most of the patients are managed conservatively with a careful reduction in immunosuppression. The addition of IVIG should be considered in patients with severe neurological deficits.

References

1. Lunemann JD, Quast I, Dalakas MC. Efficacy of intravenous immunoglobulin in neurological diseases. Neurotherapeutics. 2016;13(1):34–46.
2. Lindsey NP, Lehman JA, Staples JE, Fischer M. Division of vector-borne diseases NCfE, zoonotic infectious diseases CDC. West nile virus and other arboviral diseases–United States, 2013. MMWR Morb Mortal Wkly Rep. 2014;63(24):521–6.
3. Davis LE, DeBiasi R, Goade DE, Haaland KY, Harrington JA, Harnar JB, et al. West Nile virus neuroinvasive disease. Ann Neurol. 2006;60(3):286–300.
4. Yango AF, Fischbach BV, Levy M, Chandrakantan A, Tan V, Spak C, et al. West Nile virus infection in kidney and pancreas transplant recipients in the Dallas-Fort Worth Metroplex during the 2012 Texas epidemic. Transplantation. 2014;97(9):953–7.
5. Winston DJ, Vikram HR, Rabe IB, Dhillon G, Mulligan D, Hong JC, et al. Donor-derived West Nile virus infection in solid organ transplant recipients: report of four additional cases and review of clinical, diagnostic, and therapeutic features. Transplantation. 2014;97(9):881–9.
6. Saquib R, Randall H, Chandrakantan A, Spak CW, Barri YM. West Nile virus encephalitis in a renal transplant recipient: the role of intravenous immunoglobulin. Am J Kidney Dis. 2008;52(5):e19–21.
7. Alcendor DJ. Zika virus infection and implications for kidney disease. J Mol Med (Berl). 2018;96(11):1145–51.
8. Barzon L, Pacenti M, Franchin E, Pagni S, Martello T, Cattai M, et al. Excretion of West Nile virus in urine during acute infection. J Infect Dis. 2013;208(7):1086–92.
9. Papa A, Testa T, Papadopoulou E. Detection of West Nile virus lineage 2 in the urine of acute human infections. J Med Virol. 2014;86(12):2142–5.
10. Murray KO, Kolodziej S, Ronca SE, Gorchakov R, Navarro P, Nolan MS, et al. Visualization of West Nile virus in urine sediment using electron microscopy and Immunogold up to nine years Postinfection. Am J Trop Med Hyg. 2017;97(6):1913–9.
11. Tonry JH, Xiao SY, Siirin M, Chen H, da Rosa AP, Tesh RB. Persistent shedding of West Nile virus in urine of experimentally infected hamsters. Am J Trop Med Hyg. 2005;72(3):320–4.
12. Tonry JH, Brown CB, Cropp CB, Co JK, Bennett SN, Nerurkar VR, et al. West Nile virus detection in urine. Emerg Infect Dis. 2005;11(8):1294–6.
13. Aziz F, Saddler C, Jorgenson M, Smith J, Mandelbrot D. Epidemiology, management, and graft outcomes after West Nile virus encephalitis in kidney transplant recipients. Transpl Infect Dis. 2020;22(4):e13317.

14. Kleinschmidt-DeMasters BK, Marder BA, Levi ME, Laird SP, McNutt JT, Escott EJ, et al. Naturally acquired West Nile virus encephalomyelitis in transplant recipients: clinical, laboratory, diagnostic, and neuropathological features. Arch Neurol. 2004;61(8):1210–20.
15. Ravindra KV, Freifeld AG, Kalil AC, Mercer DF, Grant WJ, Botha JF, et al. West Nile virus-associated encephalitis in recipients of renal and pancreas transplants: case series and literature review. Clin Infect Dis. 2004;38(9):1257–60.
16. American society of transplantation. Available from https://www.myast.org/guidelines-post-kidney-transplant-management-community-setting.

Chapter 27
Early Post-Transplant Intracerebral Bacillary Angiomatosis

Arpita Basu and Stephanie Marie Pouch

Introduction

Bacillary angiomatosis (BA) is an uncommon vascular proliferative manifestation of Bartonella henselae which is even rarer in solid organ transplant recipients. In this vignette, the authors present a case of intracerebral bacillary angiomatosis seen in the early post-transplant period following a kidney transplant. Utilizing a question and answer format, the authors illustrate several aspects of the disease spectrum, including clinical features, challenges in diagnosis, and potential treatment options.

Patient History

A 55-year-old man underwent a deceased donor kidney transplant for end-stage kidney disease secondary to type 2 diabetes. This was a zero HLA mismatch transplant, and he had no preformed donor-specific antibodies. At the time of transplant, his calculated panel reactive antibody was 40%. Cytomegalovirus (CMV) serology was donor positive and recipient negative, making him a high risk for CMV. He received basiliximab induction and was placed on a maintenance

A. Basu (✉)
Division of Nephrology and Hypertension, Department of Medicine, Emory School of Medicine, Atlanta, GA, USA
e-mail: arpita.basu@emory.edu

S. M. Pouch
Division of Infectious Diseases, Department of Medicine, Emory School of Medicine, Atlanta, GA, USA
e-mail: stephanie.pouch@emory.edu

© The Author(s), under exclusive license to Springer Nature Switzerland AG 2022

F. Aziz, S. Parajuli (eds.), *Complications in Kidney Transplantation*, https://doi.org/10.1007/978-3-031-13569-9_27

immunosuppression regimen of tacrolimus (target trough 8–12 ng/mL in the first 6 months post-transplant) mycophenolate mofetil (MMF) 1000 mg twice a day, and prednisone 5 mg daily. Creatinine stabilized between 1.5 and 1.8 mg/dL. He had an unremarkable course until 6 months post-transplant when his appetite declined; he had significant weight loss, tremors, daily headaches, and gait abnormalities with subsequent multiple falls prompting hospitalization for further investigation and management. He was on prophylactic sulfamethoxazole-trimethoprim and valganciclovir at the time of presentation. Physical examination was unremarkable except for decreased strength in the left upper extremity, high-frequency, low amplitude tremor on the extension of both arms, and a hesitant, wide-based gait. Initial labs results were unremarkable.

Question 1

What is the most likely cause of the patient's presentation?

A. Opportunistic/latent infections.
B. Community-acquired infections.
C. CMV disease.
D. Post-Transplant Lymphoproliferative Disorder (PTLD).
E. Any of the above.

The correct answer is E.

Immunocompromised patients are known to be at increased risk for infections and cancers. Beyond the first month of transplant, donor-derived infections are less common. One to six months post-transplant, the effect of immunosuppression is maximal, and the risk for development of opportunistic infections or reactivation of previously latent infections, such as mycobacterium tuberculosis, is exceptionally high. CMV is known to serve as an important cofactor for several viruses, including EBV and CMV; high-risk patients are at an increased risk of EBV-associated PTLD [1].

Hospital Course

The patient had a computerized tomography (CT) of his head which showed no abnormalities. On hospitalization day 2, he developed a fever of >100.4 °F. Initial infectious workup with blood and urine cultures was unremarkable. Magnetic resonance imaging (MRI) brain done on hospital day 3 revealed several sub-centimeter enhancing lesions in the right parietal and bilateral occipital lobes, some with significant vasogenic edema surrounding the sentinel lesions concerning leptomeningeal carcinomatosis. Cerebrospinal fluid (CSF) obtained by lumbar puncture showed elevated protein, normal glucose, and lymphocytic pleocytosis. CSF biofire, testing for adenovirus, EBV, CMV, histoplasmosis, and rocky mountain spotted fever were all negative. Imaging of his chest, abdomen, and pelvis did not show any lesions concerning malignancy or disseminated infection. An echocardiogram did

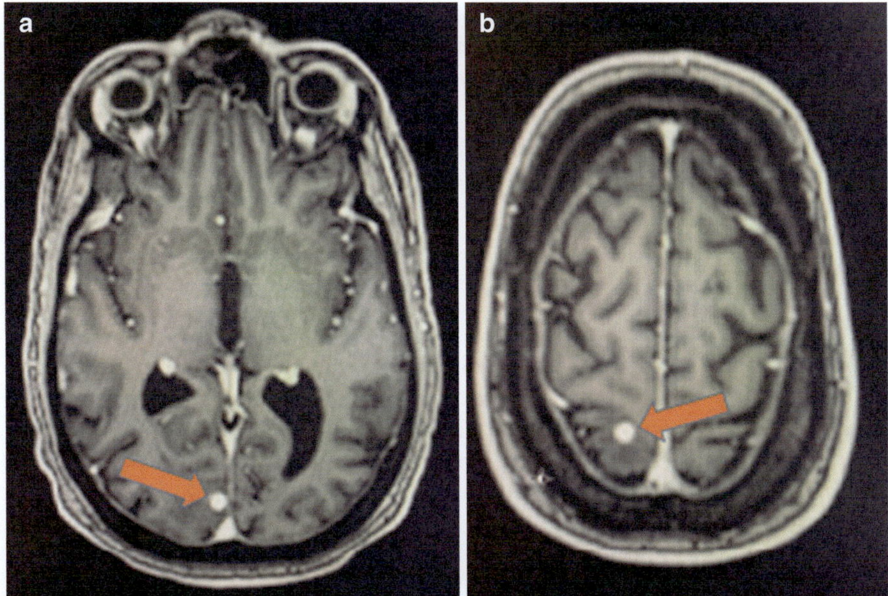

Fig. 27.1 MRI brain showing intracerebral bacillary angioma

not reveal any valvular vegetation. Serum and urine electrophoresis and kappa/ lambda free light chains were negative for paraproteins. Given the high suspicion for malignancy and negative infectious workup, no empiric antimicrobial or antiviral treatment was initiated. The patient was scheduled for a whole-body PET scan which could not be completed given poorly controlled blood sugars. With plans to pursue a possible brain biopsy, a repeat MRI brain was done on hospitalization day 12, which showed progression of enhancing disease (Fig. 27.1). The patient underwent a brain biopsy on hospitalization Day 15. The preliminary pathology read showed poorly formed abscesses with a granulomatous component. The same day Bartonella IgG titer was positive at 1:1024 and CSF Bartonella PCR is positive. The patient later admitted to having seven cats at home.

Question 2
What stain will confirm the histopathologic diagnosis?

A. Warthin–Starry stain.
B. Hematoxylin and Eosin(H&E) stain.
C. India ink stain.
D. Acid-Fast Bacilli (AFB) Stain.

The correct answer is A.

Pathology is often key to the diagnosis of Bartonella infection. The Warthin–Starry stain may show clumps, bacilli in chains, or filaments of extracellular gramnegative bacteria within areas of necrotic debris. Immunohistochemical (IHC) staining is more sensitive than Warthin–starry staining and often done in conjunction [2]. All tissue specimens are routinely stained with H&E stain to reveal the underlying tissue structures and conditions. Special stains are used to identify particular microorganisms like Indian ink stains for cryptococcus species, and AFB stains the lipid walls of acid-fast organisms such as Mycobacterium tuberculosis.

Additional Clinical Course

The patient was started on doxycycline and rifampin. MMF was discontinued, and the patient's tacrolimus goal was decreased to 3–5 ng/mL. Over the next 3 months, he improved significantly in gait, muscle strength, and mobility. He continues to have occasional headaches, though these continue to improve. Periodic imaging of his brain has shown continued radiographic improvement.

Final Diagnosis: Intracerebral Bacillary Angiomatosis due to *Bartonella henselae* (*B. henselae*).

Case Discussion

B. henselae is a zoonotic organism transmitted from scratches or bites of cats. It has a wide spectrum of clinical presentation in immunocompetent and immunocompromised hosts. A self-limited fever and regional lymphadenopathy known as Cat scratch disease is classically seen in the immunocompetent hosts, while granulomatous lesions of visceral organs or deep lymph nodes with more disseminated presentation (either necrotizing granulomatous inflammation or angioproliferative pattern) have been reported in the immunocompromised populations [2]. Bacillary angiomatosis (BA) is an uncommon vascular proliferative manifestation of *B. henselae*, first described in human immunodeficiency virus (HIV)-infected patients that frequently involve the skin and occasionally other organs, such as liver—spleen (Bacillary Peliosis—BP) respiratory tract, bone, lymph nodes, and brain [3]. The course of infection with *B. henselae* has not been well characterized in solid organ transplant recipients (SOTRs). Very limited data, primarily case reports, have been published on Bartonellosis in SOTRs. Psarros et al. identified 29 SOTRs who had Bartonella infection, of which 72% had disseminated disease presentation [4]. Morillas et al., in their literature review from 1990 to 2020, reported 14 total cases of BA/BP in the adult SOTR population, of which 10 presented with cutaneous BA/BP [5]. The reported meantime after transplantation to Bartonella infection in SOTRs ranges from 11 months to 2.7 years [4, 5]. With all forms of BA, patients have constitutional symptoms, including fever, chills, malaise, headache, and anorexia with or without weight loss [3]. The differential diagnosis for these presenting symptoms is broad, including post-transplant lymphoproliferative disease (PTLD), disseminated mycobacterial infections, invasive fungal infections, Kaposi Sarcoma, and several other etiologies.

Furthermore, diagnosing Bartonella can be challenging due to the absence of a definitive diagnostic test. Serological testing may be unreliable, particularly early in the presentation and high net state of immunosuppression status (e.g., early post-transplant), needing to be repeated in 2–4 weeks to document any subsequent rise during convalescence, especially if the initial test is negative or equivocal [5]. In patients with neurological manifestations similar to ours, CT brain is generally normal, and CSF shows mononuclear pleocytosis only in 20–30% of patients [6]. A combination of tests is necessary before a definite diagnosis can be established. Depending on the patient's clinical presentation, culture of a tissue or blood sample, Bartonella polymerase chain reaction (PCR) testing on a tissue or blood sample, and/or tissue biopsy with histopathologic examination and appropriate staining (Warthin–Starry and IHC staining) can be done to obtain a definitive diagnosis.

The optimal antibiotic regimen and treatment duration for BA have not been established. Macrolides and doxycycline are preferred antibiotics, with the addition of rifampicin or gentamycin for patients with severe disease [4–7]. The optimal duration of treatment depends on the net state of immunosuppression, the severity of disease, and the resolution of lesions on imaging studies. Data on recurrence in SOTRs is limited but known to occur. Given the likelihood of interaction of macrolides and rifampin with calcineurin Inhibitors (CNI), dose adjustments and regular monitoring of CNI drug levels are prudent. Overall reduction in immunosuppression should be considered depending on disease severity and treatment response.

In conclusion, intracerebral BA is very uncommon and, to our knowledge, has not been previously reported in SOTRs. Our case highlights the need for careful history taking and in-depth timely investigation to identify the disease early. Rapid initiation of therapy is crucial for good outcomes in this potentially fatal disease if disseminated. Further studies are needed to understand the disease process and establish treatment guidelines in SOTRs.

References

1. Mañez R, Breinig MC, Ho M, et al. Post-transplant lymphoproliferative disease in primary Epstein-Barr virus infection after liver transplantation: the role of cytomegalovirus disease. J Infect Dis. 1997;176(6):1462–7.
2. Luciani L, El Baroudi Y, Prudent E, et al. Bartonella infections diagnosed in the French reference center, 2014–2019, and focus on infections in the immunocompromised. Eur J Clin Microbiol Infect Dis. 2021;40:2407–10. https://doi.org/10.1007/s10096-021-04244-z.
3. Spach D, Kaplan S. Microbiology, epidemiology, clinical manifestations, and diagnosis of cat scratch disease. 2021. Uptodate.com. https://www.uptodate.com/contents/microbiology-epidemiology-clinical-manifestations-and-diagnosis-of-cat-scratch-disease?search=barto nella&source=search_result&selectedTitle=2~105&usage_type=default&display_rank=2. Accessed 28 Dec 2021.
4. Psarros G, Riddell J IV, Gandhi T, Kauffman CA, Cinti SK. Bartonella henselae infections in solid organ transplant recipients. Medicine. 2012;91(2):111–21. https://doi.org/10.1097/MD.0b013e31824dc07a.
5. Morillas JA, Hassanein M, Syed B, et al. Early post-transplant cutaneous bacillary angiomatosis in a kidney recipient: case report and review of the literature. Transpl Infect Dis. 2021;23:e13670. https://doi.org/10.1111/tid.13670.

                                                                      A. Basu and S. M. Pouch

6. Pischel L, Radcliffe C, Vilchez GA, Charifa A, Zhang XC, Grant M. Bartonellosis in transplant recipients: a retrospective single center experience. World J Transplant. 2021;11(6):244–53. https://doi.org/10.5500/wjt.v11.i6.244.
7. Helleberg M. Bacillary angiomatosis in a solid organ transplant recipient. IDCases. 2019;18:e00649. https://doi.org/10.1016/j.idcr.2019.e00649.

Chapter 28
BK Virus Nephropathy and Rejection

Fadee Abualrub and Vidya A. Fleetwood

Introduction

In solid organ transplants, immunosuppression is a two-edged sword. While maintaining an adequate level of immunosuppression is crucial to the well-being of the allograft, a hibernating immune system would render the patient defenseless against opportunistic infections. In this chapter, we present a complex case of polyomavirus infection to summarize the complexity of the decision-making process that a transplant physician may confront on a day-to-day basis.

Case Presentation

A 75-year-old African American female kidney transplant recipient with a history of end-stage kidney disease (ESKD) secondary to hypertension presented to the clinic 6 months post-transplant for routine follow-up. She had received a living-related donor kidney, and her creatinine had nadired at 1.3 mg/dL. Her panel reactive antibody was 0%, and she received 3 mg/kg of anti-thymocyte globulin for induction. Her maintenance immunosuppression regimen consisted of tacrolimus (tac) with a 6–8 ng/mL trough goal, mycophenolic acid (MPA) 360 mg twice daily, and low-dose prednisone. At the visit, she noted decreased appetite and mild

F. Abualrub (✉) · V. A. Fleetwood
Center for Abdominal Transplantation, Saint Louis University, St. Louis, MO, USA
e-mail: Fadee.Abualrub@health.slu.edu; Vidyaratna.fleetwood@health.slu.edu

© The Author(s), under exclusive license to Springer Nature Switzerland AG 2022
F. Aziz, S. Parajuli (eds.), *Complications in Kidney Transplantation*,
https://doi.org/10.1007/978-3-031-13569-9_28

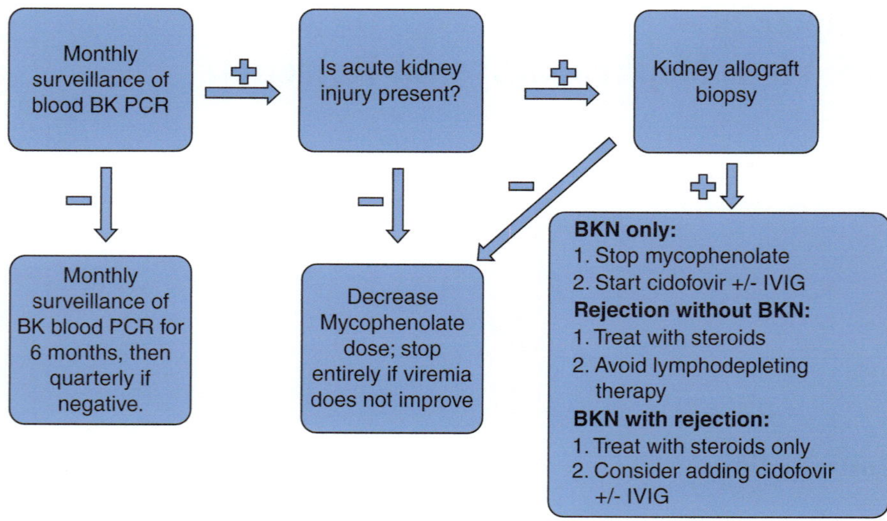

Fig. 28.1 Algorithm for screening for and treating BK nephropathy (BKN)

allograft pain. Vital signs were normal, with no fevers and systolic blood pressure of less than 140 mmHg; the physical examination was significant only for a faint bruit over the allograft. Laboratory investigations showed serum creatinine of 1.8 mg/dL, a tacrolimus trough level of 3.9 ng/dL, and a urine protein to creatine ratio of 0.9 g/g. A complete blood count (CBC) was normal. Her urine analysis (UA) showed 10–15 white blood cells with no bacteria and 0–5 squamous cells; the culture was negative. The donor-specific antibody (DSA) screen was negative. Her viral screening was negative for CMV and positive for BK at 53,211 IU/mL. A flow sheet of BK management is given in Fig. 28.1. An ultrasound doppler exam of the kidney allograft (RUS) was normal with no evidence of vascular abnormalities, hydronephrosis, or fluid collections.

Question 1

What is the most likely cause of the patient's acute kidney injury?

A. A complicated urinary tract infection (UTI).
B. Acute antibody-mediated rejection (AMR).
C. Anastomotic stenosis.
D. BK nephropathy (BKN).
E. T cell-mediated rejection (TCMR).

The correct answer is D.

A symptomatic complicated urinary tract infection (a) is likely to present with fever, leukocytosis, pyuria, and occasionally edema on RUS. A biopsy is warranted to confirm the diagnosis of BKN; although the absence of donor-specific antibodies does not rule out antibody-mediated rejection (b), it is an important diagnostic criterion. Anastomotic stenosis (c) was ruled out by RUS; the presence of a soft bruit over the allograft is considered normal. TCMR (e) cannot be ruled out here without a biopsy, but BKN (d) is more likely based on the high viral load of the polyomavirus.

Treatment Course

The patient was admitted for a biopsy, and histopathology revealed the following: moderate inflammation (i2), moderate tubulitis (t2), mild intimal arteritis(v1), mild glomerulitis (g1), and mild peritubular capillaritis (ptc1) without evidence of complement activation (C4d was negative). The staining for polyomavirus (SV40) was positive and consistent with the biopsy's inflammatory areas (Figs. 28.2 and 28.3).

Question 2
What is the most likely diagnosis?

A. Antibody-mediated rejection.
B. Combined cellular and antibody-mediated rejection.
C. T cell-mediated rejection (TCMR).
D. BK nephropathy.
E. Concomitant TCMR and BK nephropathy.

The correct answer is E.

Intimal arteritis (v1) without donor-specific antibodies and evidence of antibody reaction with the vascular endothelium is insufficient for diagnosing AMR (a, b). However, a v1 score is sufficient for the diagnosis of TCMR(c, e) with a grade of IIA, according to Banff criteria. Sample positivity for SV40 is diagnostic of BKN (e).

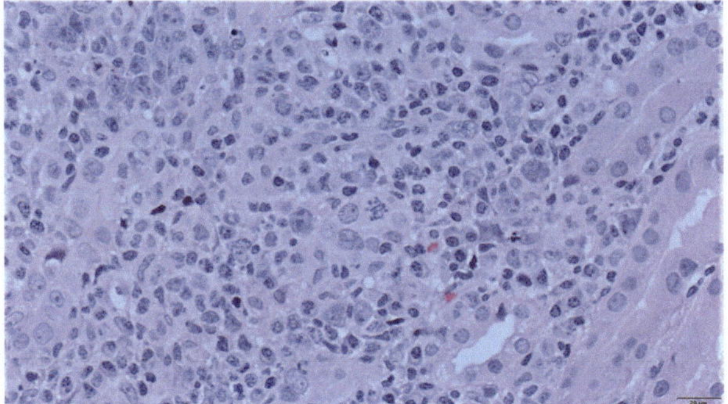

Fig. 28.2 Severe inflammation and basophilic intranuclear inclusions

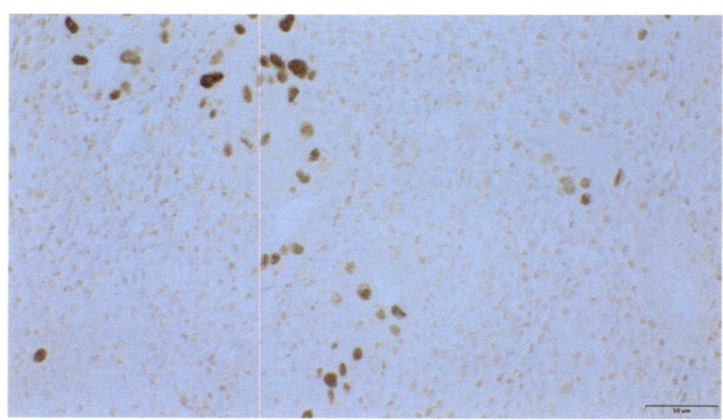

Fig. 28.3 Positive SV40 by immunochemistry

Additional Clinical Course

The patient was admitted for management of TCMR. She was treated with 500 mg of solumedrol daily for 3 days. Anti-thymocyte globulin (thymoglobulin) was withheld due to the concurrent BK nephropathy. Simultaneously, she was treated with IV cidofovir, 0.25 mg/kg, repeated every 2 weeks for five doses. The antimetabolite (MPA) was removed from the immunosuppression regimen, and her tacrolimus trough dose was maintained between 5 and 7 ng/dL. Creatinine stabilized at 1.3 mg/dL, and her BK viral load remained undetectable at 1 year.

Discussion

BK virus (BK) and JC and SV40 viruses are members of the Polyomaviridae family and can infect the uroepithelium. BK can be transmitted from the donor and reactivated after transplantation. It is commonly found in kidney transplant recipients: in one survey, pretransplantation seropositivity rate was as high as 80–88% [1]. It is believed that ischemia-reperfusion and mechanical injury during surgery can contribute to infection reactivation [2]. The infection is usually associated with high doses of immunosuppressants (tacrolimus levels >8 ng/mL) and mycophenolate mofetil (MMF) dosages (1.5–2 g/day) [3]; however, it has been reported with any combination of immunosuppressant drugs, including calcineurin inhibitors (CNI) and MMF-free regimens [3].

BK infection can lead to BK nephropathy, which is considered an ascending infection and spreads from cell to cell. It has been suggested that a BK viral load of >10,000 copies/mL is diagnostic of BKN [4]. However, while the sensitivity of this marker is 100%, the positive predictive value is only 50–85% [5]. Diagnosis of BK nephropathy relies on the allograft biopsy, the gold standard for diagnosis. It is generally indicated if the patient develops acute kidney injury (AKI) rather than a certain viral load threshold [6]. However, the biopsy is not always sensitive: BK-related inflammation can be focal and is sometimes restricted to the medulla [2]. For that reason, it is always recommended to obtain an additional medullary core for diagnosis when BKN is suspected. The pathologic findings usually include interstitial nephritis, which is not specific to BKN. The cytopathic changes and a positive SV40 stain are particular to the virus [2].

Unlike tubulitis and interstitial inflammation, arteritis is characteristic of alloimmune injury. It is a diagnostic criterion for both TCMR and AMR.

In patients with a low BK load (< 20,000 copies/mm^3), initial treatment consists of lowering immunosuppression. The antimetabolite is reduced or discontinued first, then tapering the CNI if needed. Due to the need for reduced immunosuppression in treating BK, rejection may develop while the patient is under treatment for BK, leaving the treating nephrologist "threading the needle" between maintaining sufficient immunosuppression while allowing the patient's immune system to reconstitute. Management of BKN is challenging to begin with, but when it occurs in the setting of acute rejection, it becomes even more difficult. Ordinarily, thymoglobulin is used for the treatment of advanced TCMR [7]. Lymphodepleting agents are not recommended in the setting of any active infection, especially BKN [8].

When the viral count is more severe, adjunctive agents may be necessary. In this case, we used cidofovir to counteract the immunosuppressive effect of steroids. While cidofovir, an antiviral that triggers apoptosis in the affected tubular cells, is used frequently to manage BK nephropathy, it is considered nephrotoxic and not consistently effective. We used the lowest possible dose (0.25 mg/kg) and hydrated the patient before and after infusion to minimize cidofovir nephropathy. More recently, virus-specific T-cell therapy (VST) [9], is being implemented to manage resistant viral infections, including the BK virus. This therapy depends on isolation of the primary bone marrow cells of a third-party donor, activating by incubation with specific viral epitopes, and infusion into the patient. Longer-term follow-up is needed to study risks, but a low-grade graft versus host disease has been reported with this treatment. As a common and complex pathology, more research is needed to find effective ways to treat BK nephropathy.

References

1. Gardner SD, MacKenzie EF, Smith C, Porter AA. Prospective study of the human polyomaviruses BK and JC and cytomegalovirus in renal transplant recipients. J Clin Pathol. 1984;37(5):578–86.
2. Tanabe T, Shimizu T, Sai K, Miyauchi Y, Shirakawa H, Ishida H, Honda K, Koike J, Yamaguchi Y, Tanabe K. BK polyomavirus nephropathy complicated with acute T-cell-mediated rejection in a kidney transplant recipient: a case report. Clin Transpl. 2011;25(Suppl. 23):39–43.
3. Atencio IA, Shadan FF, Zhou XJ, Vaziri ND, Villarreal LP. Adult mouse kidneys become permissive to acute polyomavirus infection and reactivate persistent infections in response to cellular damage and regeneration. J Virol. 1993;67:1424–32.
4. Rocha PN, Plumb TJ, Miller SE, Howell DN, Smith SR. Risk factors for BK polyomavirus nephritis in renal allograft recipients. Clin Transpl. 2004;18:456–62.
5. Bohl DL, Brennan DC. BK virus nephropathy and kidney transplantation. Clin J Am Soc Nephrol. 2007;2(Suppl 1):S36–46.

6. Randhawa P, Ho A, Shapiro R, Vats A, Swalsky P, Finkelstein S, Uhrmacher J, Weck K. Correlates of quantitative measurement of BK polyomavirus (BKV) DNA with clinical course of BKV infection in renal transplant patients. J Clin Microbiol. 2004;42:1176–80.
7. Sawinski D, Trofe-Clark J. BK virus nephropathy. Clin J Am Soc Nephrol. 2018;13(12):1893–6.
8. Cooper JE. Evaluation and treatment of acute rejection in kidney allografts. Clin J Am Soc Nephrol. 2020;15(3):430–8.
9. Nelson AS, Heyenbruch D, Rubinstein JD, et al. Virus-specific T-cell therapy to treat BK polyomavirus infection in bone marrow and solid organ transplant recipients. Blood Adv. 2020;4(22):5745–54.

Chapter 29
Concomitant BK Polyoma Virus and Cytomegalovirus Infection in a Kidney Transplant Recipient

Kaushik Bhunia and Kurtis J. Swanson

Introduction

Two of the most formidable viral pathogens impacting allograft and recipient outcomes after kidney transplant are BK polyomavirus (BKPyV) and cytomegalovirus (CMV). Viral co-infection is synergistic, with BKPyV and CMV promoting viral cell entry, replication, and ultimately allograft injury. Although rejection and increased net immunosuppression often can proceed viral infection, BKPyV and CMV co-infection appear to also be immunomodulatory, promoting acute rejection thereafter.

In this chapter, we will discuss a case of BK polyomavirus and cytomegalovirus co-infection in a kidney transplant recipient to illustrate how co-infection can manifest as well as provide salient points on diagnosis and management of this condition.

Patient History

A 57-year-old man with a history of ESKD secondary to diabetes mellitus underwent deceased donor kidney transplantation. At transplantation, his panel reactive antibody was 41%, and he had no preformed donor-specific antibodies. He received both depleting/non-depleting induction per protocol (total anti-thymocyte globulin dose = 2.1 mg/kg) and was maintained on tacrolimus and mycophenolate mofetil (MMF). The patient was CMV discordant at transplantation (donor positive/recipient negative) and was to receive valganciclovir prophylaxis for 6 months.

K. Bhunia · K. J. Swanson (✉)
Division of Nephrology and Hypertension, University of Minnesota, Minneapolis, MN, USA
e-mail: Bhuni005@umn.edu

© The Author(s), under exclusive license to Springer Nature Switzerland AG 2022

F. Aziz, S. Parajuli (eds.), *Complications in Kidney Transplantation*, https://doi.org/10.1007/978-3-031-13569-9_29

Post-transplant was also complicated by ureteral stenosis prompting percutaneous nephrostomy tube placement.

BK Polyoma Virus Infection

At 3 months post-transplant, the patient was found to have BK polyomavirus (BKPyV) viremia at 41,724 copies/mL. His maintenance immunosuppression at diagnosis was extended-release tacrolimus (due to tremors) and MMF. Pre-BK tacrolimus troughs were consistently running in the 11–15 ng/mL range for 3 weeks. His tacrolimus and MMF were both reduced. His BK viral load increased to 289,673 copies/mL, thereby eliciting a kidney biopsy, which was negative for BK polyomavirus nephropathy (BKPyVAN) or rejection.

Cytomegalovirus Infection

On the day of his kidney biopsy, 4 months post-transplant, he developed CMV viremia (2,412 IU/mL). We hypothesize this occurred not with standing valganciclovir prophylaxis due to (1) poor GI absorption/diarrhea and (2) under dosed valganciclovir in the context of low allograft function due to obstructive nephropathy/recurrent acute kidney injury.

Given the previous biopsy results and new CMV, his tacrolimus was switched to cyclosporine (goal 100–150), and valganciclovir was increased to the renally-adjusted treatment dose. Patient factors led to missed lab surveillance, and 1 month after initial diagnosis, his CMV viral load peaked at 459,118 IU/mL. This prompted admission for IV ganciclovir treatment. CMV antiviral resistance testing was performed due to minimal treatment response. Resistance testing demonstrated UL97 mutations consistent with ganciclovir resistance. He was switched to IV foscarnet plus weekly IV immunoglobulin (IVIG) 500 mg/kg × 3. His cyclosporine goal was reduced, MMF discontinued, and he was started on prednisone 10 mg daily.

He was treated with foscarnet, with letermovir overlap at the recommendation of transplant infectious disease. Three weeks after initiating foscarnet therapy, his CMV cleared, and he was continued on daily letermovir. MMF was restarted at 250 mg twice daily, and prednisone was reduced to 5 mg daily. He developed SARS-CoV-2 infection, and thus MMF was discontinued.

Later, he developed recurrent AKI leading to admission. He was aviremic, on letermovir as mentioned, and maintained immunosuppression with cyclosporine (goal 100–125) and prednisone 5 mg daily. His AKI improved with medical management and thus biopsy was not pursued at this time.

One month after clearing CMV, he sustained a subsequent acute kidney injury, cueing admission and an allograft biopsy. While he had cleared CMV, BK nephropathy remained a differential diagnosis for his acute kidney injury given persistent BKPyV viremia > 10 K copies and multiple infections suggesting over immunosuppression. This biopsy was consistent with BKPyVAN without clear evidence for concomitant cellular and/or antibody-mediated rejection and/or CMV nephritis.

Question 1

In a patient with BKPyVAN on tacrolimus and prednisone after anti-metabolite discontinuation, what would be a reasonable next step to reduce their immunosuppression?

A. Reduce tacrolimus by 25–50%.
B. Switch from tacrolimus to cyclosporine.
C. IVIG if hypogammaglobulinemia (i.e., IgG level < 400).
D. Any of the above would be acceptable approaches.

The correct answer is D.

No randomized controlled trial exists at this time proving that one of the afore-mentioned approaches is more effective than another. Hirsch et al. demonstrated that renal proximal tubular epithelial cells treated with cyclosporine at 1000 ng/mL across multiple time points post-infection lead to an overall decreased BKPyV load than renal proximal tubular epithelial cells treated with tacrolimus 10 ng/mL and controls, suggesting inhibitory action of BKPyV replication. This has only been shown *in vitro*, i.e., no significant clinical difference *in vivo*/in randomized control trials has been elucidated. This is shown graphically in Fig. 29.1 below based on the work of Hirsch et al. [1]

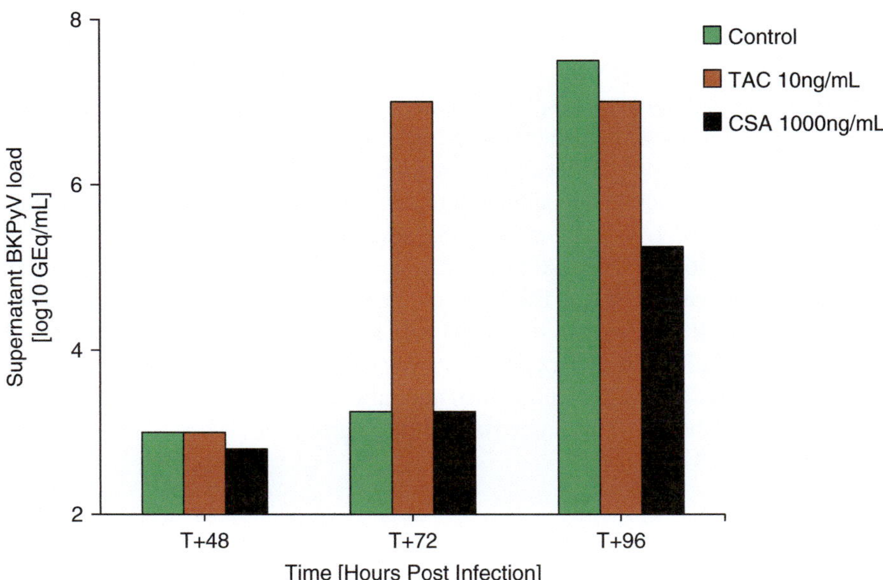

Fig. 29.1 TAC stimulates and CsA inhibits BKPyV replication

Post Biopsy Course

After diagnosis with BKPyVAN, his cyclosporine was reduced further. One week later, he experienced breakthrough CMV viremia (5500 IU/mL), prompting bringing about admission for foscarnet therapy. His IgG level was 1351 mg/dL, and IVIG was held. Interestingly, his BKPyV viremia cleared. With quick CMV response to foscarnet, low dose MMF (250 mg 2× a day) was reintroduced to his maintenance immunosuppression regimen.

Since this admission, he has had four serial serum CMV PCR and 9 BKPyV PCR measurements below the lower limit of quantification. Currently, he is on cyclosporine (goal 50–75), MMF 500 mg BID, and prednisone 5 mg daily.

Despite a complicated early post-transplant course including SARS-CoV-2 infection, persistent hydronephrosis due to ureteral stricture s/p balloon urethroplasty, vancomycin-resistant enterococcus infection, in addition to concomitant BKPyV/CMV infection, the patient is clinically stable and remains off renal replacement therapy at this time.

Question 2

What pre-transplant laboratory abnormality may predict post-transplant BKPyV and CMV infection?

A. Total protein.
B. Serum albumin.
C. White blood cell count.
D. Immunoglobulin levels.

The correct answer is B.

In their single-center retrospective study of 1717 kidney transplant recipients with serum albumin levels within 45 days of their kidney transplant, Srivastava et al. [2] showed that kidney transplant recipients with moderate (serum albumin 2.5–3.49 g/dL) and severe hypoalbuminemia (< 2.5 g/dL) incurred a higher risk for BKPyV viremia compared to recipients with normal serum albumin levels in univariate analysis (moderate hypoalbuminemia: hazard ratio [HR] = 1.5; 95% confidence interval [CI], 1.14–1.90; $p = 0.003$); severe hypoalbuminemia: HR = 2.15; 95% CI, 1.01–4.56; $p = 0.05$). Although not significant after adjustment, there was still an 18% increased risk for BKPyV viremia in those with moderate hypoalbuminemia and a 64% increase in recipients with severe hypoalbuminemia compared with the normal albumin cohort. Moderate hypoalbuminemia was also associated with a higher risk for CMV infection than normal serum albumin levels in multivariable analysis, although it was not statistically significant (HR = 1.15; 95% CI, 0.36–3.64; $p = 0.81$).

Discussion

BKPyV and CMV Co-Infection

Co-infection with BKPyV and CMV is an albeit rare but serious complication after kidney transplantation. This case shows that presumably shared risk factors (over immunosuppression, absorption of medications/diarrhea) can lead to combined infection and in due course, complicated management.

An interesting component in this patient's case is obstructive nephropathy, which not only contributed to the development of CMV via concerns surrounding his valganciclovir dosing but also was one of several causes of allograft injury facilitating the progression of BKPyV viremia to overt BKPyVAN

Though rare, several studies exist describing BKPyV and CMV co-infection as described below:

In one study of 69 adult KTRs with elevated serum creatinine, Toyoda et al. found that 6/12 (50%) patients initially with BKPyV were also CMV positive during the study, compared to only 5.3% (3/57) patients who were BKPyV negative developing CMV positivity ($p = 0.001$). *In vitro* studies have shown that (1) BK antigen can enhance CMV gene expression and promote CMV infection, (2) CMV may enhance BKPyV growth rate, and (3) CMV gene products can increase BKPyV antigen/protein and facilitate viral replication [3–5].

In another recent study from 2021, Herrera et al. present some compelling findings in regard to BKVPyV and CMV co-infection [6]. They found that in patients with BKPyV and CMV co-infection had significantly higher BKPyV viral loads compared to non-co-infected patients (3,636,210 copies/mL vs 709,853 copies/mL, $p < 0.05$). Similarly, they found that in recipients with BKPyVAN presented more frequently with CMV co-infection than those without (39% vs 19%, $p = 0.02$) and that age > 60 (OR 1.4, (95% CI 1.1–2)), CMV D+/R- serostatus (OR 4.0, (95% CI 2.5–5.3)), pancreas and kidney transplantation (OR 1.8, (95% CI 1.2–2.7)), acute rejection (OR 2.0, (95% CI 1.4–2.4)), and nephrostomy requirement (OR 2.0, (95% 1.2–3.0)) were independently associated with CMV co-infection (all $p < 0.05$).

In further support of the deleterious relationship between co-infection and allograft function, Jehn et al. in their retrospective study showed that BKPyV and CMV co-infection is significantly associated with a higher incidence of acute rejection (59.3% vs 44.1% in the BKPyV alone group and 41.5% in the CMV alone group, $p = 0.001$), and lower eGFR at 1 (40.2 ± 11.1 mL/min/1.73 m^2), 3 (40.6 ± 15.8 mL/min/1.73 m^2), and 5 years (42.9 ± 12.2 mL/min/1.73 m^2) compared to aviremic KTRs (1 year 58.4 ± 19.3 mL/min/1.73 m^2, 3 years 57.6 ± 19.0 mL/min/1.73 m^2, 5 years 54.4 ± 19.7 mL/min/1.73 m^2), CMV viremic KTRs (1 year 52.4 ± 19.6 mL/min/1.73 m^2, 3 years 51.9 ± 20.8 mL/

min/1.73 m^2, 5 years 47.8 ± 20.8 mL/min/1.73 m^2), and the BKPyV viremic group (1 year 57.6 ± 24.2 mL/min/1.73 m^2, 3 years 58.2 ± 27.2 mL/min/1.73 m^2, 5 years 52.0 ± 28.8 mL/min/1.73 m^2) (all $p < 0.05$). Interestingly, patient survival (log rank $p = 0.586$) nor death censored graft survival (long rank $p = 0.303$) were significantly reduced in the co-infected group compared to the other subgroups [7].

While the relationship between BKPyV and CMV co-infection demands further study, particularly in the context of obvious possible confounders (induction, maintenance immunosuppression), it would appear that there is some recent evidence supporting the postulate that one may beget the other and lead to adverse outcomes including acute rejection, BKPyVAN, and lower allograft function.

Therefore, vigilant surveillance for and management of allograft pathology is essential in managing kidney transplant recipients with co-infection.

References

1. Hirsch HH, Yakhontova K, Lu M, Manzetti J. BK polyomavirus replication in renal tubular epithelial cells is inhibited by Sirolimus, but activated by tacrolimus through a pathway involving FKBP-12. Am J Transplant. 2016;16(3):821–32.
2. Srivastava A, Bodnar J, Osman F, Jorgenson MR, Astor BC, Mandelbrot DA, et al. Serum albumin level before kidney transplant predicts post-transplant BK and possibly cytomegalovirus infection. Kidney Int Rep. 2020;5(12):2228–37.
3. Kristoffersen AK, Johnsen JI, Seternes OM, Rollag H, Degré M, Traavik T. The human polyomavirus BK T antigen induces gene expression in human cytomegalovirus. Virus Res. 1997;52(1):61–71.
4. Goldstein SC, Tralka TS, Rabson AS. Mixed infection with human cytomegalovirus and human polyomavirus (BKV). J Med Virol. 1984;13(1):33–40.
5. Pari GS, St Jeor SC. Human cytomegalovirus major immediate early gene product can induce SV40 DNA replication in human embryonic lung cells. Virology. 1990;179(2):785–94.
6. Herrera S, Bernal-Maurandi J, Cofan F, Ventura P, Marcos MA, Linares L, et al. BK virus and cytomegalovirus coinfections in kidney transplantation and their impact on allograft loss. J Clin Med. 2021;10(17)
7. Jehn U, Schütte-Nütgen K, Bautz J, Pavenstädt H, Suwelack B, Thölking G, et al. Clinical features of BK-polyomavirus and cytomegalovirus co-infection after kidney transplantation. Sci Rep. 2020;10(1):22406.

Chapter 30
Successful Management of Complex Primary Cytomegaloviral Disease Utilizing a Standardized Multimodal Approach

Hanna L. Kleiboeker and Margaret R. Jorgenson

Introduction

Cytomegalovirus (CMV) is the most common viral infection after solid organ transplant and remains an independent risk factor for graft loss, morbidity, and mortality. Due to the association of CMV with negative outcomes, prophylaxis is indicated to mitigate risk. If CMV disease develops, a multifaceted pharmacotherapeutic and diagnostic approach is warranted to optimize treatment response. The utility of a center-specific CMV anti-viral stewardship initiative applying the established principles and practices of antimicrobial stewardship in managing these complex patients to achieve positive outcomes is considerable. The following case demonstrates such a multimodal approach to the management of primary CMV disease.

Patient History

A 65-year-old man with a history of end-stage kidney disease secondary to type 2 diabetes mellitus on hemodialysis underwent donation after brain death kidney transplantation. At the time of transplant, his panel reactive antibody was 0%, and he had no preformed donor-specific antibodies. CMV serology was reported in UNet Organ Transplant Web Platform as donor negative and recipient negative (D−/R−). He received induction with rabbit anti-thymocyte globulin (rATG) and early steroid withdrawal. His maintenance immunosuppression included tacrolimus

H. L. Kleiboeker · M. R. Jorgenson (✉)
Department of Pharmacy, University of Wisconsin Hospital and Clinics, Madison, WI, USA
e-mail: hkleiboeker@uwhealth.org; mjorgenson@uwhealth.org

© The Author(s), under exclusive license to Springer Nature Switzerland AG 2022

F. Aziz, S. Parajuli (eds.), *Complications in Kidney Transplantation*,
https://doi.org/10.1007/978-3-031-13569-9_30

(target trough 7–8 ng/mL) and mycophenolate sodium 720 mg twice daily. Based on the reported CMV serology, he was prescribed acyclovir prophylaxis for 3 months. Seven weeks after transplant, he presented to the emergency department with a 5-day history of abdominal pain radiating bilaterally to his back, chills, mild nausea without vomiting, and constipation. Upon physical exam, he was found to be afebrile and hypertensive. Laboratory tests were notable for leukopenia (white blood cell count 2.7 K/uL), supratherapeutic tacrolimus level (22 ng/mL), BK viremia (viral load 162,181 IU/mL), and CMV viremia (viral load 691,831 IU/mL). After further review, the multidisciplinary transplant team identified that the donor's CMV serology had been inaccurately reported at the time of transplant and true CMV serology was donor positive and recipient negative (D+/R−).

Question 1

Which serostatus conveys the highest risk of CMV disease after transplant?

A. D−/R−.
B. D−/R+.
C. D+/R−.
D. D+/R+.

The correct answer is C.

The risk of CMV disease is highest in seronegative recipients who receive a latently infected organ from a seropositive donor (D+/R−) [1, 2].

Hospital Course

Given the complexity of the case and the anticipated need for prolonged therapy, the CMV Antiviral Stewardship Team was consulted. Intravenous ganciclovir, at an aggressive dose of 10 mg/kg every 12 h (renally dose adjusted), and immune globulin, at a dose of 500 mg/kg weekly for 3 weeks, were promptly initiated to treat CMV disease in an attempt to induce rapid viral clearance kinetics [3]. Immunosuppressive reduction occurred with a decrease in tacrolimus dose and discontinuation of mycophenolate. After initiation of therapy, the patient experienced a one-log decline in viral load after 2 weeks of treatment (Fig. 30.1). After 4 weeks of treatment, therapy was transitioned from intravenous ganciclovir to oral valganciclovir when the viral load fell below 10,000 IU/mL. When the delta log of viral load from treatment weeks 4–7 decreased by 0.1 log IU/mL/week, drug resistance was suspected (Fig. 30.1) [1, 2]. CMV resistance panel revealed infection with a pan-sensitive isolate. After 5 weeks of treatment, CMV-specific cell-mediated immunity (CMI) testing via intracellular cytokine staining (ICS) assay by flow cytometry (Eurofins Viracor inSIGHT™ T Cell Immunity Panel) was obtained. Results revealed that the patient had not developed CMV-specific CMI, and treatment with valganciclovir was continued.

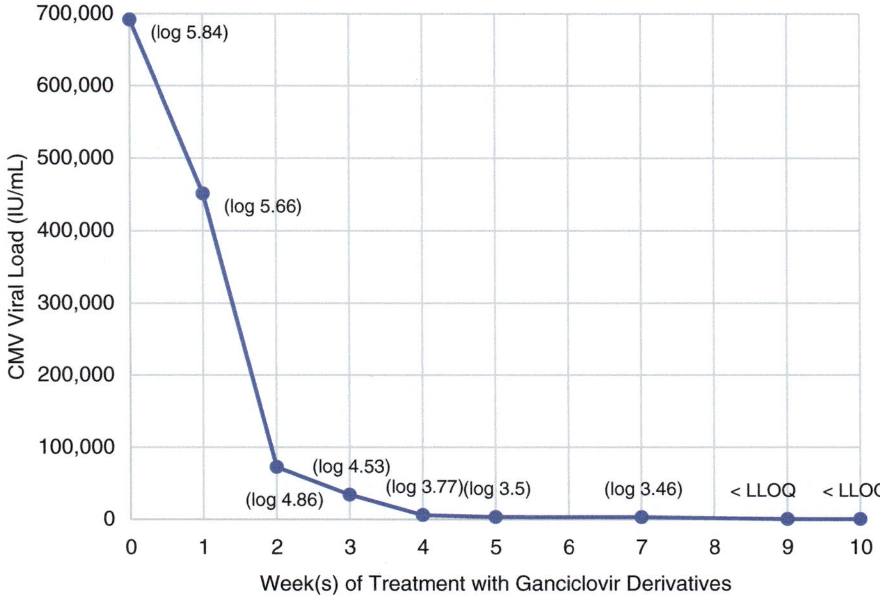

Fig. 30.1 The trend of CMV viral load after initiation of treatment. *LLOQ* lower limit of quantification

Question 2
Which of the following are risk factors for drug-resistant CMV?

A. Strongly immunosuppressive therapy.
B. Prolonged anti-viral drug exposure.
C. Lack of CMV immunity prior to transplant (D+/R−).
D. All of the above.

The correct answer is D.
These are all risk factors for drug-resistant CMV, as is inadequate anti-viral drug delivery, prolonged subtherapeutic dosing of anti-viral drugs (i.e., mini-dosing), and lung transplantation [1, 2]. Drug-resistant CMV is associated with increased mortality and morbidity. This includes prolonged time to clearance of viremia, a greater decrease in estimated Glomerular Filtration Rate (eGFR), and increased rates of allograft rejection [4].

Additional Clinical Course

After 19 weeks of treatment with (val)ganciclovir, the patient had not attained eradication of CMV viremia with persistently detectable viral loads ranging from <200 to 832 IU/mL. Concurrently, the patient had developed severe leukopenia, with absolute lymphocyte count (ALC) persistently <1000/μL. It was hypothesized that the ongoing myelosuppressive effects of (val)ganciclovir therapy were counterproductive in his ability to develop CMV-specific CMI and subsequently clear his viremia. To address this issue, the patient was transitioned from valganciclovir to letermovir 480 mg daily for secondary prophylaxis. Viral load at conversion was <200 IU/mL. Tacrolimus was empirically reduced by 50% to avoid supratherapeutic concentrations due to the potent drug interaction between these agents. His leukopenia quickly resolved with removal of the offending agent with a delta increase in white blood cell count of +1.5 K/uL and ALC +540/μL. After receiving letermovir for 4 weeks, testing for CMV-specific CMI was repeated and revealed the patient had developed CMI. While on letermovir, the patient did not experience progressive replication or breakthrough disease. Viral load at the time of demonstrated CMI was 347 IU/mL.

Discussion

CMV is a common complication after solid organ transplant and remains an independent risk factor for graft loss, morbidity, and mortality [5]. Accurate screening of donor and recipient serostatus at the time of transplant is crucial to implementing appropriate anti-viral prophylaxis after transplant. Patients at risk for CMV disease, based on donor and/or recipient seropositivity, should receive primary prophylaxis with (val)ganciclovir for 3–6 months [1, 2]. Optimal duration of primary prophylaxis is dependent upon clinical factors such as recipient serostatus, induction immunosuppression, and type of solid organ transplant performed [1, 2]. When both donor and recipient are seronegative for CMV, routine prevention of CMV is not recommended as there is minimal risk of CMV [1, 2]. Anti-viral prophylaxis against other herpesvirus infections, such as varicella and herpes simplex, is recommended with (val)acyclovir or famciclovir [1, 2].

Seronegative recipients who receive a latently infected organ from a seropositive donor (D+/R−) have the highest risk of CMV disease [1, 2, 5]. High-risk serostatus mismatch (D+/R−) is associated with viral replication kinetics with rapid doubling time as well as the tissue-invasive disease typically seen with high viral loads [6]. Because of this, prompt and aggressive treatment of CMV is indicated in patients with a high-risk serostatus mismatch.

In addition to anti-viral therapy, a dual-pronged approach involving reduction of maintenance immunosuppression is a key component of treatment. Immunosuppressive regimens consisting of two agents, compared to three agents, and lower concentrations of calcineurin inhibitors tacrolimus and cyclosporine have been associated with increased rates of early CMV eradication [7].

After initiation of management strategies, a one-log decline in viral load after 2 weeks of therapy is expected with appropriately dosed anti-viral treatment [1]. Weekly monitoring of CMV viral load should be used to modify and guide the duration of treatment [1, 2]. While there is no universally accepted viral load that necessitates intravenous ganciclovir, or one that dictates transition to oral therapy, this is often considered when the viral load falls below 10,000 IU/mL based on the VICTOR study [8]. Drug resistance can be suspected when persistent or recurrent CMV viremia or disease occurs after prolonged exposure to (val)ganciclovir (>6 weeks) or when viral load does not decrease as expected with appropriately dosed anti-viral therapy for >2 weeks [1, 2]. Genotyping of CMV is a valuable tool to identify key mutations conferring anti-viral resistance.

The interferon-gamma releasing assays (IGRAs) are newly available diagnostic testing modalities for the management of CMV. These tests, including ELISA, ELI-Spot, and ICS by flow cytometry, are assays that measure CMV-specific cell-mediated immunity (CMI). According to consensus guidelines, ICS by flow cytometry is expected to be the most clinically useful due to its ability to quantify both CD4+ and CD8+ responses. A commercially available ICS assay is available through Eurofins Viracor, known as the CMV inSIGHT™ T Cell Immunity Panel. A negative result indicates that the patient has not developed CMI and has an ongoing risk for clinically significant CMV events [9]. A positive result indicates that the patient has developed cell-mediated immunity and has a reduced risk of recurrence.

Discontinuation of anti-viral treatment is recommended after the eradication of CMV viremia. Historically this necessitated two consecutive negative viral loads at least a week apart; however, true "eradication" is difficult to define in the current era of highly sensitive molecular diagnostics, which can detect replication in latency. Furthermore, despite the presence of the World Health Organization international standard, viral loads are not directly comparable between laboratories. Finally, achievement of negativity and secondary prophylaxis has not been associated with reducing recurrence risk [1, 2]. Given these issues, attention has turned from achieving an absolute viral load goal to creating an environment conducive to the development of CMI. Indeed, negativity can be challenging to attain in the setting of persistent, low-level viral replication where prolonged therapy with (val)ganciclovir derivatives and their associated detrimental myelotoxicity become counterproductive to the development of CMI. In these situations, diagnostics such as CMV-specific CMI testing and the anti-viral drug letermovir, which utilizes a novel mechanism that does not have an associated mammalian target and thus is relatively devoid of toxicity, can be utilized to foster CMI by avoiding myelosuppressive toxicity while preventing progressive replication [10]. Furthermore, results of CMV-specific CMI testing can be used to determine the need for ongoing therapy or secondary prophylaxis.

Prevention and management of CMV disease require a multimodal approach to optimize outcomes against this common infection affecting solid organ transplant recipients. Strategies include appropriate screening and prophylaxis for donor and recipient serostatus, prompt initiation of adequately dosed anti-viral therapies, immunosuppression reduction, and use of advanced diagnostics such as resistance and cell-mediated immunity testing when indicated. A center-specific CMV anti-viral stewardship initiative utilizing the principles and practices of antimicrobial stewardship can be used to streamline management and optimize outcomes.

Disclosures H. Kleiboeker reports employment with the Department of Pharmacy at the University of Wisconsin Hospital and Clinics. M. Jorgenson reports employment with the Department of Pharmacy at the University of Wisconsin Hospital and Clinics. The authors have no conflicts of interest to disclose.

Funding None.

References

1. Razonable RR, Humar A. Cytomegalovirus in solid organ transplant recipients—guidelines of the American society of transplantation infectious diseases community of practice. Clin Transplant. 2019;33(9) https://doi.org/10.1111/ctr.13512.
2. Kotton CN, Kumar D, Caliendo AM, Huprikar S, Chou S, Danziger-Isakov L, Humar A. The transplantation society international CMV consensus group. The third international consensus guidelines on the Management of Cytomegalovirus in solid-organ transplantation. Transplantation. 2018;102(6):900–31. https://doi.org/10.1097/TP.0000000000002191.
3. Jorgenson MR, Descourouez JL, Leverson GE, Saddler CM, Smith JA, Garg N, Parajuli S, Mandelbrot DA, Odorico JS. A pilot study of an intensified ganciclovir dosing strategy for treatment of cytomegalovirus disease in kidney and/or pancreas transplant recipients. Clin Transpl. 2021; https://doi.org/10.1111/ctr.14427.
4. Fisher CE, Knudsen JL, Lease ED, et al. Risk factors and outcomes of ganciclovir-resistant cytomegalovirus infection in solid organ transplant recipients. Clin Infect Dis. 2017;65(1):57–63. https://doi.org/10.1093/cid/cix259.
5. Raval AD, Kistler KD, Tang Y, Murata Y, Snydman DR. Epidemiology, risk factors, and outcomes associated with cytomegalovirus in adult kidney transplant recipients: a systematic literature review of real-world evidence. Transpl Infect Dis. 2021;23(2):e13483. https://doi.org/10.1111/tid.13483. Epub 2020 Oct 22
6. Dioverti MV, Razonable RR. Clinical utility of cytomegalovirus viral load in solid organ transplant recipients. Curr Opin Infect Dis. 2015;28(4):317–22. https://doi.org/10.1097/QCO.0000000000000173.
7. Asberg A, Jardine AG, Bignamini AA, Rollag H, Pescovitz MD, Gahlemann CC, Humar A, Hartmann A, VICTOR Study Group. Effects of the intensity of immunosuppressive therapy on outcome of treatment for CMV disease in organ transplant recipients. Am J Transplant. 2010;10(8):1881–8. https://doi.org/10.1111/j.1600-6143.2010.03114.x.
8. Åsberg A, Humar A, Rollag H, Jardine AG, Mouas H, Pescovitz MD, Sgarabotto D, Tuncer M, Noronha IL, Hartmann A. Oral valganciclovir is noninferior to intravenous ganciclovir for the treatment of cytomegalovirus disease in solid organ transplant recipients. Am J Transplant. 2007;7(9):2106–13. https://doi.org/10.1111/j.1600-6143.2007.01910.x.
9. Rogers R, Saharia K, Chandorkar A, Weiss ZF, Vieira K, Koo S, Farmakiotis D. Clinical experience with a novel assay measuring cytomegalovirus (CMV)-specific CD4+ and CD8+ T-cell immunity by flow cytometry and intracellular cytokine staining to predict clinically significant CMV events. BMC Infect Dis. 2020;20(1):58. https://doi.org/10.1186/s12879-020-4787-4. Erratum in: BMC Infect Dis. 2020;20(1):122.
10. Goldner T, Hewlett G, Ettischer N, et al. The novel anticytomegalovirus compound AIC246 (Letermovir) inhibits human cytomegalovirus replication through a specific anti-viral mechanism that involves the viral terminase. J Virol. 2011;85:10884–93.

Chapter 31
Beyond Transplantation: Urinary Infectious Complications and Malignancy Risk in Autosomal Dominant Polycystic Kidney Disease

Judy Hindi and Emily Joachim

Introduction

Polycystic kidney disease is the most common genetic kidney disorder; the autosomal dominant form accounts for 10% of cases of end-stage kidney disease (ESKD). The disease, which is attributed to mutations in PKD1 and PKD2 genes, is not only limited to the kidney but involves the formation of cysts in the liver, pancreas and seminal vesicles, vascular malformations in the brain and cardiovascular system and increased incidence of diverticulitis [1]. Kidney manifestations of the disease include rupture of cysts, presenting as hematuria or flank pain, nephrolithiasis, recurrent urinary tract infection, and chronic kidney disease with progression to ESKD. Kidney transplantation offers patients with ESKD the ability to recover their kidney function and alleviate symptoms associated with advanced kidney disease. However, the structural abnormalities associated with multi-organ cystic formations and vascular malformations are complications that persist post-transplant and must be periodically monitored. In this book chapter, we present a case highlighting the morbidity associated with recurrent urinary tract infections in autosomal dominant polycystic kidney disease (ADPCKD) patients post-transplantation and discuss the need for close monitoring of cystic malformations in the native kidneys given the increased risk for renal cell carcinoma (RCC) in this patient population.

J. Hindi · E. Joachim (✉)
Division of Nephrology, Department of Medicine, Medical College of Wisconsin, Milwaukee, WI, USA
e-mail: jhindi@mcw.edu; ejoachim@mcw.edu

© The Author(s), under exclusive license to Springer Nature Switzerland AG 2022
F. Aziz, S. Parajuli (eds.), *Complications in Kidney Transplantation*,
https://doi.org/10.1007/978-3-031-13569-9_31

Patient History

A 57-year-old female with chronic kidney disease stage 5 secondary to ADPCKD, hypertension, rheumatoid arthritis, obesity status-post Roux-en-Y, and hypothyroidism underwent a preemptive living unrelated kidney transplant. At the time of transplant, her panel reactive antibody was 0%, and she had no preformed donor-specific antibodies. Her CMV serology was donor negative and recipient positive, and her EBV serology was donor and recipient positive. She received induction with anti-thymocyte globulin and steroids. Her maintenance immunosuppression included tacrolimus (target trough 8–10 ng/mL), prednisone 5 mg, and mycophenolate mofetil 1000 mg BID. She received prophylaxis with valganciclovir for 3 months and trimethoprim/sulfamethoxazole 400 mg/80 mg daily for 1 year. Her serum creatinine 4 weeks post-transplant was 0.9 mg/dL.

Before transplant, she had a history of several kidney cyst ruptures associated with back, pelvic and flank pain, hematuria, and nausea. She also had a long history of recurrent urinary tract infections (UTI), averaging two infections per year. Eight months before the transplant, she developed resistant extended-spectrum beta-lactamase (ESBL) *E. coli* urinary tract infections and had two infections within 2 months. After treatment, she was started on weekly fosfomycin for prophylaxis before transplant. At the time of transplant, she received intravenous ertapenem peri-operatively (7 days before surgery and continued for 4 days after) given screening urine culture was positive for multi-drug resistant (MDR) *E. coli,* and her double J stent was removed at 2 weeks rather than 4 weeks post-operatively.

Simultaneous bilateral native nephrectomy at the time of transplant was considered. However, this was ultimately not undertaken given concern for hemodynamic instability intra-operatively and to minimize the risk of surgical complications at the time of organ transplantation.

Question 1

What is the most common microorganism causing urinary tract infections post-kidney transplant?

A. E. coli.
B. Pseudomonas.
C. Staph aureus.
D. Klebsiella.
E. Enterococcus.

The correct answer is A.

Similar to non-immunocompromised patients, *E. coli* remains the most frequently isolated microorganism found on urine cultures accounting for more than 80% of UTIs. This is likely secondary to virulence adhesion structures intrinsic to the bacteria.

Clinical Course

She presented to the emergency department at 5 weeks post-transplant with fever, chills, malaise, nausea, and vomiting. Her labs on presentation revealed an acute kidney injury with a serum creatinine of 1.19 mg/dL, urinalysis was indicative of a urinary tract infection, and a urine culture subsequently demonstrated >100,000 MDR *E. coli*. She completed a 10-day course of IV ertapenem and was placed on nitrofurantoin for suppression. Two months later, she had an episode of cyst rupture associated with hematuria, back pain, nausea, and vomiting, which resolved with no associated febrile illness. The decision was made to undergo elective bilateral native nephrectomies given recurrent urinary tract infections despite suppressive therapy, as well as ongoing cyst rupture.

She ultimately underwent bilateral nephrectomy 4 months post-transplant, with no post-surgical complications. Pathology showed bilaterally enlarged kidneys with multiple large cysts consistent with ADPKD. The left kidney demonstrated focal microabscess with calcification and urate crystals. There were incidentally noted tubulopapillary adenomas in both kidneys (2 mm on the right and 2.5 mm on the left) (Fig. 31.1).

She was maintained on suppressive antibiotic therapy with nitrofurantoin for additional 3 months after bilateral nephrectomy. She has had no documented urinary tract infections since.

Question 2
Which diagnostic modality is recommended to screen for renal cell cancer in the native kidneys post-kidney transplantation?

A. CT scan of the abdomen and pelvis.
B. MRI of the abdomen and pelvis.
C. Urine cytology.

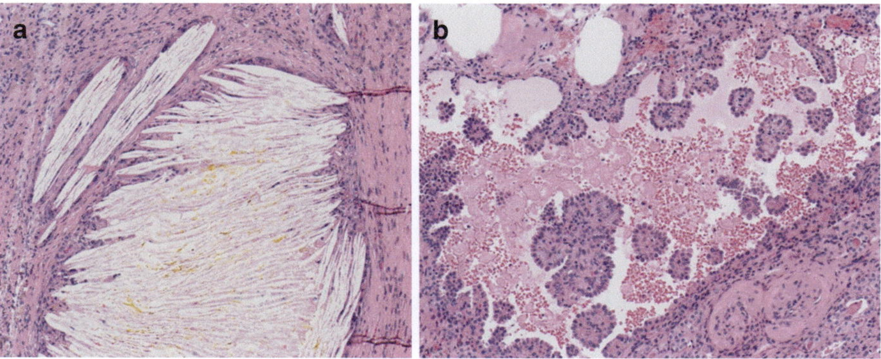

Fig. 31.1 Pathology of native kidneys post native nephrectomy (**a**) Aggregates of interstitial needle-shaped crystals with surrounding granulomatous reaction in areas of prior hemorrhage and tissue injury (**b**) Small papillary adenoma composed of fibrovascular cores lined by neoplastic epithelial cells

D. Ultrasonography.
E. None of the above.

The correct answer is E.

The incidence of renal cell carcinoma is increased in patients post-kidney transplantation, particularly those who have been on dialysis for longer periods prior to transplantation and have acquired cystic disease in their native kidneys. However, there is currently no evidence for the efficacy of a particular screening modality, nor there is a consensus on the frequency of screening that is indicated.

Discussion

UTIs are the most commonly occurring infection in kidney transplant (KT) recipients, with a wide range of prevalence between 20 and 80%. This variable reported incidence is in part due to the lack of uniform diagnostic criteria and the use of prophylactic antibiotics post-transplantation [2]. Notably, the peak incidence appears to be in the first 6 months post-transplant [3], which could be attributed to the use of induction immunosuppression and peri-operative instrumentation. The leading risk factors for UTI in KT recipients include advanced age, female gender, structural or anatomical abnormalities in the urinary tract system, diabetes mellitus, prior history of UTI, instrumentation, and intensity of immunosuppression [4]. Like non-transplanted patients, most UTIs are due to Gram-negative bacteria, with *E. coli* being the most frequently isolated microorganism on urine cultures.

Furthermore, the rate of occurrence of multi-drug resistant organisms (MDRO) has increased in recent years, with a study by Velioglu et al. reporting a rate of around 68% [5]. Interestingly, up to 85% of these isolates were resistant to sulfamethoxazole/trimethoprim (TMP-SMX), the most common antibiotic used for prophylaxis against Pneumocystis jirovecii post-transplantation. This is particularly concerning as UTIs due to MDROs have a threefold increased risk of recurrence in KT patients [6].

ADPKD patients have an increased risk of UTIs inherent to the anatomic abnormalities associated with enlarged cysts. A study comparing ADPCKD patients to non-diabetic patients found that the former had a significantly higher rate of post-transplant UTI (42.5% compared to the control group at 26%), and they were more likely to experience lethal infections [7]. On the other hand, a longitudinal study looking at 15-year outcomes of 534 ADPCKD patients compared to 4779 non-ADPCKD patients found that despite the increased prevalence of urinary tract infections in the ADPCKD arm, this was not statistically significant [8]. Rozanski et al. found similar patient and graft outcomes post-transplant in ADPCKD patients with pretransplant unilateral nephrectomies compared to those transplanted with intact native kidneys [9]. These results suggest that routine pretransplant nephrectomy in ADPCKD is not indicated, but an individualized approach must be considered for each patient based on their symptoms and inherent risk factors for UTIs.

In a single-center study of patients with ADPCKD who underwent native nephrectomy, UTI was the most common indication for native nephrectomy (45%), with most nephrectomies being performed post-transplant (71%) although the number of patients in this study was small [10]. Overall, nephrectomy for recurrent UTI in these patients was quite successful; of the 14 patients who underwent nephrectomy for UTI, 11 had resolution of their recurrent UTIs [10].

Patients with ADPCKD have been shown to have an increased risk of renal cell cancer that is independent of kidney function, as shown in a cohort study performed by Yu et al. of PCKD patients without CKD [11]. Aside from recurrent infections, native nephrectomy in patients with ADPCKD is indicated in cases with a concern for malignancy. A recent meta-analysis reported an incidence of 0.7% of de novo RCC in the native kidney and 0.2% in the transplanted kidney in kidney transplant recipients in general compared to an incidence of 0.005% in the general population [12]. Another study by Hajj et al. found that the prevalence of renal cell carcinoma in ADPCKD patients with chronic kidney failure was as high as 8.3%, and this increased to 12% when the authors accounted for patients who had been on dialysis for more than 1 year or had received kidney transplantation [13]. The latter, however, may be related to the development of acquired cystic disease rather than a direct association with the original underlying disease. Of note, the authors diagnosed RCC based on pathologic examination of kidneys following native nephrectomies for non-cancer-related indications.

Interestingly, the authors found that 36% of kidneys with RCC were also associated with papillary adenomas, which was present in our patient. Therefore, a high degree of suspicion should be kept for the development of RCC post-kidney transplantation, particularly in patients with ADPCKD as an underlying etiology of their kidney failure. However, there is no consensus on the optimal screening frequency and modality. This is left up to provider discretion.

Acknowledgments We would like to thank Dr. Alexander Gallan for providing the slides illustrating the nephrectomy histopathology and summarizing the findings.

References

1. Torres VE, Harris PC, Pirson Y. Autosomal dominant polycystic kidney disease. Lancet. 2007;369(9569):1287–301. ISSN 0140-6736
2. Goldman JD, Julian K. Urinary tract infections in solid organ transplant recipients: guidelines from the American Society of Transplantation infectious diseases Community of Practice. Clin Transpl. 2019;33(9):e13507.
3. Alangaden G. Urinary tract infections in renal transplant recipients. Curr Infect Dis Rep. 2007;9:475–9.
4. Ariza-Heredia EJ, Beam EN, Lesnick TG, Kremers WK, Cosio FG, Razonable RR. Urinary tract infections in kidney transplant recipients: role of gender, urologic abnormalities, and antimicrobial prophylaxis. Ann Transplant. 2013;18:195–204.
5. Velioglu A, Guneri G, Arikan H, Asicioglu E, Tigen ET, et al. Incidence and risk factors for urinary tract infections in the first year after renal transplantation. PLoS One. 2021;16(5):e0251036.

6. Michail A, Dimitrios N, Eleftherios M. Urinary tract infections caused by ESBL-producing Enterobacteriaceae in renal transplant recipients: a systematic review and meta-analysis. Transpl Infect Dis. 2017;19(6)
7. Stiasny B, Ziebell D, Graf S, Hauser IA, Schulze BD. Clinical aspects of renal transplantation in polycystic kidney disease. Clin Nephrol. 2002;58(1):16–24.
8. Jacquet A, Pallet N, Kessler M, Hourmant M, Garrigue V, Rostaing L, Kreis H, Legendre C, Mamzer-Bruneel MF. Outcomes of renal transplantation in patients with autosomal dominant polycystic kidney disease: a nationwide longitudinal study. Transpl Int. 2011;24(6):582–7.
9. Rozanski J, Kozlowska I, Myslak M, Domanski L, Sienko J, Ciechanowski K, Ostrowski M. Pretransplant nephrectomy in patients with autosomal dominant polycystic kidney disease. Transplantation Proceedings. 2005;37(2) ISSN 0041-1345
10. Patel P, Horsfield C, Compton F, Taylor J, Koffman G, Olsburgh J. Native nephrectomy in transplant patients with autosomal dominant polycystic kidney disease. Ann R Coll Surg Engl. 2011;93(5):391–5.
11. Yu TM, Chuang YW, Yu MC, Chen CH, Yang CK, Huang ST, Lin CL, Shu KH, Kao CH. Risk of cancer in patients with polycystic kidney disease: a propensity-score matched analysis of a nationwide, population-based cohort study. Lancet Oncol. 2016;17(10):1419–25. https://doi.org/10.1016/S1470-2045(16)30250-9. Epub 2016 Aug 20
12. Chewcharat A, Thongprayoon C, Bathini T, et al. Incidence and mortality of renal cell carcinoma after kidney transplantation: a meta-analysis. J Clin Med. 2019;8(4):530. https://doi.org/10.3390/jcm8040530. Published 2019 Apr 17
13. Hajj P, Ferlicot S, Massoud W, Awad A, Hammoudi Y, Charpentier B, Durrbach A, Droupy S, Benoît G. Prevalence of renal cell carcinoma in patients with autosomal dominant polycystic kidney disease and chronic renal failure. Urology. 2009;74(3):631–4. https://doi.org/10.1016/j.urology.2009.02.078. Epub 2009 Jul 18. PMID: 19616833

Chapter 32
Disseminated Cryptococcal Infection in Kidney Transplant Recipients

Venkata Manchala and Fahad Aziz

Introduction

Cryptococcosis is a severe fungal infection caused by pathogenic encapsulated yeasts in the genus Cryptococcus. This disease primarily affects immunocompromised patients with cellular immune deficiency. It affects mainly the lungs and central nervous system but can disseminate to any organ in immunocompromised individuals such as organ transplant patients. The diagnosis can be frequently delayed due to various clinical presentations. Definitive diagnosis of cryptococcosis is made by isolation of Cryptococcus from a clinical specimen. In immunocompromised individuals with Cryptococcus isolated from the lung or other sterile body site, a lumbar puncture to rule out CNS disease should be considered, regardless of a patient's symptoms or serum antigen titer results. Liposomal amphotericin B (L-AmB) and flucytosine (5-FC) as the combination therapy are recommended for primary induction in cryptococcal meningitis or severe pulmonary cryptococcosis. Consolidation and maintenance treatment is typically done with fluconazole. Drug interactions between fluconazole and immunosuppressive agents should be anticipated owing to CYP3A4 inhibition, and a preemptive reduction in calcineurin inhibitors should be considered. Management of immunosuppression in the setting of cryptococcal infection requires a stepwise reduction in immunosuppression, and the approach should be individualized for each patient. Along with the optimization of antifungal therapy, increased intracranial pressure management is critically important in cryptococcal meningoencephalitis.

V. Manchala (✉) · F. Aziz
Department of Medicine, University of Wisconsin—Madison School of Medicine and Public Health, University of Wisconsin Hospital and Clinics, Madison, WI, USA
e-mail: vrmanchala@wisc.edu; faziz@wisc.edu

© The Author(s), under exclusive license to Springer Nature Switzerland AG 2022

199

F. Aziz, S. Parajuli (eds.), *Complications in Kidney Transplantation*,
https://doi.org/10.1007/978-3-031-13569-9_32

Case Presentation

A 65-year-old female with amyloidosis s/p autologous bone marrow transplant with end-stage kidney disease (ESKD) from amyloidosis received a preemptive living unrelated kidney transplant. At the time of transplant, her panel reactive antibody was 0%, and she had no preformed donor-specific antibodies. Cytomegalovirus (CMV) serology was donor positive and recipient negative. She received induction with anti-thymocyte globulin. Her maintenance immunosuppression includes prednisone 10 mg daily, mycophenolate 540 mg BID, tacrolimus with a trough goal of 5–7. About 4 years post-transplant, she presented to the emergency room (ER) with shortness of breath, weakness, diarrhea, headache, weight loss of 30lbs in the past 3 months. Physical examination revealed an ill-appearing female in no acute distress. Her baseline Cr was around 2–2.5 mg/dL. When she presented, she had AKI with Cr of 3.21 mg/dL. Chest X-ray revealed right upper lobe nodules. She was admitted for further studies and management.

Question 1
What is the most likely cause of the patient's presentation?

A. Pulmonary tuberculosis.
B. Cryptococcosis.
C. CMV pneumonitis.
D. Lung malignancy.

The correct answer is B.

Our patient is an immunocompromised individual presenting with pulmonary symptoms, unexplained weight loss, AKI, and lung nodules, pointing towards cryptococcal infection. The patient did not have any exposure to mycobacterium, making this option less likely (option A). Although CMV pneumonitis can present with a similar clinical picture, it usually does not have nodules (option C). This presentation is also less likely to be from lung malignancy (option D).

Hospital Course

CT chest (Fig. 32.1) confirmed lung nodules. Infectious workup sent with histoplasma antigen, Blastomyces antigen, Beta 1, 3 glucan, galactomannan, AFB, cryptococcal antigen, coccidiosis antibodies, and CMV PCR. She was started empirically on broad-spectrum antibiotics. CMV PCR was less than 250. Cryptococcal antigen returned positive. The infectious disease team was consulted. Lumbar puncture was done, and CSF was positive for cryptococcal antigen at >1:2560. CSF cultures were returned positive for cryptococcus neoformans. She was diagnosed with disseminated Cryptococcus with meningitis.

Fig. 32.1 Computed Tomography Chest: Focal area of ground glass with a tiny cluster of underlying nodules in the right upper lobe suspicious for granulomatous infection

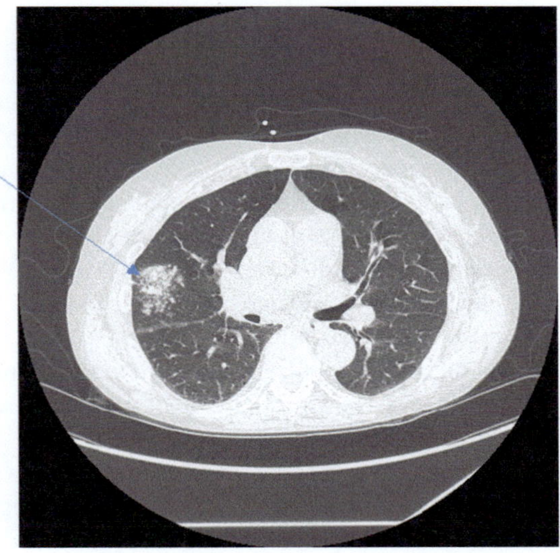

Question 2

How would you treat this patient?

A. Antifungal therapy with IV liposomal amphotericin B and oral flucytosine.
B. Reduction of immunosuppression.
C. Both A and B.
D. Do not initiate treatment until further microbiological data is available.

The correct answer is C.

This patient should be treated with a combination of antifungal agents active against cryptococci along with a reduction of baseline immunosuppression (option A & B). Waiting for microbiological data can be associated with increased mortality, so the empiric treatment should be started with the suspicion of fungal pneumonia (option D).

Further Hospital Course

She was started on induction treatment with IV liposomal amphotericin B at 3 mg/ kg daily with pre and post hydration and PO flucytosine 25 mg/kg BID. Due to complaints of headaches, she required serial lumbar punctures to normalize the intracranial pressures. Her immunosuppression was adjusted with a new tacrolimus goal of 4–6 ng/mL and prednisone decreasing to 10 mg daily along with discontinuation of mycophenolate. With the antifungal treatment, CSF crypto titers were eventually reduced over 3 weeks to 1:320. Infectious disease service recommended transitioning the patient to the consolidation therapy with PO fluconazole 600 mg daily with liver function test and electrocardiogram monitoring periodically. Kidney function returned to her baseline.

Discussion

Cryptococcosis is a severe fungal infection caused by pathogenic encapsulated yeasts in the genus Cryptococcus. The majority of the infections are caused by Cryptococcus neoformans. Cryptococcosis primarily affects immunocompromised patients with cellular immune deficiency, in particular, HIV-positive patients [1]; however, with the use of highly active antiretroviral therapy (HAART), cryptococcosis is now more often reported in HIV-negative patients, especially solid organ transplant (SOT) recipients, which account for 20–60% of cryptococcosis cases among HIV-negative individuals [2].

Cryptococcosis represents the third most common fungal infection in SOT recipients after invasive candidiasis and aspergillosis, with approximately half of the cases involving the central nervous system [3].

The diagnosis is frequently delayed due to a wide array of clinical presentations and the absence of a systematic screening strategy. The respiratory tract serves as the most important portal of entry for Cryptococcus. It affects mainly the lungs and central nervous system. However, it can widely disseminate and infect most organs in severely immunosuppressed patients. In transplant patients, cryptococcal pneumonia is usually symptomatic and in some cases can progress rapidly to acute respiratory distress syndrome, even in the absence of CNS involvement [4].

In immunocompromised individuals with Cryptococcus isolated from the lung or other sterile body site, a lumbar puncture to rule out CNS disease should be considered, regardless of a patient's symptoms or serum antigen titer results. Clinical manifestations of CNS cryptococcosis include a myriad of signs and symptoms, such as headache, fever, cranial neuropathies, altered mentation, lethargy, memory loss, and signs of meningeal irritation [5]. Symptoms usually develop over several weeks. In severely immunocompromised, the burden of fungal organisms is usually high and may consequently have a shorter onset of signs and symptoms, greater CSF polysaccharide antigen titers, and higher intracranial pressures than other immunocompetent individuals [1]. Definitive diagnosis of cryptococcosis is made by isolating Cryptococcus from a clinical specimen or direct detection of the fungus using India ink staining of body fluids. Cryptococcus can be cultured readily from biologic samples such as CSF, sputum, and skin biopsy on routine fungal and bacterial culture media [6]. The diagnosis of cryptococcosis improved significantly with the development of serologic tests for the cryptococcal polysaccharide capsular antigen (CrAg), which is shed during infection. Latex agglutination and enzyme immunoassay techniques to detect CrAg have been widely available (using both serum and CSF) with overall sensitivities and specificities of 93–100% and 93%–98%, respectively [7]. Baseline cryptococcal polysaccharide antigen titers in serum and CSF correlate with fungal burden and carry prognostic significance in patients with cryptococcal meningitis. However, there is limited value in serial monitoring of antigen titers acutely in assessing treatment response because the kinetics of antigen clearance is a slower and less predictable marker of treatment response than quantitative culture [8].

Liposomal amphotericin B (L-AmB) and flucytosine (5-FC) as the combination therapy are recommended for primary induction in cryptococcal meningitis or severe pulmonary cryptococcosis. This combination represents the most potent fungicidal regimen, with faster CSF sterilization, fewer relapses, and lower attributable mortality. The antifungal treatment is complicated by the nephrotoxicity of liposomal amphotericin B (L-AmB) in patients with impaired renal function, but also by drug–drug interactions between fluconazole and calcineurin inhibitors [9]. A 3-stage regimen of induction, consolidation, and maintenance is the standard treatment for cryptococcal meningitis in all patients, irrespective of host risk factors [10].

Consolidation and maintenance treatment is typically done with fluconazole. Drug interactions between fluconazole and immunosuppressive agents should be anticipated owing to CYP3A4 inhibition, and a preemptive reduction in calcineurin inhibitors should be considered. Management of immunosuppression in the setting of cryptococcal infection requires a stepwise reduction in immunosuppression, and the approach should be individualized for each patient. Along with optimizing antifungal therapy, increased intracranial pressure management is critically important in cryptococcal meningoencephalitis. Intracranial imaging should be performed before lumbar puncture if impaired mentation or focal neurologic deficits are present. A baseline CSF opening pressure should be obtained in all patients. Aggressive attempts to control increased intracranial pressure should occur when patients are symptomatic with serial lumbar punctures and may need lumbar drain insertion, ventriculostomy, or ventriculoperitoneal shunt if obstructive hydrocephalus develops [11].

References

1. Maziarz EK, Perfect JR. Cryptococcosis. Infect Dis Clin N Am. 2016;30(1):179–206.
2. Neofytos D, Fishman JA, Horn D, Anaissie E, Chang C-H, Olyaei A, et al. Epidemiology and outcome of invasive fungal infections in solid organ transplant recipients. Transpl Infect Dis Off J Transplant Soc. 2010;12(3):220–9.
3. Wu G, Vilchez RA, Eidelman B, Fung J, Kormos R, Kusne S. Cryptococcal meningitis: an analysis among 5521 consecutive organ transplant recipients. Transpl Infect Dis. 2002;4(4):183–8.
4. Brizendine K, Baddley J, Pappas P. Pulmonary cryptococcosis. Semin Respir Crit Care Med. 2011;32(6):727–34.
5. Perfect JR, Casadevall A. Cryptococcosis. Infect Dis Clin N Am. 2002;16:837–74.
6. Sato Y, Osabe S, Kuno H, et al. Rapid diagnosis of cryptococcal meningitis by microscopic examination of centrifuged cerebrospinal fluid sediment. J Neurol Sci. 1999;164:72–5.
7. Tanner DC, Weinstein MP, Fedorciw B, et al. Comparison of commercial kits for detection of cryptococcal antigen. J Clin Microbiol. 1994;32:1680–4.
8. Kabanda T, Siedner M, Klausner J, et al. Point-of-care diagnosis and prognostication of cryptococcal meningitis with the cryptococcal lateral flow assay on cerebrospinal fluid. Clin Infect Dis. 2014;58(1):113–6.
9. Day JN, Chau T, Wolbers M, et al. Combination antifungal therapy for cryptococcal meningitis. N Engl J Med. 2013;368:1291–30.

10. Perfect JR, Dismukes WE, Dromer F, et al. Clinical practice guidelines for the Management of Cryptococcal Disease: 2010 update by the infectious disease Society of America. Clin Infect Dis. 2010;50:291–322.
11. Graybill JR, Sobel J, Saag M, et al. Diagnosis and management of increased intracranial pressure in patients with AIDS and cryptococcal meningitis. The NIAID mycoses study group and AIDS cooperative treatment groups. Clin Infect Dis. 2000;30(1):47–54.

Chapter 33
Pulmonary Nocardiosis Post-Kidney Transplantation

Safaa Azzouz and Shaifali Sandal

Introduction

Solid organ transplant (SOT) recipients are at risk of opportunistic infections. Pulmonary nocardiosis (PN) is an infrequent but severe infection caused by *Nocardia* species; however, it is associated with high morbidity and mortality. Herein, we describe the case of a 77-year-old kidney transplant recipient who developed PN. We discuss the incidence, risk factors, clinical manifestations, diagnostics, therapeutics, outcomes, and prophylactic options of PN.

Case

A 77-year-old male patient with a second deceased donor kidney transplantation 2 years prior presented with a three-day history of fever, chest pain, fatigue, and non-productive cough. He had a history of diabetic nephropathy, and the first transplant failed due to chronic rejection. His calculated panel reactive antibody (cPRA) was 99% when he received a crossmatch negative kidney transplant with

S. Azzouz
Department of Medicine, McGill University Health Centre, Research Institute of the McGill University Health Centre, Montreal, QC, Canada
e-mail: safaa.azzouz@mail.mcgill.ca

S. Sandal (✉)
Division of Nephrology, Department of Medicine, McGill University Health Centre, Montreal, QC, Canada

Royal Victoria Hospital Glen Site, Montreal, QC, Canada
e-mail: shaifali.sandal@mcgill.ca

© The Author(s), under exclusive license to Springer Nature Switzerland AG 2022
F. Aziz, S. Parajuli (eds.), *Complications in Kidney Transplantation*,
https://doi.org/10.1007/978-3-031-13569-9_33

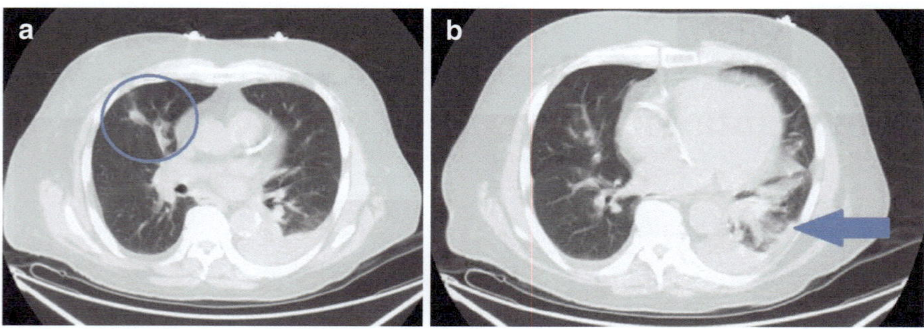

Fig. 33.1 CT thorax of the patient diagnosed with pulmonary nocardiosis. (**a**) Peribronchovascular nodular opacities in the right middle lobe and lower lobe. (**b**) Arrow pointing to the left lower lobe parenchymal opacity and small left pleural effusion

alemtuzumab and methylprednisolone induction. Thereafter, maintenance immunosuppression included tacrolimus (target trough level 4–8 ng/mL), mycophenolate mofetil (720 mg twice a day), and prednisone 5 mg daily. He had good graft function with a baseline creatinine of 1.2–1.4 mg/dL. His past medical history included hypertension, dyslipidemia, and benign prostatic hyperplasia.

On presentation, he had a temperature of 39 °C, oxygen saturation was 96% on room air, and an elevated WBC count (17×10^9/L with a left-sided shift). He was initially started on broad-spectrum intravenous antibiotics. Most of the initial microbiology workup (respiratory virus PCR, legionella antigen, and blood cultures) was negative. A chest CT revealed a moderate left pleural effusion and left lower lobe basilar consolidation. Several poorly defined peribronchovascular and perifissural nodular opacities in the right lung were noted, raising concerns for opportunistic infection (Fig. 33.1). Diagnostic bronchoalveolar lavage and thoracentesis were performed, and no organism was isolated initially, although the pleural effusion was exudative. Given clinical improvement, he was discharged 4 days later with amoxicillin/clavulanic acid and azithromycin treatment. Concerns for *Nocardia* were raised, and laboratory staff was made aware. 2 weeks after presentation, *Nocardia* species were isolated from his bronchoalveolar lavage specimen and eventually were identified to be *N. beijingensis*.

Question 1

Which of the following tests should be pursued following PN diagnosis?

A. MRI brain.
B. Whole body PET scan.
C. Lung biopsy.
D. No further testing is indicated.

The correct answer is A.

In solid organ transplant recipients with PN, CNS involvement is common even in the absence of neurological symptoms. Thus, brain imaging is recommended. A whole body PET scan is routinely not recommended. There is no added need for a lung biopsy due to the identification of *Nocardia* species.

Clinical Course

Following the identification of *Nocardia*, no CNS involvement was confirmed with MRI. Based on the provincial susceptibility data, the patient was started on doxycycline and ceftriaxone. Dual therapy was continued for 6-months, followed by another 6 months of doxycycline alone. A 6-month chest CT confirmed the resolution of all acute findings. No prophylactic treatment was pursued thereafter, and he was monitored for recurrence.

Question 2

Which of the following statements concerning pulmonary nocardiosis is incorrect?

A. A high index of suspicion is needed to diagnose it.
B. It is a rare disease in kidney transplant recipients and may be more frequent in lung transplant recipients.
C. Antimicrobial therapy is the mainstay of therapy.
D. There is strong evidence to support secondary prophylaxis after treatment is completed to prevent recurrent disease.

The correct answer is D.

Secondary prophylaxis is recommended once therapy is stopped, but evidence supporting it is poor. Nocardiosis recurrence in SOT recipients is 2–6.1%, and secondary prophylaxis is not entirely protective. All the other statements are correct, as mentioned in the discussion below.

Three years post-diagnosis of PN, his graft function has stayed stable, and there has been no recurrence of PN.

Discussion

Nocardia species belong to the aerobic actinomycetes group of bacteria, with more than 85 identified species and more than 40 being associated with human infections [1, 2]. They are found worldwide in soil, fresh- and salt-water, and decaying vegetation [2]. Infections can occur due to inhalation, through abraded skin, or are hospital-acquired [1, 3]. Thus, the clinical presentation is predominantly pulmonary or cutaneous, but bacteremia and disseminated nocardiosis can occur [1].

PN is an infrequent but severe infection caused by *Nocardia* species that can present as pneumonia, lung abscess, and cavitary lesions [1]. A high index of suspicion in susceptible patients is needed for a timely diagnosis. We will now summarize the current literature on PN; however, we caution the reader that due to the rarity of this disease, much of the current literature report findings on all *Nocardia* infections that include less futile cases of skin and soft tissue infections to more severe cases where there is CNS involvement are limited. In addition, in the transplant literature, findings in all SOT recipients are often cumulatively reported.

Incidence

The incidence of nocardiosis in SOT recipients is increasing and is likely driven by improved diagnostics, an increase in the number of SOT recipients, and more potent immunosuppression [2, 3]. The reported incidence of *Nocardia* infections in SOT ranges from 0.4 to 2.65%, and PN is the most common disease [2–4]. It typically presents in the late post-transplant period, although the onset varies from 1 month to many years post-transplantation [2–5]. Before the availability of sophisticated molecular tools, most *Nocardia* strains were reported to be due to *N. asteroids* [5]. More recently, amongst all cases of *Nocardia* in the United States, the species most commonly identified were *N. nova*, *N. brasiliensis*, and *N. farcinica* [6].

Risk Factors

Immunosuppression or immunocompromised status and impairment of lung defenses are risk factors for PN [5, 7]. Male sex and co-morbid diseases, such as diabetes, are also risk factors [1, 7]. In SOT recipients, other risk factors include recipients of lung transplantation, higher levels of calcineurin inhibitor levels, use of tacrolimus and high-dose steroids, age of the recipient, and cytomegalovirus disease [2–5].

Clinical Manifestation

PN can present as an acute, subacute, or chronic disease, and clinical symptoms are non-specific [2, 5, 7, 8]. Symptoms usually include fever and cough; however other respiratory symptoms, such as increased sputum, dyspnea, chest pain, hemoptysis, and constitutional symptoms, can occur [2, 5, 7]. Of note, *Nocardia* can disseminate to any organ, and rates of extrapulmonary dissemination in SOT are reported to be 20–71% [2]. CNS involvement is common even in the absence of neurologic symptoms; thus, brain imaging is recommended in any SOT recipient with PN [2, 4, 9].

Diagnosis

A high index of suspicion is needed for diagnosing PN as clinical presentation and imaging findings are non-specific. Chest CT findings include lung infiltrates with consolidation, excavations, pleural effusion, ground-glass opacities, and septal thickening [2, 5]. In SOT recipients, the most common finding is lung nodule(s) [4]. Regardless, the diagnosis of PN relies on identifying the microorganism from respiratory samples, such as the sputum, bronchial aspirate, and pleural fluid [5]. Bronchoalveolar lavage or transbronchial or fine-needle biopsy should therefore be pursued. Modified acid-fast staining using 1% sulfuric acid as a decolorizer can demonstrate the pink-colored filamentous branching bacilli [1]. The culture of *Nocardia* species requires prolonged incubation periods for isolation; a visible growth may take more than 1 week for some species [1, 3]. Thus, laboratory and microbiology staff must be informed to take the necessary steps to isolate, identify, and determine the sensitivity pattern [1, 3].

Treatment

Antimicrobials are the mainstay of therapy, and sulfonamides are the initial antimicrobial of choice. However, the selection of treatment must account for the *Nocardia* species involved, local susceptibility data, site(s) of infection, presence of co-pathogens, adverse effects, intolerabilities, and drug interactions [2, 3]. Current recommendations in SOT recipients are to use antibiotics active against a broad spectrum of *Nocardia* species, such as sulfamethoxazole-trimethoprim, amikacin, third-generation cephalosporins, carbapenem, or linezolid [10]. A 10-year retrospective evaluation of the epidemiology and identification of *Nocardia* isolates demonstrated that 61% of the isolates were resistant to sulfamethoxazole, and 42% were resistant to sulfamethoxazole-trimethoprim [6]. Thus, antibiotic combinations are recommended in severe cases of nocardiosis [2, 5, 10].

Other things to consider include reducing the immunosuppressive drugs [5]. Surgical options should be considered in the presence of abscesses and cases that are resistant to therapy. In terms of duration, the American Society of Transplantation suggests at least 6 months of antimicrobial therapy for PN and 6–12 months for disseminated disease [2]. However, the exact duration should depend on the response to treatment, resolution of disease, and degree of immunosuppression [2, 3].

Outcomes/Prognosis

In general mortality rate of PN exceeds that of community-acquired pneumonia and is similar to that of invasive mycotic diseases, the disseminated disease has a worse prognosis [7]. Mortality from PN ranges from 39 to 100% depending on whether the disease is disseminated and whether there is concurrent CNS involvement [7]. In SOT, overall mortality rates of 16–32% have been reported from nocardiosis [3, 8]. Additionally, concurrent infections may also carry significant morbidity and mortality [3]. In a case-control study involving 117 SOT recipients, 1 year mortality was found to be 10-fold higher in patients with nocardiosis than in control transplant recipients [8]. Delays in diagnosis and early discontinuation of therapy are suspected to be driving these numbers [2, 8].

Primary and Secondary Prevention

In SOT recipients, preventative strategies are not well known [5]. Daily sulfamethoxazole-trimethoprim to prevent *Pneumocystis jirovecii* pneumonia in the first 6 months post-transplantation is thought to reduce the rate of nocardial infections [2]. However, in 171 SOT recipients with *Nocardia* infections, this was not protective against the occurrence of nocardiosis in a multivariate analysis [4]. The authors speculated a low dose of sulfamethoxazole-trimethoprim as contributory. In those with nocardiosis, once therapy is stopped, the role of secondary prophylaxis is not known either. Rates of recurrence following primary therapy range from 2.0 to 6.1% [11]. Thus, the American Society of Transplantation recommends secondary prophylaxis with sulfamethoxazole-trimethoprim, one double-strength tablet daily [2]. However, a retrospective cohort study found this not completely protective [11]. Efficacy of primary and secondary prophylaxis may depend on antimicrobial resistance, post-transplant immunosuppression, and comorbidities [2]. Regardless, monitoring for nocardiosis recurrence should continue for up to 1 year after the discontinuation of therapy [2].

Acknowledgments there are no acknowledgments listed.

References

1. Human KV. Nocardia Infections: a review of pulmonary Nocardiosis. Cureus. 2015;7(8):e304.
2. Restrepo A, Clark NM. Nocardia infections in solid organ transplantation: guidelines from the infectious diseases Community of Practice of the American Society of Transplantation. Clin Transpl. 2019;33(9):e13509.
3. Hemmersbach-Miller M, Catania J, Saullo JL. Updates on Nocardia skin and soft tissue Infections in solid organ transplantation. Curr Infect Dis Rep. 2019;21(8):27.
4. Coussement J, Lebeaux D, van Delden C, Guillot H, Freund R, Marbus S, et al. Nocardia infection in solid organ transplant recipients: a multicenter European case-control study. Clin Infect Dis. 2016;63(3):338–45.
5. Lebeaux D, Morelon E, Suarez F, Lanternier F, Scemla A, Frange P, et al. Nocardiosis in transplant recipients. Eur J Clin Microbiol Infect Dis. 2014;33(5):689–702.
6. Uhde KB, Pathak S, McCullum I Jr, Jannat-Khah DP, Shadomy SV, Dykewicz CA, et al. Antimicrobial-resistant nocardia isolates, United States, 1995-2004. Clin Infect Dis. 2010;51(12):1445–8.
7. Martínez Tomás R, Menéndez Villanueva R, Reyes Calzada S, Santos Durantez M, Vallés Tarazona JM, Modesto Alapont M, et al. Pulmonary nocardiosis: risk factors and outcomes. Respirology. 2007;12(3):394–400.
8. Lebeaux D, Freund R, van Delden C, Guillot H, Marbus SD, Matignon M, et al. Outcome and treatment of Nocardiosis after solid organ transplantation: new insights from a European study. Clin Infect Dis. 2017;64(10):1396–405.
9. Anagnostou T, Arvanitis M, Kourkoumpetis TK, Desalermos A, Carneiro HA, Mylonakis E. Nocardiosis of the central nervous system: experience from a general hospital and review of 84 cases from the literature. Medicine (Baltimore). 2014;93(1):19–32.

10. Clark NM, Reid GE. Nocardia infections in solid organ transplantation. Am J transplant. 2013;13(Suppl 4):83–92.
11. Yetmar ZA, Wilson JW, Beam E. Recurrent nocardiosis in solid organ transplant recipients: an evaluation of secondary prophylaxis. Transpl Infect Dis. 2021;23(6):e13753.

Chapter 34
Post-Transplant Adenovirus Infection

Angelie Santos and Fahad Aziz

Introduction

Adenovirus, a double-stranded DNA virus that typically causes mild respiratory, gastrointestinal, and conjunctival illnesses in healthy persons, has been an emerging pathogen in solid organ transplant (SOT) recipients, causing significant morbidity and mortality in immunocompromised hosts. Adenovirus causes a variety of clinical syndromes ranging from asymptomatic infection to life-threatening disseminated disease, with a reported incidence of 5–22% in SOT recipients, most reported early after transplant when immunosuppression is intense. Adenovirus infection frequently presents with hemorrhagic cystitis, fever, and dysuria in kidney transplant recipients. Although adenovirus infection is usually self-limiting in immunocompetent hosts, there are no generally accepted treatment guidelines for adenovirus infection in SOT recipients. This chapter highlights a case of adenovirus infection in a patient with a history of simultaneous pancreas and kidney transplants.

Patient History

A 49-year-old male with a history of End-Stage Kidney Disease (ESKD) secondary to diabetes mellitus type 1 underwent a deceased donor simultaneous pancreas and kidney transplantation. He received induction with anti-thymocyte globulin. His maintenance immunosuppression included tacrolimus twice a day (target trough

A. Santos (✉) · F. Aziz
Department of Medicine, University of Wisconsin—Madison School of Medicine and Public Health, University of Wisconsin Hospital and Clinics, Madison, WI, USA
e-mail: asantos@uwhealth.org; faziz@wisc.edu

© The Author(s), under exclusive license to Springer Nature Switzerland AG 2022

F. Aziz, S. Parajuli (eds.), *Complications in Kidney Transplantation*,
https://doi.org/10.1007/978-3-031-13569-9_34

6–8 ng/mL), mycophenolate sodium 360 mg three times a day, and prednisone 10 mg daily. He achieved a baseline creatinine of 1.5–1.8 mg/dL. Two years after the transplant, the patient started experiencing fever, nausea, vomiting, and abdominal pain. With these symptoms, he was admitted to the hospital, where he was also found to have acute kidney injury. Urinalysis showed turbid amber urine with large blood, >300 protein, 21–50 white blood cells (WBCs), packed red blood cells (RBCs), and 1+ bacteria. Urine microscopy was significant for sheets of RBCs, with very few dysmorphic RBCs and no actual cast appreciated. Computed Tomography (CT) of the abdomen revealed fat stranding around the transplanted kidney and ureter; otherwise, no mass or hydronephrosis. He was admitted for suspected pyelonephritis and was started on broad-spectrum antibiotics. On hospital day 3, the patient remained febrile with rigors and a temperature ranging between 101 and 103 °F. Urine, stool, and blood cultures were negative for any growth. Chest CT was unremarkable.

Question 1

What other diagnostic studies must be done at this time?

A. Fungal culture.
B. Adenovirus/RSV/flu panel.
C. ANA.
D. Transplant kidney biopsy.
E. All of the above.

The correct answer is E.

The patient was diagnosed with a fever of unknown origin (FUO) given several days of infectious evaluation with negative results on commonly used imaging and microbiologic tests. It is appropriate to broaden the differential diagnosis, including fungal, parasitic, and viral etiologies. Non-infectious causes such as autoimmune diseases should also be ruled out. A kidney biopsy would also be warranted as important findings such as allograft rejection can also present with fever and hematuria.

Further Course

The patient underwent a kidney allograft biopsy, negative for rejection (t0, g0, ptc0, cg0, c4d0). It revealed mild interstitial fibrosis and tubular atrophy. Most of his viral serologies were unremarkable. However, he was positive for adenovirus infection with 1.3 million copies on polymerase chain reaction (PCR). His autoimmune work-up, which included antinuclear antibody (ANA), antineutrophil cytoplasmic antibody (ANCA), and anti-glomerular basement membrane, was negative. Infectious work-up, including fungal and parasitic serologies, was also negative. Based on these findings, he was diagnosed with adenovirus hemorrhagic cystitis, which was the cause of his fever and hematuria.

Question 2
What will be the next best step in managing a patient's adenovirus hemorrhagic cystitis?

A. Observation.
B. Reduction of immunosuppression.
C. Cidofovir.
D. Urology consult for further evaluation of hematuria.

The correct answer is B.

There is no consensual therapeutic approach for adenovirus infection. Treatment strategies have been based on case reports or case series. In all these cases, the most crucial component of therapy remains supportive care and decreased immunosuppression [1–3]. As in many cases, reduction of immunosuppression leads to resolution of the infection; therefore, mainly observing the patient and continuing their current immunosuppressive regimen would not be a good option. Cidofovir has shown to have the best evidence of all proposed antiviral agents, but it has been associated with significant nephrotoxicity and neutropenia [4]. Urology consult for hematuria evaluation with cystoscopy can be considered if infectious and non-infectious work-up remains negative. However, in this case, a high suspicion for adenovirus infection is likely in transplant patients presenting with fevers and hematuria.

Additional Clinical Course

Due to concern for nephrotoxicity, cidofovir was not started. The patient's immunosuppressive medications were changed, including discontinuation of the mycophenolate, prednisone was slightly increased from 5 to 10 mg daily, and tacrolimus with the same target trough of 6–8 ng/mL. In addition, he received weekly Intravenous Immunoglobulin (IVIG) infusions. He was subsequently discharged from the hospital and was followed up weekly with adenovirus quantitative PCR, which was done to monitor disease progression.

Discussion

Patients with acquired immunodeficiency have grown steadily in the last few decades, partly because of the increasing number of patients receiving solid organ transplants. With newer and more potent immunosuppressive regimens being offered, patients are given a chance to have longer survival times but also increase the frequency of opportunistic infections. Adenoviruses, which are nonenveloped, linear, double-stranded DNA molecules from a large group of viruses, represented by at least 52 serotypes, take advantage of this impaired immunologic response in immunocompromised hosts [5]. These infections are common, have a worldwide distribution, and frequently occur in the pediatric population when they are self-limited. Although they can be asymptomatic in immunocompromised patients, adenovirus infections can cause life-threatening multiorgan disease and impact morbidity, mortality, and graft survival [1].

There is no consensus on adenovirus infection and disease definitions, but for this chapter, the most common descriptions will be used, as they have been in other studies. Asymptomatic adenovirus infection is defined as detecting adenovirus in patients from stool, blood, urine, or upper airway specimens (by viral culture, antigen tests, or PCR) in the absence of signs and symptoms. On the other hand, adenovirus disease is defined by organ-specific signs and symptoms with virus detection in biopsy specimens by immunohistochemical stain, or from bronchoalveolar lavage or cerebrospinal fluid culture antigen detection, or PCR, in the absence of another diagnosis. Adenovirus disease is considered disseminated if two or more organs are involved, not including viremia [1, 4].

Clinical manifestations vary with the sites affected and type of transplanted organ, with the allograft frequently involved. In kidney transplant recipients, hemorrhagic cystitis and graft dysfunction are described more often. In a study by Watcharananan et al. (Table 34.1), the primary clinical presentations were dysuria/urinary urgency with 88.2% of patients and fever with 82.4% of patients presenting with such symptoms [2]. In a review of literature by Kolankiewicz et al., where they analyzed 11 cases of renal transplant-related adenoviral nephritis, patients commonly presented with gross hematuria and dysuria (91%), fever (82%), and acute renal failure (82%) [3].

Table 34.1 Case series reviews of some treatment strategies used in a transplant recipient with adenovirus disease

Studies	No of patients	Treatment strategy	Outcome	Toxicity
Watcharananan et al. [2]	17	Baseline immunosuppression reduction	All patients cleared adenovirus	N/A
Ljungman et al. [4]	45	Cidofovir	31 patients—Cleared adenovirus 10 patients—Failed the treatment 4 patients—Early death from other causes	28 patients—No toxicity 14 patients—Kidney toxicity 2 patients—Bone marrow suppression 1 patient—Liver toxicity
Florescu et al. [6]	13	Brincidofovir	Marked improvement in adenovirus PCR in patients receiving Brincidofovir	No
Lankester et al. [7]	4	Ribavirin	None of the patients responded	No

Conventional and molecular methods are available for direct detection of the virus. These include viral culture, direct antigen detection, molecular techniques, and histopathology. The method chosen would depend on the site of infection and the available sample collected [8]. Although cell culture remains the gold standard, limitations include insensitivity with clinical samples (i.e., blood), prolonged results, and contamination. In recent years, molecular methods using amplification and detection of the viral genome using PCR have increased the sensitivity and provided a more rapid diagnosis [5, 8]. Serial quantitative PCR levels provide utility regarding a decision to initiate therapy and monitoring response to therapy [1, 9, 10].

The first step in managing adenovirus infection in transplant recipients is reducing the immunosuppressive regimen [1, 2, 5, 8, 11]. The role of immune recovery should not be undervalued as many cases have shown resolution of infection with reduction of immunosuppression [1, 12]. It remains unclear how much of the recovery can be attributed to additional antiviral therapy as it is not well studied. The need for antiviral medication to treat adenovirus disease has been reported in several cases but has not been supported by prospective randomized clinical trials. Of all the antiviral agents used to treat adenovirus infections, cidofovir has the most data to support its use but is associated with significant side effects, including nephrotoxicity (up to 50% of patients), neutropenia (up to 20% of patients), and uveitis [1, 4, 8].

Adenovirus infections in solid organ transplant recipients are increasingly recognized as a significant cause of morbidity and mortality. Although our understanding of the disease remains limited, as with other serious infections, immunosuppression should be reduced as much as possible. Antiviral agents, such as cidofovir, have shown data supporting their clinical application in patients with adenovirus disease but significant toxicity risk. There remain many uncertainties regarding adenovirus infection in the setting of renal transplantation. Further studies are needed to understand the disease's natural history, identify specific risk factors, whether the monitoring of viral load is reliable to assess response to therapy, whether adenovirus prophylaxis is warranted, and lastly, the treatment of the disease that remains to be further studied.

References

1. Florescu D, Hoffman J, et al. Adenovirus in Solid Organ Transplant. Am J Transplant. 2013;13:206–11.
2. Watcharananan SP, Avery R, et al. Adenovirus disease after kidney transplantation: course of infection and outcome in relation to blood viral load and immune recovery. America Journal of Transplantation. 2011;11(6):1308–14.
3. Kolankiewicz, LM., Pullman J., et al. Adenovirus nephritis and obstructive uropathy in a renal transplant recipient: case report and literature review. NDT Plus 2010; 3(4): 388–392.
4. Ljungman P, Ribaud P, Eyrich M, et al. Cidofovir for adenovirus infections after allogeneic hematopoietic stem cell transplantation: a survey by the infectious diseases working Party

of the European Group for blood and marrow transplantation. Bone Marrow Transplant. 2003;31:481–6.

5. Echavarria M. Adenoviruses in immunocompromised hosts. Clin Microbiol Rev. 2008;21(4):704–15.

6. Gray G, McCarthy T. Genotype prevalence and risk factors for severe clinical adenovirus infection, United States 2004-2006. Clin Infect Dis. 2007;45(9):1120–31.

7. Parasuraman R, Zhang P. Severe necrotizing adenovirus Tubulointerstitial nephritis in a kidney transplant recipient. Case Reports in Transplantation. 2013; https://doi.org/10.1155/2013/969186.

8. Florescu M, Miles C, et al. What do we know about adenovirus in renal transplantation? Nephrol Dial Transplant. 2013;28:2003–10.

9. Leruez-Ville M, Minard V, Lacaille F, et al. Real-time blood plasma polymerase chain reaction for management of disseminated adenovirus infection. Clin Infect Dis. 2004;38:45–52.

10. Seidemann K, Heim A, Pfister ED, et al. Monitoring of adenovirus infection in pediatric transplant recipients by quantitative PCR: report of six cases and review of the literature. Am J Transplant. 2004;4:2102–8.

11. Hatlen T, Mroch H. Disseminated adenovirus nephritis after kidney transplantation. Kidney Int Rep. 2018;3:19–23.

12. Ison MG. Adenovirus infections in transplant recipients. Clin Infect Dis. 2006;43:331–9.

Chapter 35
Post-Transplant Parvovirus B19 Infection

Hasan Nadeem and Fahad Aziz

Introduction

Parvovirus B19 (PV-B19) is a single-stranded DNA virus replicating within human erythroid progenitor cells. Infection in immunocompromised patients can cause a prolonged impairment of erythropoiesis, which manifests as anemia and reticulocytopenia due to red cell aplasia [1]. Though less common, chronic PV-B19 infection in immunocompromised hosts can also present with leukopenia and thrombocytopenia [2].

Kidney transplant recipients are one such group of immunosuppressed patients susceptible to chronic PV-B19 infection. While the infection is rare, viremia in post-kidney transplant recipients may be underestimated [3]. In this chapter, we highlight a case of chronic PV-B19 infection in a post-kidney transplant recipient with persistent anemia.

Patient History

A 44-year-old male with a history of stage 5 chronic kidney disease due to focal segmental glomerulosclerosis (FSGS) underwent a living, unrelated kidney transplant. He received anti-thymocyte globulin induction therapy and maintenance immunosuppression with tacrolimus (goal trough 8–10 ng/mL), mycophenolate sodium 720 mg BID, and prednisone 5 mg. He also received prophylaxis of trimethoprim-sulfamethoxazole (TMP-SMX), valganciclovir, and nystatin. He

H. Nadeem (✉) · F. Aziz
Department of Medicine, University of Wisconsin—Madison School of Medicine and Public Health, University of Wisconsin Hospital and Clinics, Madison, WI, USA
e-mail: hnadeem1@uw.edu; faziz@wisc.edu

© The Author(s), under exclusive license to Springer Nature Switzerland AG 2022

F. Aziz, S. Parajuli (eds.), *Complications in Kidney Transplantation*,
https://doi.org/10.1007/978-3-031-13569-9_35

achieved a baseline creatinine of 1.5 mg/dL with eGFR of 45 mL/min/1.73m². At a 6-week post-transplant follow-up visit, he was found to have symptomatic anemia with hemoglobin of 7.7 g/dL. Over the next 2 weeks, his hemoglobin dropped to 5.6 g/dL.

Question 1

What is the most common cause of early post-transplant anemia in kidney transplant recipients?

A. Chronic inflammation.
B. Iron deficiency.
C. Adverse effect due to immunosuppressive or prophylactic medications.
D. Impaired graft function.

The correct answer is B.

Early post-transplant anemia (PTA) is defined as anemia within the first 6 months of transplantation. The most common cause is iron deficiency anemia, which can occur due to insufficient iron stores before transplantation, depletion of iron stores with the onset of post-transplant erythropoiesis, significant blood loss during surgery, or poor post-operative nutrition [4, 5]. Conversely, late PTA is defined as anemia that occurs more than 6 months after transplant and can be caused by chronic inflammation, impaired graft function, renal insufficiency, and immunosuppressive medications that affect the renin—angiotensin—aldosterone system (RAAS) (e.g., trimethoprim-sulfamethoxazole, valganciclovir, mycophenolate sodium).

Further Course

After administration of 4 units of PRBCs, the patient's hemoglobin increased to 7.9 g/dL. Mycophenolate, TMP-SMX, and valganciclovir were held, and the patient's anemia was further evaluated with iron studies, erythropoietin (EPO) level, viral PCR panel, and analysis of the peripheral blood smear. Iron studies and EPO levels were within normal limits; however, the peripheral smear showed a near absence of reticulocytes. This prompted further investigation via bone marrow aspiration and biopsy. A review of the bone marrow with hematopathology was notable for hypocellular marrow with erythroid hypoplasia, features consistent with pure red cell aplasia due to chronic PV-B19 infection. This diagnosis was corroborated by detecting parvovirus nucleic acids on qualitative PCR.

Question 2

What is chronic parvovirus B-19 infection management in post-renal transplant patients?

A. Hold all immunosuppression.
B. PRBC transfusions and/or filgrastim as needed.
C. Erythropoiesis stimulating agent (ESA).

D. Intravenous immunoglobulin (IVIG).
E. Observation.

The correct answer is D.

According to the American Society of Transplantation Guidelines for human PV-B19 infection in solid organ transplant (SOT) recipients, the recommended treatment is the administration of IVIG and reduction of immunosuppression if possible [6]. Withholding all immunosuppression is not recommended to treat chronic PV-B19 infection in SOT patients. Treatment with PRBCs, filgrastim, or ESAs are temporizing measures that do not address the underlying cause of infection. Observation is not recommended in immunosuppressed patients with symptomatic PV-B19 infection.

Additional Clinical Course

The patient's tacrolimus dose was reduced, and he was treated with a 5-day course of IVIG 2 g/kg. His hemoglobin and reticulocyte count increased favorably to 10 g/dL and 80 K/uL, respectively, but his parvovirus viremia persisted. To prevent potential pure red cell aplasia relapse, it was recommended that the patient undergoes IVIG maintenance therapy of 400 mg/kg every 4 weeks until clearance of parvovirus viremia is achieved (Fig. 35.1). Post-transplant, the patient received 10 cycles of IVIG infusion therapy, which resulted in a reduction of viral titers from 3.5 to 2.3 log units/mL and stabilization of hemoglobin.

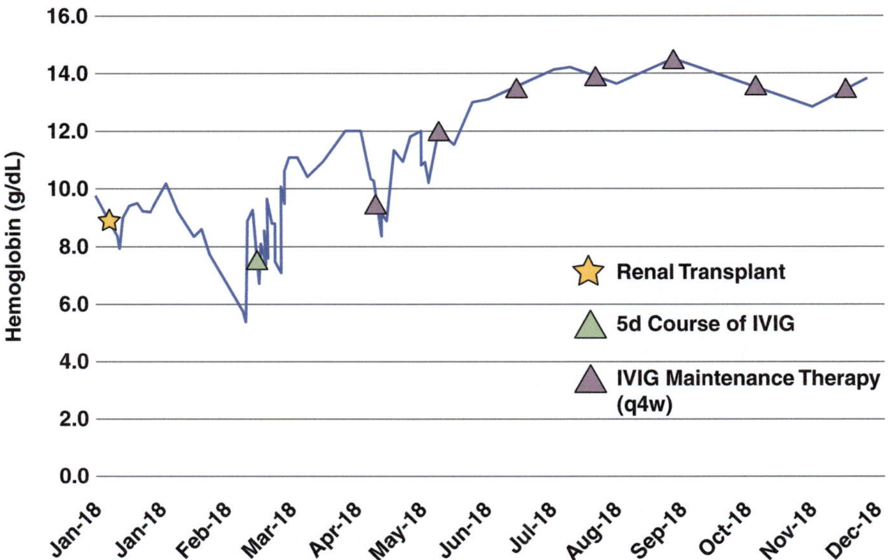

Fig. 35.1 Hemoglobin Values During Year 1 Post-Transplant

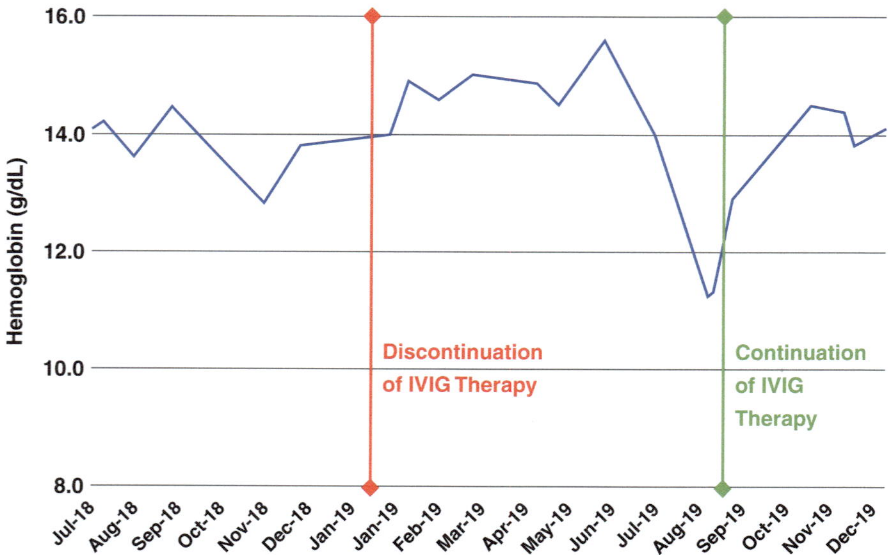

Fig. 35.2 Hemoglobin Values During Maintenance IVIG Therapy and Therapy Hiatus

After 10 treatment cycles with IVIG, the patient elected to discontinue treatment due to adverse effects. Seven months after discontinuing IVIG, the patient presented with an increased viral titer of PV-B19 by quantitative PCR and a drop in hemoglobin from 14 to 11.2 g/dL. He was subsequently restarted on IVIG therapy, which reduced viral titers to previously low levels and stabilized his hemoglobin to >12 g/dL (Fig. 35.2). The patient continues to be maintained on monthly, prophylactic IVIG therapy with consistently low PV-B19 viral titers and hemoglobin values >12 g/dL.

Discussion

PV-B19 is a single-stranded DNA virus that was first described by Yvonne Cossart in 1975 [7]. Since then; much has been learned about PV-B19 infection. The virus utilizes the primary receptor globoside (Gb4), which is found most commonly on cells of erythroid lineage, platelets, and cells of the heart, liver, lung, kidneys, endothelium, and synovium [2, 8, 9]. Replication of the virus occurs primarily within human erythroid progenitor cells, and the direct cytotoxic damage caused by viral replication inhibits erythropoiesis. Infection is ultimately terminated via IgG or IgM antibodies, though if patients are immunocompromised or immunosuppressed, production of these antibodies will not occur, and persistent infection can ensue [10, 11].

In transplant recipients with chronic PV-B19 infection, the most common presenting symptom is persistent anemia (98.8%), followed by leukopenia (37.5%) and thrombocytopenia (21.0%) [12]. As such, a patient with normal iron studies and anemia refractory to product support or ESA therapy warrants evaluation for potential PV-B19 infection.

Testing for PV-B19 infection can be done via serology, nucleic acid detection, or bone marrow aspiration and biopsy [12]. PV-B19 serology may remain negative early on in the disease course due to the inability of immunosuppressed patients to produce a detectable quantity of antibodies. Nucleic acid testing via PCR is the most sensitive for diagnosing chronic PV-B19, and quantitative PCR can be used to monitor for clearance of the disease. The gold standard for diagnosing chronic PV-B19 infection is bone marrow biopsy and aspiration, which shows giant pronormoblasts and hypocellular marrow with red cell aplasia.

Chronic PV-B19 infection is treated with IVIG and reduction of immunosuppression [6, 12]. Many patients are treated with a dose of 400 mg/kg/day for 5 days, but the exact recommendation for dosage and length of treatment with IVIG has not been determined. IVIG therapy does not always result in clearance of viremia, and in these patients, discontinuation of therapy can result in relapse [13].

In summary, the burden of PV-B19 infection in renal transplant patients may be underestimated. The most common manifestation of this disease is persistent anemia that may be accompanied by leukopenia and/or thrombocytopenia. This is likely due to the cytotoxic effects of viral replication, mainly within erythroid progenitor cells. IVIG therapy is the primary treatment of chronic PV-B19 infection in renal transplant patients. Despite treatment, some patients may harbor a low level of viremia that is asymptomatic but has the potential to result in a relapse of pure red cell aplasia if IVIG treatments are discontinued.

Note

The initial 5-day course of IVIG was dosed at 2 g/kg. Maintenance therapy with IVIG is dosed at 500 mg/kg.

References

1. Cassinotti P, Burtonboy G, Fopp M, Siegl G. Evidence for persistence of human parvovirus B19 DNA in bone marrow. J Med Virol. 1997;53(3):229–32. https://doi.org/10.1002/(SICI)1096-9071(199711)53:3<229::AID-JMV8>3.0.CO;2-A.
2. Florea AV, Ionescu DN, Melhem MF. Parvovirus B19 infection in the immunocompromised host. Arch Pathol Lab Med. 2007;131(5):799–804. https://doi.org/10.5858/2007-131-799-PBIITI.
3. Porignaux R, Vuiblet V, Barbe C, et al. Frequent occurrence of parvovirus B19 DNAemia in the first year after kidney transplantation. J Med Virol. 2013;85(6):1115–21. https://doi.org/10.1002/jmv.23557.
4. Teruel JL, Lamas S, Vila T, et al. Serum ferritin levels after renal transplantation: a prospective study. Nephron. 1989;51(4):462–5. https://doi.org/10.1159/000185376.
5. Gafter-Gvili A, Gafter U. Posttransplantation anemia in kidney transplant recipients. Acta Haematol. 2019;142(1):37–43. https://doi.org/10.1159/000496140.
6. Eid AJ, Ardura MI, AST Infectious diseases Community of Practice. Human parvovirus B19 in solid organ transplantation: guidelines from the American society of transplantation infectious

diseases community of practice. Clin Transpl 2019;33(9):e13535. https://doi.org/10.1111/ctr.13535.

7. Cossart YE, Field AM, Cant B, Widdows D. Parvovirus-like particles in human sera. Lancet Lond Engl. 1975;1(7898):72–3. https://doi.org/10.1016/s0140-6736(75)91074-0.

8. Bieri J, Ros C. Globoside is dispensable for parvovirus B19 entry but essential at a Postentry step for productive infection. J Virol. 2019;93(20):e00972–19. https://doi.org/10.1128/JVI.00972-19.

9. Corcoran A, Doyle S. Advances in the biology, diagnosis and host–pathogen interactions of parvovirus B19. J Med Microbiol. 2004;53(6):459–75. https://doi.org/10.1099/jmm.0.05485-0.

10. Flunker G, Peters A, Wiersbitzky S, Modrow S, Seidel W. Persistent parvovirus B19 infections in immunocompromised children. Med Microbiol Immunol (Berl). 1998;186(4):189–94. https://doi.org/10.1007/s004300050063.

11. Pure Red-Cell Aplasia of 10 Years' Duration Due to Persistent Parvovirus B19 Infection and Its Cure with Immunoglobulin Therapy. NEJM. https://www-nejm-org.ezproxy.library.wisc.edu/doi/10.1056/NEJM198908243210807. Accessed 3 February 2022

12. Eid AJ, Brown RA, Patel R, Razonable RR. Parvovirus B19 infection after transplantation: a review of 98 cases. Clin Infect Dis. 2006;43(1):40–8. https://doi.org/10.1086/504812.

13. Gosset C, Viglietti D, Hue K, Antoine C, Glotz D, Pillebout E. How many times can parvovirus B19-related anemia recur in solid organ transplant recipients? Transpl Infect Dis. 2012;14(5):E64–70. https://doi.org/10.1111/j.1399-3062.2012.00773.x.

Chapter 36
Checkpoint Inhibitors in Kidney Transplant Recipients and the Potential Risk of Rejection

Mohamed M. Ibrahim and Tarek Alhamad

Introduction

The immune system utilizes checkpoints to maintain self-tolerance or to prevent collateral tissue damage during an immune response. The immune system recognizes and eliminates cancer cells; however, cancers can develop multiple strategies to suppress this immune response. Cancers can alter the normal control mechanisms used to enforce peripheral self-tolerance, such as cytotoxic T-lymphocyte-associated protein 4 (CTLA4)-mediated suppression by regulatory T cells. They can also mitigate chronic inflammation through programmed cell death protein-1 (PD1)-mediated exhaustion of antitumor cytotoxic T lymphocytes.

Checkpoint inhibitors are a group of immunotherapy agents used for the treatment of malignancies that are not responsive to standard chemotherapeutic regimens. They are primarily used to treat metastatic skin cancers, renal cell carcinoma, and non-small-cell lung cancer. They mainly include anti-CTLA4 (ipilimumab) and anti- PD1 (pembrolizumab, nivolumab). They are effective in tumor regression for multiple malignancies in the general population; however, they are not thoroughly studied in kidney transplant recipients who are on lifelong immunosuppressive therapy.

The checkpoint inhibitors have the potential to upregulate a kidney transplant recipient's alloimmune response, which can lead to allograft rejection and even loss; thus, the benefits of treatment versus the potential risk of allograft rejection and loss should be considered carefully.

M. M. Ibrahim (✉) · T. Alhamad
Division of Nephrology, Department of Medicine, Washington University School of Medicine, St. Louis, MO, USA
e-mail: Mohamed.Ibrahim@som.umaryland.edu; talhamad@wustl.edu

© The Author(s), under exclusive license to Springer Nature Switzerland AG 2022

F. Aziz, S. Parajuli (eds.), *Complications in Kidney Transplantation*,
https://doi.org/10.1007/978-3-031-13569-9_36

Patient History

A 63-year-old man with a history of end-stage kidney disease due to hypertension underwent a deceased donor kidney transplantation. This was a 1A, 1B, and 2DR HLA mismatch. His maintenance immunosuppression medications were cyclosporine, azathioprine, and prednisone. Post-transplant, he developed multiple cutaneous squamous cell carcinoma (SCC) and melanoma that were surgically excised. Five years post-transplantation, he was diagnosed with SCC of unknown primary with notable metastases to the lungs and bone.

Question 1

What is the most likely risk factor of his cutaneous manifestations?

A. Azathioprine.
B. Supratherapeutic cyclosporine dose.
C. Prednisone.
D. Induction immunosuppression.

The correct answer is A.

Azathioprine photosensitizes the skin and causes the production of mutagenic reactive oxygen species. It increases the risk of squamous cell carcinoma and other skin cancers in organ transplant recipients [1]. The risk is increased with a longer duration of treatment and a higher cumulative dose of azathioprine [2].

Cyclosporine is another risk factor for skin cancers; however, the risk is not as high as azathioprine (choice B) [3]. There are no studies that show that long-term prednisone use is associated with skin cancers (choice C) [4]. Induction immunotherapy is less likely to be the cause of cancer in this patient given the timing of development of the complication (choice D).

His azathioprine was discontinued, and his cancer was treated with carboplatin and paclitaxel with complete regression of the metastatic lesions.

Clinical Course

Ten years later, he developed metastatic melanoma with unresectable inguinal, iliac, and aortocaval adenopathy. Biopsy of the inguinal node confirmed metastatic melanoma, and no BRAF mutation was detected. Cyclosporine was discontinued, and the patient was treated with four doses of ipilimumab (CTLA4 antibody), 3 mg/kg every 3 weeks.

Restaging showed interval progression with an increase in the size of retroperitoneal and inguinal adenopathy. Two weeks after the last dose of ipilimumab, pembrolizumab (PD1 antibody) was initiated with a stable baseline serum creatinine of 1.1 mg/dL. He experienced diarrhea that resolved after 3 days. Three weeks later and prior to the second dose of pembrolizumab, his serum creatinine increased to 8.7 mg/dL.

Question 2

What is the most likely cause of the increase in serum creatinine?

A. Diarrhea.
B. Acute BK nephropathy.
C. Acute rejection due to checkpoint inhibitors.
D. Acute interstitial nephritis.

The correct answer is C.

The rise in serum creatinine is likely due to acute rejection in the setting of immunosuppression withdrawal and the use of checkpoint inhibitors. The effect of checkpoint inhibitors is not directed only against malignant cells but also against other cells expressing foreign antigen such as the transplanted kidney. This could lead to acute cellular rejection and also activate pathways that lead to antibody-mediated rejection, especially in the setting of immunosuppression withdrawal.

Blockade of anti-CTLA4 and anti-PD1 increases the activation of T cells, not only against malignant cells but also against other cells expressing foreign antigen such as the transplanted kidney. This T cell activation could lead to acute cellular rejection. The activated CD4 T cells might lead to B cell proliferation and activation through costimulatory ligands (e.g., CD40L) and cytokines leading to antibody-mediated rejection, especially in the setting of immunosuppression withdrawal. B cells can also be activated as a direct effect on memory B cells expressing PD1 if there were prior sensitization of the transplanted organ or a decrease in immunosuppressive medications.

Diarrhea has resolved after 3 days; hence it is less likely to cause increased creatinine (choice A). Acute BK nephropathy (choice B) is a potential etiology of the increased creatinine; however, it should have improved with decreasing the immunosuppression with anticipated improvement in creatinine, which was not the case. Acute interstitial nephritis is a reported complication of checkpoint inhibitors; however, the patient is already on corticosteroids, and rejection is more likely to be the cause of his increased creatinine (choice D).

Further Clinical Course

A kidney allograft biopsy revealed mixed acute cellular rejection (severe tubulitis [t3], severe interstitial inflammation [i3], and intimal arteritis [v1]); Banff grade IIa with and areas of cortical necrosis. (Fig. 36.1).

Question 3

What is the next step in managing his rejection based on the biopsy findings?

A. Resume cyclosporine and antimetabolite with a higher cyclosporine peak level.
B. Give intravenous thymoglobulin 6 mg/kg.
C. Do plasmapheresis followed by intravenous immunoglobulins (IVIG).
D. Give intravenous methylprednisolone.

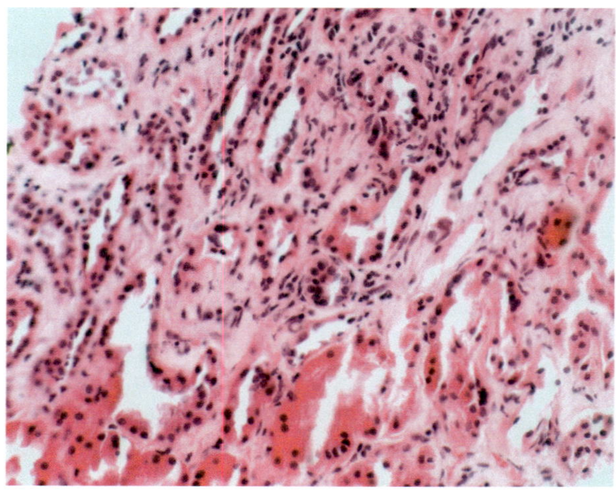

Fig. 36.1 Brightfield microphotograph of the kidney allograft biopsy. (Image courtesy of Parker Wilson, MD, PhD)

The correct answer is D.

The biopsy findings are consistent with rejection due to checkpoint inhibitor antibodies use; thus, managing the patient with more aggressive immunosuppression (choices A and B) would not be appropriate, especially in the setting of active malignancy. Doing plasmapheresis followed by IVIG would be appropriate in the setting of antibody-mediated rejection, which is not consistent with the biopsy findings (choice C).

The patient was treated with methylprednisolone 500 mg for three doses, and low-dose once-a-day tacrolimus was started. Kidney function slightly improved initially, but the patient eventually required the initiation of hemodialysis.

Discussion

The incidence of skin cancer is high in kidney transplant recipients compared to the general population, with higher morbidity and mortality [5]. This is mainly due to immunosuppression that increases ultraviolet-induced DNA damage. The most common skin cancer in transplant recipients is SCC.

The use of checkpoint inhibitor antibodies has resulted in significant improvements and demonstrated significant clinical benefits in tumor regression and prolonged stabilization of non-small cell lung cancer, melanoma, and renal cell cancer [6].

Checkpoint inhibitor antibodies are lifesaving treatments against many tumors. However, the benefits of treatment versus the potential risk of allograft rejection and loss should be considered carefully. According to one study, rejection reportedly developed at a median of 24 days after initiation of checkpoint inhibitor antibodies, and 80% of all rejection episodes occurred within the first 60 days following initiation [7]. The mechanism of checkpoint inhibitors and site of action of different check inhibitor antibodies are illustrated in Fig. 36.2.

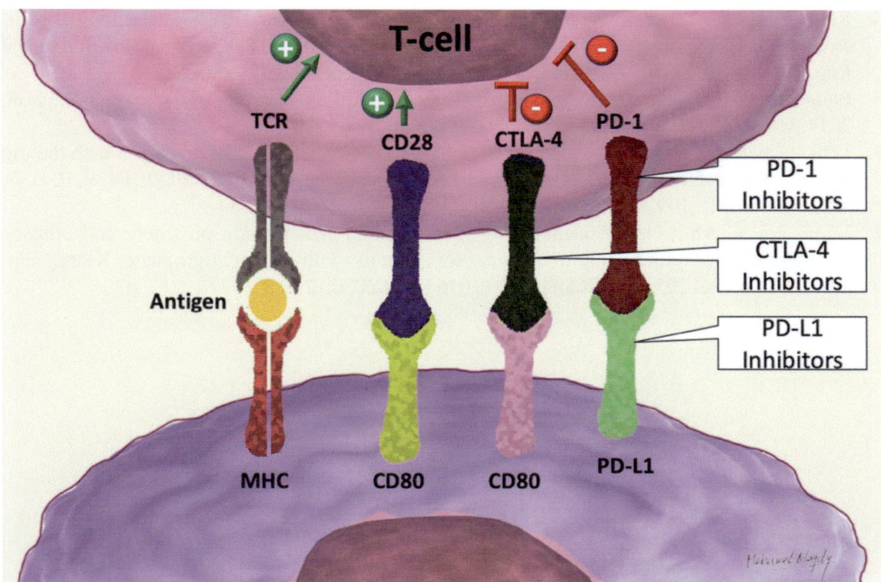

Fig. 36.2 Mechanism of checkpoint inhibitors

There are no specific recommendations to manage recipients receiving checkpoint inhibitors. Current suggested strategies include: (1) holding checkpoint inhibitors during acute kidney injury with possible reintroduction after creatinine has normalized and (2) increasing or restarting corticosteroids. As for the maintenance immunosuppression during checkpoint inhibitor therapy, some approaches include dual treatment of low calcineurin inhibitor dose and prednisone or switching to everolimus and higher dose prednisone. The limited studies we have so far demonstrated poor outcomes of kidney transplant recipients with metastatic cancer receiving checkpoint inhibitors.

References

1. Jiyad Z, Olsen CM, Burke MT, Isbel NM, Green AC. Azathioprine and risk of skin cancer in organ transplant recipients: systematic review and meta-analysis. Am J Transplant. 2016;16(12):3490–503. https://doi.org/10.1111/ajt.13863.
2. van den Reek JM, van Lümig PP, Janssen M, et al. Increased incidence of squamous cell carcinoma of the skin after long-term treatment with azathioprine in patients with auto-immune inflammatory rheumatic diseases. J Eur Acad Dermatol Venereol. 2014;28(1):27–33. https://doi.org/10.1111/jdv.12041.
3. Muellenhoff MW, Koo JY. Cyclosporine and skin cancer: an international dermatologic perspective over 25 years of experience. A comprehensive review and pursuit to define safe use of cyclosporine in dermatology. J Dermatolog Treat. 2012;23(4):290–304. https://doi.org/10.3109/09546634.2011.590792.

4. Ratib S, Burden-Teh E, Leonardi-Bee J, Harwood C, Bath-Hextall F. Long-term topical corticosteroid use and risk of skin cancer: a systematic review. JBI Database System Rev Implement Rep. 2018;16(6):1387–97. https://doi.org/10.11124/JBISRIR-2017-003393.
5. Ponticelli C, Cucchiari D, Bencini P. Skin cancer in kidney transplant recipients. J Nephrol. 2014;27(4):385–94. https://doi.org/10.1007/s40620-014-0098-4.
6. Venkatachalam K, Malone AF, Heady B, Santos RD, Alhamad T. Poor outcomes with the use of checkpoint inhibitors in kidney transplant recipients. Transplantation. 2020;104(5):1041–7. https://doi.org/10.1097/TP.0000000000002914.
7. Murakami N, Mulvaney P, Danesh M, et al. A multi-center study on safety and efficacy of immune checkpoint inhibitors in cancer patients with kidney transplant. Kidney Int. 2021;100(1):196–205. https://doi.org/10.1016/j.kint.2020.12.015.

Chapter 37
Angiotensin Type 1 Receptor Antibody-Mediated Rejection in a Kidney Transplant Recipient

Bonnie Ann Sarrell and Beatrice P. Concepcion

Introduction

Antibody-mediated rejection of a kidney allograft can be caused by non-human leukocyte antigen (HLA) antibodies such as Angiotensin Type 1 Receptor (AT1R) antibodies. AT1R antibodies are associated with an increased risk of early rejection and reduced long-term allograft survival. Although infrequent, a high index of suspicion for AT1R antibody-mediated rejection is warranted when there is histologic evidence of antibody-mediated injury in the allograft but no identified donor-specific HLA antibody. Treatment options for AT1R antibody-mediated rejection include the use of angiotensin receptor blockade in addition to other antibody-directed therapies.

Clinical History

A 46-year-old male with end-stage kidney disease due to hypertension and human immunodeficiency virus-associated nephropathy underwent deceased donor kidney transplantation. Transplant characteristics included a Kidney Donor Profile Index 13%, panel reactive antibody 0%, 3-antigen ABDR mismatch, and cytomegalovirus IgG donor positive/CMV IgG recipient negative. He received induction with basiliximab and intravenous (IV) methylprednisolone. The post-transplant course was complicated by delayed graft function. Ultrasound showed elevated resistive indices

B. A. Sarrell · B. P. Concepcion (✉)
Division of Nephrology and Hypertension, Vanderbilt University Medical Center, Nashville, TN, USA
e-mail: bonnie.a.sarrell@vumc.org; Beatrice.p.concepcion@vumc.org

© The Author(s), under exclusive license to Springer Nature Switzerland AG 2022

F. Aziz, S. Parajuli (eds.), *Complications in Kidney Transplantation*,
https://doi.org/10.1007/978-3-031-13569-9_37

but no other abnormalities. Donor-specific antibodies were not detected. Allograft biopsy on post-op day 11 showed one large artery with endothelialitis, two interlobular arteries with fibrinoid necrosis, severe microcirculation inflammation with severe peritubular capillaritis, and rare foci of interstitial hemorrhage. There was no glomerulitis, and C4d staining was negative. These biopsy findings were consistent with acute vascular rejection and antibody-mediated rejection. Testing for non-HLA antibodies revealed an elevated level of AT1R antibodies of 22 U/mL.

Question 1

AT1R antibodies are associated with what histologic type of rejection?

A. Cellular rejection.
B. Vascular rejection.
C. Antibody-mediated rejection.
D. Both B and C.

The correct answer is D.

The AT1R is a G-protein coupled receptor on endothelial cell surfaces. It is hypothesized that these receptors become exposed when damage occurs to the endothelium, allowing AT1R antibody formation and attachment. Once attached, the antibodies cause unchecked and sustained activation of the AT1R leading to vasoconstriction, matrix remodeling, and immune cell migration. The combined effect of these processes is accelerated HTN, reduced blood flow, fibrosis, and rejection [1]. The rejection may have histologic qualities of antibody-mediated rejection and/or vascular rejection and usually demonstrates low levels of complement deposition [2].

Question 2

Which antibody status portends the *worst* allograft survival?

A. No antibodies.
B. HLA antibodies alone.
C. Non-HLA antibodies alone.
D. HLA and non-HLA antibodies.

The correct answer is D.

The presence of donor-specific HLA antibodies correlates with reduced allograft survival. Studies also show that AT1R antibodies lead to higher rates of rejection (especially early rejection within the first 4–6 months) and decreased long-term allograft survival. For example, Giral et al. [3] showed that kidney transplant recipients with pre-transplant AT1R antibody titers > 10 U/mL had a higher risk of acute rejection within the first 4 months post-transplant, as well as a 2.6-fold higher risk of graft failure beyond 3 years. Lefaucher et al. [4] also supported the finding that AT1R antibodies are an independent risk factor for antibody-mediated rejection and vascular rejection lesions at 1 year. This study also showed a synergistic effect of AT1R antibodies and donor-specific HLA antibodies. Recipients with both types of antibodies present had the lowest 7-year allograft survival compared to recipients with no antibodies or with either type of antibody alone.

Question 3

Which of the following may be a treatment option for AT1R antibody-mediated rejection?

A. Rabbit anti-thymocyte globulin (rATG).
B. Plasma exchange.
C. Angiotensin receptor blockade.
D. Intravenous immunoglobulin (IVIG).
E. All of the above.

The correct answer is E.

There is very little evidence to guide the treatment of AT1R antibody-mediated rejection. A suggested approach is shown in Fig. 37.1. One specific therapy that may be beneficial is angiotensin receptor blocking medication that can competitively bind to the AT1R and reduce the binding of pathogenic antibodies. Other strategies that have been reported include induction with rATG, plasma exchange, and IVIG. In one study by Carrol et al. [5], 14 patients with AT1R antibody titers > 17.5 U/mL were treated with rATG induction (rather than anti-IL-2R alpha antibodies) and pre- and post-operative candesartan; plasma exchange was also performed pre-and post-operatively if AT1R antibody titers were > 25 U/mL. These patients experienced fewer rejection episodes compared to a similar cohort of patients prior to the use of these treatments. One case report [6] described successful desensitization for a patient with an AT1R antibody titer >40 U/mL. Therapy

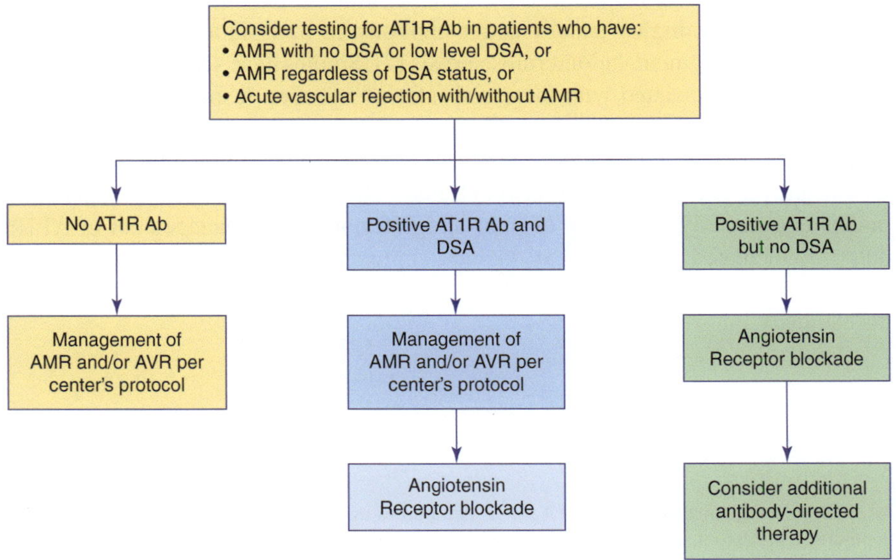

Fig. 37.1 Approach to the diagnosis and treatment of AT1R antibody-mediated rejection

consisted of pre-operative plasma exchange and IVIG followed by a few sessions of post-operative plasma exchange; allograft function was reasonable at 1-year post-transplant with a creatinine of 1.6 mg/dL.

Clinical Course

Our patient was treated for combined antibody-mediated and vascular rejection with IV methylprednisolone, plasma exchange, IVIG, rituximab, and rATG. Urine output improved, and creatinine down trended from 9.8 to 3.2 mg/dL by the time of hospital discharge. He was started on angiotensin receptor blockade. His creatinine continued to improve to a baseline of 1.4–1.6 mg/dL where it has remained nearly 1-year post-transplant.

Discussion

Anti-endothelial cell antibodies (AECA), such as AT1R antibodies, cause damage at the interface of the immune system and the transplanted organ—the vasculature/endothelial cells. AECAs were described as early as the 1980s in cases of rejection in HLA-identical pairs and when no identifiable donor-specific antibodies were present. AT1R antibodies seem to be more common in patients with younger age (44 years or less), higher panel reactive antibody, re-transplant, male gender, and history of focal segmental glomerulosclerosis [7]. Studies have suggested that AT1R antibodies are associated with increased rates of rejection (especially early rejection) and reduced long-term allograft survival. Many of these rejections are histologically consistent with vascular and/or antibody-mediated rejection but may be C4d negative. The combination of AT1R antibodies and donor-specific HLA antibodies is especially predictive of poor allograft outcomes. Management of AT1R antibody-mediated rejection may include angiotensin receptor blockade, plasma exchange, IVIG, rATG, or other therapies; there is a dearth of evidence to support a best strategy.

References

1. Philogene M, Johnson T, Vaught A, et al. Antibodies against angiotensin II type 1 and endothelin a receptors: relevance and pathogenicity. Hum Immunol. 2019;80:561–7. https://doi.org/10.1016/j.humimm.2019.04.012.
2. Dragun D, Muller D, Brasen J, et al. Angiotensin II type 1-receptor activating antibodies in renal allograft rejection. N Engl J Med. 2005;352:558–69.
3. Giral M, Foucher Y, Dufay A, et al. Pretransplant sensitization against angiotensin II type 1 receptor is a risk factor for acute rejection and graft loss. Am J Transplant. 2013;13:2567–76. https://doi.org/10.1111/ajt.12397.

4. Lefaucher C, Viglietti D, Bouatou Y, et al. Non-HLA agonistic anti-angiotensin II type 1 receptor antibodies induce a distinctive phenotype of antibody-mediated rejection in kidney transplant recipients. Kidney Int. 2019;96:189–201. https://doi.org/10.1016/j.kint.2019.01.030.
5. Carrol R, Riceman M, Hope C, et al. Angiotensin II type-1 receptor antibody (AT1Rab) associated with humoral rejection and the effect of peri operative plasma exchange and candesartan. Hum Immunol. 2016;77:1154–8. https://doi.org/10.1016/j.humimm.2016.08.009.
6. Karpel H, Ali N, Lawson N, et al. Successful A2 to B deceased donor kidney transplant after desensitization for high-strength non-HLA antibody made possible by utilizing a hepatitis C positive donor. Case Reports in Transplantation. 2020; https://doi.org/10.1155/2020/3591274.
7. Philogene M, Zhou S, Lonze B, et al. Pre-transplant screening for non-HLA antibodies: who should be tested? Hum Immunol. 2018;79:195–202. https://doi.org/10.1016/j.humimm.2018.02.001.

Chapter 38
Donor-Derived Cell-Free DNA

Neetika Garg

Introduction

Antibody-mediated rejection (ABMR) is the most common cause of late kidney allograft failure. Early diagnosis is critical to limiting the damage rejection does to the allograft. However, due to the compensatory adaptive ability of the kidney, changes in serum creatinine or proteinuria are usually late findings in the disease process. Kidney allograft biopsy provides only a one-time assessment. These considerations underscore the importance of non-invasive biomarkers for screening kidney transplant recipients for rejection and monitoring for response to the therapy. Donor-derived cell-free DNA (dd-cfDNA) is one such biomarker data that is rapidly emerging.

Patient History

A 49-year-old woman with a history of IgA nephropathy and multiple pregnancies underwent a deceased donor transplant. Her calculated panel reactive antibody was 100%, and her virtual crossmatch was positive for DR10 donor-specific antibody (DSA) at a mean fluorescent intensity (MFI) of approximately 3500. Her 3-month protocol biopsy did not show any evidence of rejection. She received anti-thymocyte globulin for induction immunosuppression, and her maintenance immunosuppression regimen consisted of tacrolimus with goal trough levels of 6–8 ng/mL,

N. Garg (✉)
Division of Nephrology, Department of Medicine, University of Wisconsin School of Medicine and Public Health, Madison, WI, USA
e-mail: ngarg@medicine.wisc.edu

© The Author(s), under exclusive license to Springer Nature Switzerland AG 2022
F. Aziz, S. Parajuli (eds.), *Complications in Kidney Transplantation*,
https://doi.org/10.1007/978-3-031-13569-9_38

mycophenolic acid 720 mg twice daily, and prednisone 5 mg once daily. Her renal function was excellent and stable, with a serum creatinine of 1.1 mg/dL and no detectable proteinuria. Her DSA levels remain unchanged with MFI around 3000. Given significant anxiety surrounding procedures and chronic pain history, the patient questioned the need for 1-year protocol biopsy. A dd-cfDNA was obtained using the AlloSure® assay (CareDx, Inc., Brisbane CA), which resulted at 2.4%.

Question 1

What is the most appropriate next step in management?

A. Continue to monitor dd-cfDNA.
B. Kidney allograft biopsy.
C. Treat with steroids.
D. Treat with steroids, intravenous immunoglobulin, and rituximab.

The correct answer is B.

Dd-cfDNA is a non-invasive biomarker increasingly used to monitor and screen kidney transplant recipients for rejection. However, although better for ABMR than T-cell mediated rejection (TCMR), the test's performance characteristics are modest [1]. Since dd-cfDNA is neither fully sensitive nor specific for the diagnosis of rejection; an allograft biopsy is usually performed to confirm the diagnosis. Monitoring dd-cfDNA (option A) would not be appropriate as it may lead to a delay in diagnosis of rejection. Treating without biopsy (options C and D) is also not appropriate as the dd-cfDNA result does not provide information regarding the type and severity of rejection or the health of the underlying parenchyma, which are relevant to making treatment decisions.

Clinical Course

The patient underwent a kidney allograft biopsy which revealed g2 ptc2 lesions, consistent with a diagnosis of ABMR.

Question 2

Which of the following is true about dd-cfDNA testing is correct?

A. It is 100% sensitive for ABMR.
B. It is 100% sensitive for TCMR.
C. It is more sensitive for ABMR than TCMR.
D. It is more sensitive for TCMR than ABMR.

The correct answer is C.

Multiple studies show that the dd-cfDNA levels are lower in TCMR than in ABMR. Dd-cfDNA is neither fully sensitive nor fully specific for either type of rejection. One plausible explanation is that endothelial injury in the form of glomerulitis or peri-tubular capillaritis is the hallmark of ABMR, and the dd-cfDNA is released from the endothelial cells directly into the circulation. Inflammation in

TCMR, especially in the lower grade lesions, is restricted to the tubulointerstitial compartment. Consequently, the dd-cfDNA is not instantly released into the bloodstream leading to lower measured fractions.

Discussion

Cf-DNA is non-encapsulated fragmented DNA that is continuously shed into the circulation as a result of cell turn-over [2]. Dd-cfDNA, usually expressed as a percentage, represents the proportion of cf-DNA originating from foreign tissue such as an allograft. Panels of single nucleotide polymorphisms (SNPs) with a high probability of being non-identical between any two individuals regardless of their ancestral origin are used to detect and quantify dd-cfDNA [3]. Higher levels suggest increased cell turnover and death. Half-life is only 30–90 min, making it ideal for longitudinal monitoring of the allograft for rejection.

Data on the use of dd-cfDNA for kidney transplant recipient surveillance is rapidly emerging. The Circulating Donor-Derived Cell-Free DNA in Blood for Diagnosing Active Rejection in Kidney Transplant Recipients (DART) Study prospectively evaluated the diagnostic performance of AlloSure for dd-cfDNA assessment in a sample of 107 biopsies with matched dd-cfDNA samples [1]. The area under the curve (AUC) for diagnosis of any rejection was 0.74, compared with an AUC of 0.54 for serum creatinine. Using the 1% cut-off to define test positivity, AlloSure had a sensitivity of 59%, specificity of 85%, positive predictive value (PPV) of 61%, and negative predictive value (NPV) of 84%. For ABMR diagnosis, the AUC was higher at 0.87, and the 1% threshold yielded a sensitivity of 81%, specificity of 83%, PPV of 44%, and NPV of 96%. Similarly, modest performance characteristics of AlloSure were confirmed in another single-center study by Huang et al. [4] The currently available version of AlloSure evaluates 405 SNPs with low linkage, distributed over 22 chromosomes. Prospera® (Natera, Inc., San Carlos) is another dd-cfDNA assay that uses 13,392 SNPs concentrated across four chromosomes. Sigdel et al. showed in a retrospective study of 217 biopsy-matched dd-cfDNA samples, 38 of which had active rejection, that the 1% threshold provided sensitivity, specificity, PPV, and NPV of 89%, 73%, 52%, and 95%, respectively [5]. A noteworthy difference for Prospera compared to the previously discussed AlloSure studies was that the median dd-cfDNA by Prospera did not differ between ABMR (2.2%), TCMR (2.7%), and mixed rejection (2.6%) groups ($p = 0.855$). AlloSure and Prospera are covered by Medicare, the insurance provider for the majority of transplant recipients in the United States. Transplant Rejection Allograft Check (TRAC)® (Viracor Eurofins, Inc., Lee's Summit, MO) is another available assay that analyses approximately 70,000 SNPs. Data on the utility of TRAC is emerging; the ongoing TRULO (TruGraf Long Term Clinical Outcomes) Study investigates the role of a combination of a gene expression assay named TruGraf and TRAC dd-cfDNA in kidney transplant recipients beyond the first year.

There are several reasons a biopsy is still needed after dd-cfDNA assessment becomes available. First, dd-cfDNA is not fully sensitive to rejection. Dd-cfDNA levels in TCMR are lower than in ABMR [6]. This is especially the case for border-line and Banff 1a TCMR lesions. Secondly, dd-cfDNA is not specific for rejection and can be elevated in several other diagnoses, including BK nephropathy, pyelone-phritis, etc. [1, 7] Additionally, dd-cfDNA does not provide important information regarding the type of rejection, the severity of rejection, and chronic changes in the renal parenchyma, which are important variables factoring into decision-making regarding treatment.

Approximately, a-tenth of the kidney transplant recipients in the United States have prior transplants, and due to sensitization, these patients are at increased risk of rejection. One investigation showed that while repeat recipients have somewhat higher baseline dd-cfDNA levels than first-time recipients (0.29% vs. 0.19%; $p < 0.001$), the fraction in both groups was still significantly lower than the 1% cut-off. Although limited by a small sample size, these data support the use of this test in repeat transplant recipients [8]. Interpretation in kidney allograft recipients with concomitant functioning non-kidney allografts is also challenging and depends on the type of allografts. Mean dd-cfDNA fractions of 0.19% and 0.52% have been documented in studies of stable simultaneous kidney-pancreas transplant recipients and stable heart kidney transplant recipients, respectively [9, 10]. On the other hand, due to high cell turnover in the liver, patients with liver and liver-kidney transplants are expected to have high levels even in the absence of pathology.

In summary, dd-cfDNA is an important biomarker that can assist in the earlier diagnosis of rejection and monitoring response to therapy. Further studies are needed to further understand its role in clinical management. In particular, the value of using dd-cfDNA concomitantly with other invasive and non-invasive tests needs to be explored.

References

1. Bloom RD, Bromberg JS, Poggio ED, Bunnapradist S, Langone AJ, Sood P, et al. Cell-free DNA and active rejection in kidney allografts. J Am Soc Nephrol. 2017;28:2221–32. https://doi.org/10.1681/ASN.2016091034.
2. Beck J, Urnovitz HB, Riggert J, Clerici M, Schutz E. Profile of the circulating DNA in apparently healthy individuals. Clin Chem. 2009;55:730–8. https://doi.org/10.1373/clinchem.2008.113597.
3. Grskovic M, Hiller D, Woodward RN. Performance of donor-derived cell-free DNA assays in kidney transplant patients. Transplantation. 2020;104:e135. https://doi.org/10.1097/TP.0000000000003084.
4. Huang E, Sethi S, Peng A, Najjar R, Mirocha J, Haas M, et al. Early clinical experience using donor-derived cell-free DNA to detect rejection in kidney transplant recipients. Am J Transplant. 2019;19:1663–70. https://doi.org/10.1111/ajt.15289.
5. Sigdel TK, Archila FA, Constantin T, Prins SA, Liberto J, Damm I, et al. Optimizing detection of kidney transplant injury by assessment of donor-derived cell-free DNA via massively multiplex PCR. J Clin Med. 2018;8 https://doi.org/10.3390/jcm8010019.

6. Wijtvliet V, Plaeke P, Abrams S, Hens N, Gielis EM, Hellemans R, et al. Donor-derived cell-free dna as a biomarker for rejection after kidney transplantation: a systematic review and meta-analysis. Transpl Int. 2020; https://doi.org/10.1111/tri.13753.
7. Goussous N, Xie W, Dawany N, Scalea JR, Bartosic A, Haririan A, et al. Donor-derived cell-free DNA in infections in kidney transplant recipients: case series. Transplant Direct. 2020;6:e568. https://doi.org/10.1097/TXD.0000000000001019.
8. Mehta SG, Chang JH, Alhamad T, Bromberg JS, Hiller DJ, Grskovic M, et al. Repeat kidney transplant recipients with active rejection have elevated donor-derived cell-free DNA. Am J Transplant. 2019;19:1597–8. https://doi.org/10.1111/ajt.15192.
9. Olaitan OKLS, Hetterman E, Peev V, Saltzberg S, Hertl M, Dholakia S. Donor-derived cell-free DNA for surveillance in simultaneous pancreas and kidney transplant recipients, can we extrapolate from kidney transplant alone? [abstract]. Am J Transplant. 2019;
10. Al-Saffar F, Hsu J, Fuentes J, Smith J, Fraschilla S, Stimpson E, et al. Combined AlloSure and AlloMap testing in multi-organ heart transplantation rejection surveillance. J Heart Lung Transplant. 2020;39:S260–1.

Chapter 39
Isolated Vascular Lesions in Renal Allograft Biopsy: How Do I Treat it?

Abd Assalam Qannus, Erika Bracamonte, and Bekir Tanriover

Introduction

Isolated vascular lesion (IvL) is an infrequent finding in allograft kidney biopsies, but it poses a challenge in terms of understanding its underlying pathophysiology and treatment decisions. In the following case, a discussion will cover these challenges and answer some related questions in light of recently published literature.

Patient History

A 74-year-old Caucasian man with advanced chronic kidney disease (CKD) presumed secondary to hypertension underwent a preemptive living unrelated kidney transplant in August 2021. The post-surgery course was unremarkable, and the patient had excellent allograft function (serum creatinine leveled off around 1 mg/dL). His pre-transplant calculated panel reactive antibody (cPRA) was 0%, and both T cell and B cell flow cross matches were negative. He received thymoglobulin (total 3 mg/kg) induction and was then maintained on triple immunosuppressive medications (tacrolimus, mycophenolic acid, and prednisone); he was slowly transitioned from tacrolimus to belatacept due to worsening tremors.

A. A. Qannus (✉) · B. Tanriover
Division of Nephrology, The University of Arizona, College of Medicine, Tucson, AZ, USA
e-mail: aqannus@arizona.edu; btanriover@arizona.edu

E. Bracamonte
Department Pathology, The University of Arizona, College of Medicine, Tucson, AZ, USA
e-mail: erikab@pathology.arizona.edu

© The Author(s), under exclusive license to Springer Nature Switzerland AG 2022
F. Aziz, S. Parajuli (eds.), *Complications in Kidney Transplantation*,
https://doi.org/10.1007/978-3-031-13569-9_39

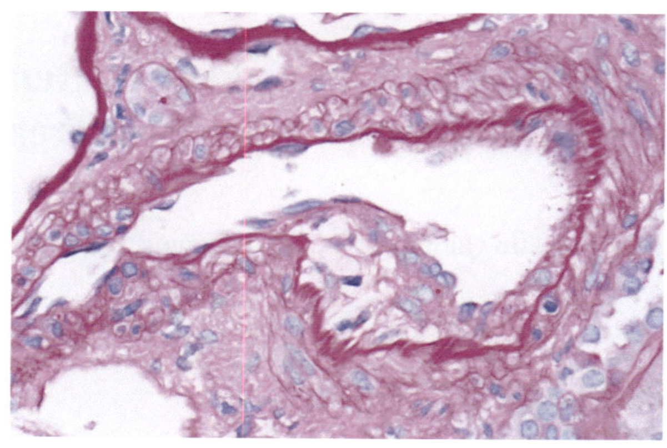

Fig. 39.1 A muscular artery shows reactive endothelial cells with edema, nuclear enlargement,and an activated lymphocyte beneath the cell surface (PAS, 400× magnification)

Four months after transplant, he was hospitalized with dyspnea, lower extremity edema, and worsening allograft function, which had developed 2 weeks prior. The patient was diagnosed with asthma exacerbation and congestive heart failure (based on abnormal BNP, chest XR, and ECHO-2D findings). The serum creatinine (Scr) on admission was 2 mg/dL and peaked at 3.2 mg/dL by day 7. Physical exam was remarkable for bibasilar crackles and lower extremities 3+ pitting edema, otherwise was normal. The patient was treated initially with low-dose solumedrol, fluticasone/salmeterol discus, and intravenous bumetanide. The basic workup revealed a urine analysis with 3–10 RBCs and spot urine protein/creatine ratio < 0.2 g/day. The renal allograft sonogram was negative for hydronephrosis, is a CMV, and BK blood PCRs testing was negative.

We suspected the possibility of acute rejection; thus, an allograft kidney biopsy was obtained, which showed isolated V1 lesions (see Fig. 39.1), focal endotheliitis, consistent with vascular rejection. Reported Banff scoring consisted of i0, t0, g0, v1, ci0, ct0, cg0, cv1, mm0, ah0, ptc0, C4d0.

Question 1

What is the differential diagnosis for the isolated V lesions?

A. Acute cellular rejection (ACR) Banff type 2A or above.
B. Antibody-mediated rejection (AMR).
C. A benign phenotype of acute rejection/or non-rejection phenomenon.
D. ANCA vasculitis.
E. Viral infection (COVID 19 vasculitis).
F. All the above.

The correct answer is F.

Isolated V lesions (IvL) could be a manifestation of any of the above choices.

As per the 2017 Banff classification, this lesion could be a part of findings in acute T cell mediated rejection (TCMR) type 2 and above, or AMR. The absence of other criteria of acute TCMR (like tubulitis or interstitial inflammation) or AMR (like glomerulitis, peritubular capillaritis, C4d staining) makes them less likely and requires more workup to prove the diagnosis.

The benign and mild course of some IvL cases and complete resolution intimal arteritis with steroid treatment made transplant physicians consider it as a benign phenotype of acute rejection or non-rejection phenomenon that happens in the setting of hidden ischemia-reperfusion phenomenon, especially if an injury happens early in the course after the transplant.

The debate about the nature and significance of this lesion is a challenging one; one school of thought considers the response to antirejection (steroid and T cell depleting) treatment as absolute evidence for the classic rejection etiology, whereas others argue that IvL represents a benign phenotype of acute rejection/or non-rejection phenomenon based on unconvincing tissue transcriptome analysis and resolution of the lesions with steroid treatment alone.

ANCA vasculitis (lack of pauci-immune necrotizing and crescentic glomerulo-nephritis) and vasculitis secondary to systemic viral infections are low on the list, but they should always be ruled out, especially in the COVID-19 pandemic, as there are several reports describing different forms of vasculitis affecting organ systems.

Question 2
What test would you order to diagnose the underlying disease?

A. Donor specific antibody (DSA).
B. Tissue gene expression with allograft biopsy.
C. ANCA panel.
D. Respirator viral panel (including COVID-19).
E. All the above.

The correct answer is E.

All the above. DSA should always be ordered when assessing any acute kidney injury (AKI) with suspicion of acute rejection (a Banff criterion for diagnosing AMR).

Tissue gene expression "transcriptome analysis" usually shows remarkable selected gene upregulation in TCMR. ANCA serology and a respiratory viral panel including COVID 19 PCR will help to rule out systemic causes of vasculitis.

Back to our Patient

The rest of the workup, including DSA, ANCA panel, and respiratory viral panel including COVID-19 PCR, was negative. No samples were sent for transcriptome analysis due to inpatient status (reimbursement related restrictions).

Question 3

How should we treat isolated V lesions?

A. Monitor renal function and re-biopsy in 2 weeks.
B. Pulse steroids alone.
C. Pulse steroids IV and thymoglobulin.
D. Plasmapheresis, IVIG, and steroids.

The correct answer is C.

Most cases are still treated as an acute TCMR. The type and intensity of treatment (pulse steroids vs. thymoglobulin) should be guided by the severity of AKI, the timing of the injury, and patient characteristics. Some cases show complete clinical and pathological resolution with pulse steroids only. Number 1 could have been correct if the lesions found on protocol biopsies did not show AKI. Number 4 could have been correct if the IvL was found in the setting of AMR.

Patient Hospital Course

We decided to treat our patient, given the severity of AKI, with thymoglobulin and IV steroids. He received about 4.5 mg/kg over 4 days. His Scr started to improve 3 days into the treatment and returned to baseline after 10 days. A repeat kidney biopsy 7 days later showed complete resolution of the IvL (Fig. 39.2). His hospital course was complicated with partial small bowel obstruction after completing the thymoglobulin course, which required exploratory laparotomy for lysis of adhesions, delaying discharge 2 weeks. His post-rejection treatment donor-derived cell-free DNA (dd cf-DNA) was 0.12% (normal < 1%) in February 2022, his baseline post-transplant dd cf-DNA in October 2021 was 0.16%.

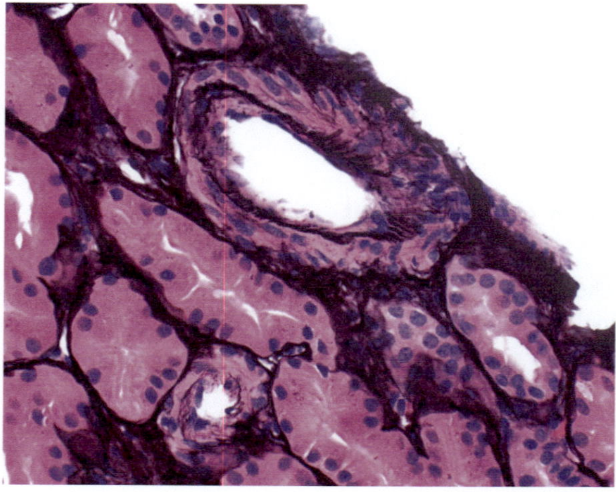

Fig. 39.2 Muscular arteries and arterioles show decreased endothelial cell reactivity, and no inflammation (Jones silver, 400× magnification)

Discussion

Isolated vascular lesions (IvL) were first described in 2009 [1] as intimal arteritis or endotheliitis in the absence of other or any tissue's rejection criteria. It should be distinguished from classical acute vascular rejection, which could a part of cellular (TCMR II and III) [2] or humoral rejection (AMR) (Banff 2013), which represents a poor prognosis of the renal allograft [3].

Vascular lesions could be seen in three major phenotypes of acute vascular rejection (AMR, TCMR, and isolated v-lesion) [4, 5]. Recent studies showed that the IvL phenotype has the most favorable outcome among the three [5, 6]. The IvL could result from allograft intimal injury rather than a classical acute rejection, especially in cases early after transplant without DSA [7]. It is important to note that patients with IvL still have a higher risk of allograft failure than patients without rejection [8].

The absence of other pathological findings on allograft biopsy, negative DSA, the minimal or no activity on the transcriptomic analysis, and the quick response to steroid treatment are clues to IvL non-rejection benign pathology. Some still believe that the IvL is because of hidden ischemia-reperfusion injury [7]. However, they could not provide good evidence to support it.

We recommend sending extended workup for vasculitis, including ANCA serology [9], respiratory viral panel [10], COVID-19 PCR [11], tissue gene expression testing [7, 12]. However, it should be done on fresh allograft tissue, and not all centers do it routinely on biopsies due to insurance coverage and reimbursement concerns.

Although IvL could be a benign and self-limited injury, we believe it should be treated, especially if associated with AKI and found on a cause biopsy. The treatment could be milder than the one used for classical AMVR and TCMR, and pulse steroids or a reduced dose of thymoglobulin could be enough [13]. The decision on which one to use should be based on the patient's characteristics, the severity of IvL V2 and V3 [14], and the risk of adverse events. Incidental IvL found on protocol biopsies without AKI can be monitored closely with Scr, dd cf-DNA testing, blood gene expression testing, and/or follow-up the allograft biopsy to document the resolution of the lesions [15].

References

1. Sis B, Mengel M, Haas M, Colvin RB, Halloran PF, Racusen LC, Solez K, Baldwin WM 3rd, Bracamonte ER, Broecker V, Cosio F, Demetris AJ, Drachenberg C, Einecke G, Gloor J, Glotz D, Kraus E, Legendre C, Liapis H, Mannon RB, Nankivell BJ, Nickeleit V, Papadimitriou JC, Randhawa P, Regele H, Renaudin K, Rodriguez ER, Seron D, Seshan S, Suthanthiran M, Wasowska BA, Zachary A, Zeevi A. Banff '09 meeting report: antibody-mediated graft deterioration and implementation of Banff working groups. Am J Transplant. 2010;10(3):464–71. https://doi.org/10.1111/j.1600-6143.2009.02987.x. Epub 2010 Jan 29
2. Racusen LC, Solez K, Colvin RB, Bonsib SM, Castro MC, Cavallo T, Croker BP, Demetris AJ, Drachenberg CB, Fogo AB, Furness P, Gaber LW, Gibson IW, Glotz D, Goldberg JC, Grande J, Halloran PF, Hansen HE, Hartley B, Hayry PJ, Hill CM, Hoffman EO, Hunsicker LG,

Lindblad AS, Yamaguchi Y, et al. The Banff 97 working classification of renal allograft pathology. Kidney Int. 1999;55(2):713–23. https://doi.org/10.1046/j.1523-1755.1999.00299.x.

3. Haas M, Sis B, Racusen LC, Solez K, Glotz D, Colvin RB, Castro MC, David DS, David-Neto E, Bagnasco SM, Cendales LC, Cornell LD, Demetris AJ, Drachenberg CB, Farver CF, Farris AB 3rd, Gibson IW, Kraus E, Liapis H, Loupy A, Nickeleit V, Randhawa P, Rodriguez ER, Rush D, Smith RN, Tan CD, Wallace WD, Mengel M. Banff meeting report writing committee. Banff 2013 meeting report: inclusion of c4d-negative antibody-mediated rejection and antibody-associated arterial lesions. Am J Transplant. 2014;14(2):272–83. https://doi.org/10.1111/ajt.12590. Erratum in: Am J Transplant. 2015 Oct;15(10):2784. Rangel, Erika [corrected to Rangel, Erika B]

4. Shimizu T, Tanabe T, Shirakawa H, Omoto K, Ishida H, Tanabe K. Acute vascular rejection after renal transplantation and isolated v-lesion. Clin Transpl. 2012;26(suppl 24):2–8.

5. Rabant M, Boullenger F, Gnemmi V, Pellé G, Glowacki F, Hertig A, Brocheriou I, Suberbielle C, Taupin JL, Anglicheau D, Legendre C, Duong Van Huyen JP, Buob D. Isolated v-lesion in kidney transplant recipients: characteristics, association with DSA, and histological follow-up. Am J Transplant. 2018;18(4):972–81. https://doi.org/10.1111/ajt.14617. Epub 2018 Jan 12

6. Mikhail D, Chan E, Sharma H, Kleinsteuber D, Wei J, Rim C, Henein M, Sener A, Jevnikar AM, Gabril M, Moussa M, Luke PP. Clinical significance of isolated V1 arteritis in renal transplantation. Transplant Proc. 2021;53(5):1570–5. https://www.sciencedirect.com/science/article/pii/S0041134521002207. https://doi.org/10.1016/j.transproceed.2021.03.027.

7. Wohlfahrtova M, Hruba P, Novotny M, Klema J, Krejcik Z, Stranecky V, Honsova E, Vichova P, Viklicky O. Isolated v-lesion early after kidney transplantation may not truly represent a rejection. Transplantation. 2018;102:S267–8. https://doi.org/10.1097/01.tp.0000542958.03051.ea.

8. Sis B, Bagnasco SM, Cornell LD, Randhawa P, Haas M, Lategan B, Magil AB, Herzenberg AM, Gibson IW, Kuperman M, Sasaki K, Kraus ES, Banff Working Group. Isolated endarteritis and kidney transplant survival: a multicenter collaborative study. J Am Soc Nephrol. 2015;26(5):1216–27. https://doi.org/10.1681/ASN.2014020157. Epub 2014 Nov 7. PMID: 25381427; PMCID: PMC4413758

9. Cosmes PG, Gómez PF, Lewczuk K, González MR, Ferreras ER, Fernández GT. Recurrence of ANCA-associated vasculitis in a patient with kidney trasplant. Nefrología (English Edition). 2016;36(2):176–80. https://doi.org/10.1016/j.nefroe.2016.03.006.

10. Choucair J. Infectious Causes of vasculitis. In: Sakkas LI, Katsiari C, editors. Updates in the Diagnosis and Treatment of Vasculitis [Internet]. London: IntechOpen; 2013 [cited 2022 Feb 15]. Available from: https://www.intechopen.com/chapters/42990. https://doi.org/10.5772/55189.

11. Kronbichler A, Geetha D, Smith RM, Egan AC, Bajema IM, Schönermarck U, Mahr A, Anders HJ, Bruchfeld A, Cid MC, Jayne DRW. The COVID-19 pandemic and ANCA-associated vasculitis–reports from the EUVAS meeting and EUVAS education forum. Autoimmun Rev. 2021;20(12):102986. https://doi.org/10.1016/j.autrev.2021.102986. Epub 2021 Oct 28. PMID: 34718165; PMCID: PMC8552556

12. Mueller TF, Einecke G, Reeve J, Sis B, Mengel M, Jhangri GS, Bunnag S, Cruz J, Wishart D, Meng C, Broderick G, Kaplan B, Halloran PF. Microarray analysis of rejection in human kidney transplants using pathogenesis-based transcript sets. Am J Transplant. 2007;7(12):2712–22. https://doi.org/10.1111/j.1600-6143.2007.02005.x.

13. Reeve J, Sellarés J, Mengel M, Sis B, Skene A, Hidalgo L, de Freitas DG, Famulski KS, Halloran PF. Molecular diagnosis of T cell-mediated rejection in human kidney transplant biopsies. Am J Transplant. 2013;13(3):645–55. https://doi.org/10.1111/ajt.12079. Epub 2013 Jan 28

14. Wu K, Budde K, Lu H, et al. The severity of acute cellular rejection defined by Banff classification is associated with kidney allograft outcomes. Transplantation. 2014;97(11):1146–54.

15. Moinuddin I, Thajudeen B, Sussman A, Madhrira M, Bracamonte E, Popovtzer M, Kadambi PV. Early posttransplant isolated v1 lesion does not need to be treated and does not lead to increased fibrosis. Case Reports in Transplantation. 2016;2016:3.

Chapter 40
Post-Transplant Idiopathic Immune Complex Glomerulonephritis

Keshvi Chauhan and Fahad Aziz

Introduction

Membranoproliferative Glomerulonephritis (MPGN) is one of the important causes of end-stage kidney disease (ESKD), leading to kidney transplants. Moreover, the occurrence of MPGN in kidney allograft negatively impacts its survival. The reclassification of MPGN with immunofluorescence has transformed the way we diagnose and treat the condition in kidney transplant recipients. The optimal treatment of post-transplant idiopathic immune complex-mediated MPGN (IC-MPGN) is not established. In this chapter, we have attempted to highlight a classic case of de novo idiopathic IC-MPGN in a kidney allograft recipient. He achieved successful remission with rituximab and appropriate up-titration of immunosuppression.

Patient History

A 53-year-old male with a history of chronic kidney disease stage 5, due to membranous nephropathy, underwent a deceased donor kidney transplantation. At the time of transplant, his panel reactive antibody (PRA) was 0%, and he had no preformed donor-specific antibodies (DSA). He received induction with anti-thymocyte globulin. His maintenance immunosuppression included tacrolimus twice a day (target trough 6–8 ng/mL), mycophenolate sodium 720 mg twice a day, and prednisone 5 mg daily. He achieved a baseline creatinine of 1.2 mg/dL with eGFR of

K. Chauhan (✉) · F. Aziz
Department of Medicine, University of Wisconsin—Madison School of Medicine and Public Health, University of Wisconsin Hospital and Clinics, Madison, WI, USA
e-mail: kchauhan@uwhealth.org; faziz@wisc.edu

© The Author(s), under exclusive license to Springer Nature Switzerland AG 2022

F. Aziz, S. Parajuli (eds.), *Complications in Kidney Transplantation*,
https://doi.org/10.1007/978-3-031-13569-9_40

60 mL/min/1.73m^2. His post-transplant course was unremarkable. Nine years after the transplant, he developed new proteinuria. His urine protein-creatinine ratio was more than 1 g/g. His creatinine and eGFR stayed at the baseline. He presented for further management.

Question 1
what should be the next step in the management?

A. Start lisinopril.
B. Steroid pulse.
C. Transplant kidney biopsy.
D. Start spironolactone.

The correct answer is C.

There can be multiple reasons for late proteinuria in kidney transplant recipients, including recurrence of glomerulonephritis, transplant glomerulopathy (TG), acute antibody-mediated rejection, and chronic antibody-mediated rejections. The treatment should be focused on the histological diagnosis. Though the addition of lisinopril and spironolactone can help reduce proteinuria, they would not treat the underlying disease process.

Further Course

The patient underwent a biopsy of the kidney allograft. His biopsy was negative for rejection (t0, g0, ptc0, cg0, c4d0) but showed glomerular hypercellularity on light microscopy (Fig. 40.1). However, the electron microscopy showed segmental mild endocapillary hypercellularity and segmental basement membrane double contours. There were small mesangial electron-dense deposits, segmental subendothelial deposits, and scattered subepithelial deposits (Fig. 40.2). The immunofluorescence showed granular staining for IgG, IgM, IgA, C3, and C1q.

With the diagnosis of immune complex-mediated glomerulonephritis (IC-MPGN), he underwent an extensive workup to look for infections, autoimmune disease, and monoclonal gammopathies as a cause of IC-MPGN. The workup showed normal antinuclear antibody (ANA), double standard DNA (dsDNA), C3 and C4 levels. Infectious workup for hepatitis, HIV, CMV, BKV, EBV, and adenovirus was negative. The workup was negative for monoclonal gammopathies, including serum protein electrophoresis (SPEP) and urine protein electrophoresis (UPEP). With a negative workup, it was labeled as idiopathic IC-MPGN.

Fig. 40.1 Hypercellularity of glomerulus on light microscopy

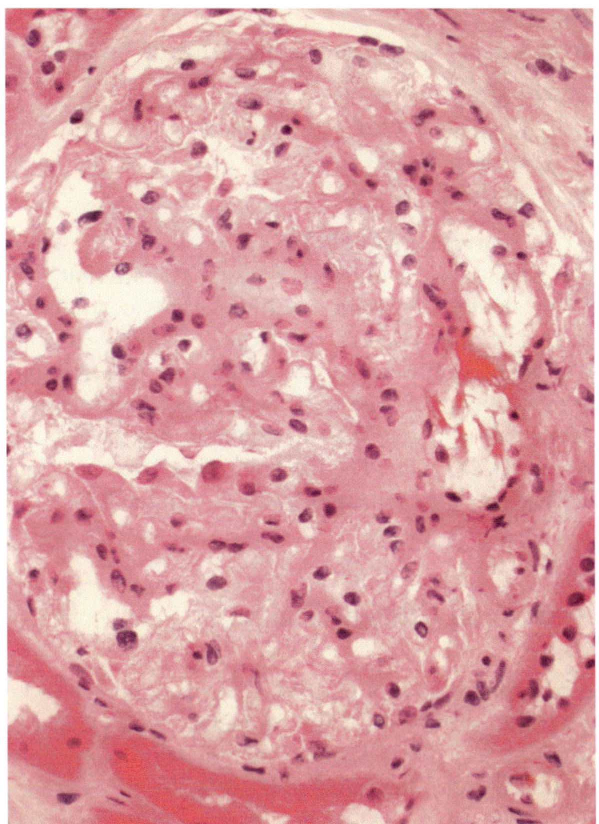

Fig. 40.2 Election microscopy showing mesangial electron-dense deposits, segmental subendothelial deposits, and scattered subepithelial deposits

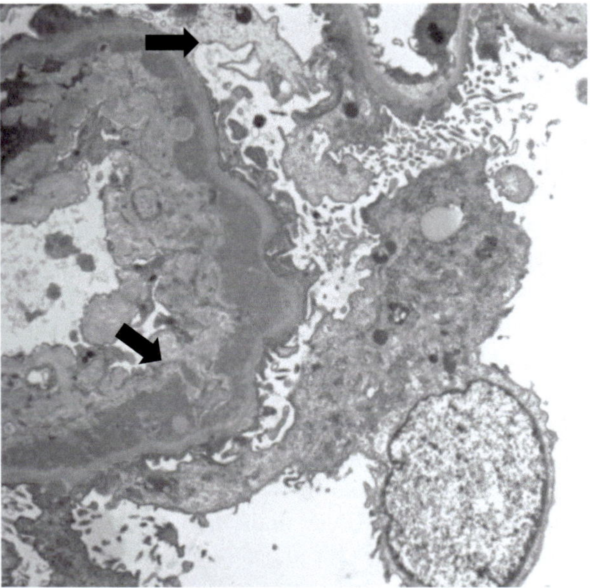

Question 2

What will be the next step in managing IC-MPGN?

A. Observe.
B. Rituximab.
C. Lisinopril.
D. Belatacept.

The correct answer is B.

The optimal treatment of de novo or recurrent IC-MPGN is not known. However, a few studies suggested that treating this condition with rituximab may improve graft outcomes [1]. The recurrence of MPGN or idiopathic MPGN is associated with significantly worse graft outcomes. Observation alone would not be a good option (option A). Similarly, an increase in immunosuppression by adding belatacept is not shown to improve the graft outcomes in patients with recurrence or de novo MPGN (option D). The addition of lisinopril can improve proteinuria, but it is not the primary treatment of MPGN (Option C).

Additional Clinical Course

After the diagnosis of IC-MPGN, the patient received two doses of rituximab 1 gm 2 weeks apart to treat ICGN of unclear etiology, and the baseline immunosuppression was increased. Within 3 months after receiving rituximab, his urine protein-creatinine ratio decreased to 0.2 g/g. At 1 year follow-up after the diagnosis of ICGN, the patient had stable creatinine at 1.2 mg/dL with eGFR of 60 mL/min/m^2 and urine protein-creatinine ratio of 0.1 g/g.

Discussion

MPGN is a disease defined by a pattern of glomerular injury observed by light microscopy. MPGN was traditionally classified as type I MPGN (idiopathic), type II MPGN, and type III MPGN (secondary due to infection or autoimmune disease) [2]. However, a newer classification of MPGN has been proposed by Sethi et al. [3]. It classifies MPGN based on immunofluorescence into immune complex GN and complement-mediated GN. Most of the studies in post-transplant MPGN are based on the older classification of MPGN. Both type I and type II MPGN in the older classification can be a complement-mediated disease that is more likely to recur post-transplant. Idiopathic MPGN and MPGN from complement dysregulation can reoccur in transplant kidneys in 19–48% of patients with MPGN as the primary cause of their renal failure [4–9]. The reported incidence is even higher in children [10]. Idiopathic IC-MPGN in the transplanted kidney is not well described in the literature. Risk factors for idiopathic IC-MPGN, treatment, and graft outcomes are also unknown.

Recurrence or de novo MPGN in the transplanted kidney is reported to have significant deleterious effects on graft survival, especially in the presence of crescents [11, 12]. Alasfar et al. retrospectively reviewed 34 cases of MPGN who underwent a kidney transplant. In this cohort, 89% of patients with pre-transplant MPGN had immune complex-mediated, and 11% had complement-mediated MPGN. Recurrence was detected in 45% of the patients. Half of the patients with recurrence lost their allografts [1]. In another series of 68 patients who underwent kidney transplants for MPGN as the primary cause of ESKD, one-fourth of the patients had a recurrence of MPGN, and 56% of the patients with recurrence lost their allografts [13]. In contrast, only 27% of patients had glomerulonephritis as the cause of their ESKD, but none of them had MPGN as the cause of their ESKD. In our series, 34% of patients lost their allograft. Several other reports found that post-transplant MPGN diagnosis occurs 1–2 years post-transplant [1, 14, 15].

The optimal treatment of de novo or recurrent IC-MPGN is not known. Treatment of recurrent idiopathic MPGN was disappointing in the past, with recurrence usually associated with graft loss [15]. In the series by Alasfar et al., 14 out of 18 patients received treatment. Four patients received steroids alone, and only 25% of them responded. Eight patients received rituximab with or without plasmapheresis, and only 37.5% responded to the treatment [1]. However, in our experience, the treatment with rituximab is associated with significantly better graft outcomes. We also found a trend toward improved outcomes in patients treated with steroids alone.

Although not well described in the literature, post-transplant idiopathic IC-MPGN is an important cause of kidney allograft dysfunction. Aggressive treatment of the IC-MPGN with rituximab and appropriate up-titration in the immunosuppression can improve graft outcomes. Further, studies are needed to determine the risk factors, diagnosis, management, and long-term outcomes in kidney allograft recipients with IC-MPGN.

References

1. Alasfar S, Carter-Monroe N, Rosenberg AZ, Montgomery RA, Alachkar N. Membranoproliferative glomerulonephritis recurrence after kidney transplantation: using the new classification. BMC Nephrol. 2016;17:7.
2. RJ G. Membranoproliferative glomerulonephritis. In: Molony DA CJ, editor. Evidence-based nephrology. London: Wiley-Blackwell; 2009. p. 183–96.
3. Sethi S, Fervenza FC. Membranoproliferative glomerulonephritis: pathogenetic heterogeneity and proposal for a new classification. Semin Nephrol. 2011;31(4):341–8.
4. Denton MD, Singh AK. Recurrent and de novo glomerulonephritis in the renal allograft. Semin Nephrol. 2000;20(2):164–75.
5. Floege J. Recurrent glomerulonephritis following renal transplantation: an update. Nephrol Dial Transplant. 2003;18(7):1260–5.
6. Mathew TH. Recurrence of disease following renal transplantation. Am J Kidney Dis. 1988;12(2):85–96.
7. Cameron JS. Glomerulonephritis in renal transplants. Transplantation. 1982;34(5):237–45.
8. Glicklich D, Matas AJ, Sablay LB, Senitzer D, Tellis VA, Soberman R, et al. Recurrent membranoproliferative glomerulonephritis type 1 in successive renal transplants. Am J Nephrol. 1987;7(2):143–9.

9. Andresdottir MB, Assmann KJ, Hoitsma AJ, Koene RA, Wetzels JF. Recurrence of type I membranoproliferative glomerulonephritis after renal transplantation: analysis of the incidence, risk factors, and impact on graft survival. Transplantation. 1997;63(11):1628–33.

10. Habib R, Antignac C, Hinglais N, Gagnadoux MF, Broyer M. Glomerular lesions in the transplanted kidney in children. Am J Kidney Dis. 1987;10(3):198–207.

11. Little MA, Dupont P, Campbell E, Dorman A, Walshe JJ. Severity of primary MPGN, rather than MPGN type, determines renal survival and post-transplantation recurrence risk. Kidney Int. 2006;69(3):504–11.

12. Allen PJ, Chadban SJ, Craig JC, Lim WH, Allen RDM, Clayton PA, et al. Recurrent glomerulonephritis after kidney transplantation: risk factors and allograft outcomes. Kidney Int. 2017;92(2):461–9.

13. Moroni G, Casati C, Quaglini S, Gallelli B, Banfi G, Montagnino G, et al. Membranoproliferative glomerulonephritis type I in renal transplantation patients: a single-center study of a cohort of 68 renal transplants followed up for 11 years. Transplantation. 2011;91(11):1233–9.

14. Green H, Rahamimov R, Rozen-Zvi B, Pertzov B, Tobar A, Lichtenberg S, et al. Recurrent membranoproliferative glomerulonephritis type I after kidney transplantation: a 17-year single-center experience. Transplantation. 2015;99(6):1172–7.

15. Lorenz EC, Sethi S, Leung N, Dispenzieri A, Fervenza FC, Cosio FG. Recurrent membranoproliferative glomerulonephritis after kidney transplantation. Kidney Int. 2010;77(8):721–8.

Chapter 41
Recurrent Thrombotic Microangiopathy in a Kidney Transplant Recipient

Jefferson L. Triozzi and Saed Shawar

Introduction

The development of thrombotic microangiopathy (TMA) in the kidney allograft may be related to various primary or secondary causes. These include thrombotic thrombocytopenic purpura, drug-induced TMA, infection-associated TMA, antibody-mediated rejection, and complement-mediated TMA, among others. Thrombotic microangiopathy is a histopathologic diagnosis of the microvasculature, including vessel wall thickening, platelet thrombosis, and luminal obstruction. Clinically, this histopathologic process may be limited to the kidney or may result in systemic manifestations such as microangiopathic hemolytic anemia, thrombocytopenia, and end-organ damage. In the minority of cases, thrombotic microangiopathy in the kidney allograft represents recurrence of the disease affecting the native kidney. In most cases, thrombotic microangiopathy develops de novo. In this case of recurrent thrombotic microangiopathy in a kidney transplant recipient, the evaluation and treatment of post-transplant TMA are reviewed.

Clinical History

A 25-year-old woman initially presented with preeclampsia at 31 weeks of gestation with hypertension, proteinuria, and acute kidney injury requiring hemodialysis. The patient underwent an emergency cesarean section with an improvement in her blood

J. L. Triozzi · S. Shawar (✉)
Division of Nephrology and Hypertension, Vanderbilt University Medical Center1161 21st Ave S, Nashville, TN, USA
e-mail: Jefferson.triozzi@vumc.org; Saed.h.shawar@vumc.org

© The Author(s), under exclusive license to Springer Nature Switzerland AG 2022

F. Aziz, S. Parajuli (eds.), *Complications in Kidney Transplantation*,
https://doi.org/10.1007/978-3-031-13569-9_41

pressure. However, her acute kidney injury did not improve post-partum, and she subsequently underwent a kidney biopsy. This revealed thrombotic microangiopathy, which was attributed to hypertension and preeclampsia. She remained on dialysis for 6 months until she received a living-related donor kidney transplant. The transplant had immediate graft function, and she was discharged on standard maintenance immunosuppression with tacrolimus and mycophenolate mofetil. She remained in good health with a baseline serum creatinine of 0.8–1 mg/dL until 5 months after her transplant, when she presented with severe anemia and acute kidney injury. She was afebrile and hypertensive to 155/115 mmHg with normal oxygen saturation on room air. She was well-appearing and had a normal cardiopulmonary examination. A basic metabolic profile was notable for a serum creatinine of 14.8 mg/dL.

A complete blood count was notable for a white blood cell count of 1200/μL, hemoglobin of 3.8 g/dL, and platelet count of 94/μL. A peripheral blood smear demonstrated 4+ schistocytes per high-powered field. Lactate dehydrogenase was 950 U/L, haptoglobin < 8 mg/dL, fibrinogen 509 mg/dL, reticulocyte count 7.2%. Complement factor 3 (C3) was decreased, and complement factor 4 (C4) was normal. Vitamin B12 and folate levels, Coombs test, G6PD activity, and ADAMTS13 activity were normal. A kidney biopsy was planned.

Question 1

What is the most likely finding on kidney biopsy?

A. Focal and segmental glomerulosclerosis.
B. Glomerulitis and peritubular capillaritis.
C. Interstitial lymphocytic infiltrate and tubulitis.
D. Microvascular thrombosis.

The correct answer is D.

The patient's prior history of thrombotic microangiopathy (TMA), along with the presence of hemolytic anemia and thrombocytopenia, is highly suspicious for TMA. TMA is defined by a histopathological lesion of the microvasculature which includes vessel wall thickening, platelet thrombosis, and luminal obstruction [1]. TMA causes platelet consumption and red blood cell shearing in the microvasculature resulting in a clinical triad of thrombocytopenia, microangiopathic hemolytic anemia with schistocyte formation, and end-organ damage with acute kidney injury.

Additional Clinical History

A repeat kidney biopsy was performed and demonstrated recurrence of thrombotic microangiopathy without evidence of cellular or antibody-mediated allograft rejection.

Question 2
What is the most likely cause of TMA in this patient?

A. Complement-mediated TMA.
B. Hemolytic uremic syndrome.
C. Thrombotic thrombocytopenic purpura.
D. Chronic allograft nephropathy.

The correct answer is A.

The recurrence of TMA after kidney transplantation raises suspicion for an underlying abnormality of complement activity [2]. There are primary and secondary forms of TMA, which are indistinguishable by histopathologic findings alone [3]. Primary causes of TMA include thrombotic thrombocytopenic purpura (TTP), hemolytic uremic syndrome (HUS), and complement-mediated TMA (also known as atypical HUS). Secondary causes of TMA include a range of acute and chronic conditions, including hypertension, infection, malignancy, autoimmune disease, pregnancy, preeclampsia, and drugs [4]. Some secondary causes of TMA are related to kidney transplantation, including calcineurin inhibitors, antibody-mediated rejection, and ischemia-reperfusion injury of solid organ transplantation itself. However, it is thought that secondary causes of TMA may trigger an underlying complement abnormality [5]. Advancements in TMA genetic testing allow for identifying specific complement factor mutants in approximately two-thirds of patients with complement-mediated TMA. However, it is important to remember that mutations are not detected in 40–50% of cases; hence the absence of an identified mutation does not exclude complement-mediated TMA.

Additional Clinical History

Genetic testing for complement mutations, antibodies, and activity was sent. The patient was initially started on empiric treatment with steroids and therapeutic plasma exchange. Given her clinical presentation and the previous native renal biopsy result, she was suspected of having an underlying complement dysregulation, and eculizumab was started.

Discussion

Thrombotic microangiopathy (TMA) is a group of disorders defined by a common histopathologic finding of endothelial damage leading to microvascular thromboses. Clinically, it is a syndrome characterized by microangiopathic hemolytic anemia (MAHA), thrombocytopenia, and end-organ damage from microvascular thrombi causing acute kidney injury with or without neurological symptoms and gastroenterology symptoms. TMA in the setting of kidney transplantation can commonly

(40%) present without any systemic manifestations. This renal-limited TMA is usually found after a renal allograft biopsy is performed for allograft dysfunction or on routine post-transplant protocol biopsies even with stable renal function [6].

Epidemiology

Post-transplant TMA (PT-TMA) occurs in 0.8–14% of cases after kidney transplantation. PT-TMA can occur either as a recurrence of the disease involving the native kidney (accounts for ~10% of cases) or as de novo disease (accounts for ~90% of cases) [7]. De novo PT-TMA is caused by various pathogenic mechanisms, which could be either due to any of the etiologies that cause TMA in the general population or may be related to the transplantation (Fig. 41.1). Recurrent TMA has an underlying dysregulation of the alternative complement pathway which caused both the pretransplant TMA and the recurrence after transplantation (hence the name complement-mediated TMA or aHUS) [8]. The incidence of aHUS recurrence depends upon the individual mutation, with estimates of recurrence varying from 15

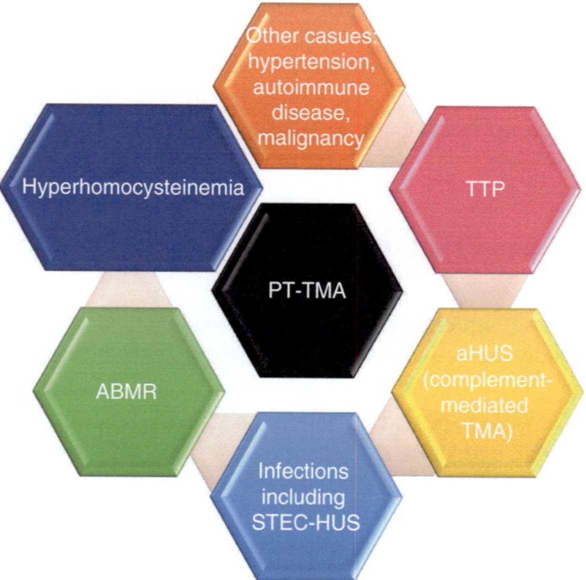

Fig. 41.1 Major causes of post-transplant TMA (PT-TMA) include the following: thrombotic thrombocytopenic purpura (TTP) either inherited or acquired disorders, complement-mediated TMA (aHUS) either inherited or acquired disorders, infections such as cytomegalovirus, *Streptococcus* pneumonia, human immunodeficiency virus, parvovirus B19, Shiga toxin *E. coli*-mediated hemolytic uremic syndrome (STEC-HUS), drug-induced TMA mainly calcineurin inhibitors, vascular endothelial growth factor [VEGF] inhibitors, mammalian target of rapamycin inhibitors (mTORi), ABMR: antibody-Mediated rejection, hyperhomocysteinemia secondary to cobalamin deficiency, other causes like malignancies, pregnancy, malignant hypertension, and autoimmune diseases (systemic lupus erythematosus, antiphospholipid syndrome, scleroderma, and vasculitis)

to 100% depending on the mutation affected, as will be discussed. The recurrence usually presents within 1 year from transplantation and often within days to weeks after transplantation [9].

Diagnostic Workup

Once TMA has been suspected, it is important to formulate an accurate differential diagnosis and send an efficient workup due to the high morbidity and mortality associated with untreated TTP and aHUS (Table 41.1). It is crucial to determine the cause of the patient's original renal disease by reviewing the patient's history and the native kidney biopsy if one was performed.

Major Causes and Treatment of Post-Transplant TMA (PT-TMA)

The major causes of PT-TMA are shown in Fig. 41.1.

1. *Thrombotic Thrombocytopenic Purpura (TTP)* is related to either a congenital abnormality with mutation encoding for ADAMTS13 protein (5% of TTP cases) or immune-mediated due to autoantibodies that inhibit plasma ADAMTS13 activity (95% of TTP cases). Once the diagnosis of TTP is suspected, plasma-

Table 41.1 Workup for post-transplant TMA

For all PT-TMA patients:	Based on the underlying pathogenic mechanism:
• CBC, BMP, LFT, LDH, reticulocyte count, PT/PTT, haptoglobin, blood smear, direct antiglobulin test, urinalysis with spot urine protein-to-creatinine • ADAMTS13 activity and inhibitor • Homocysteine level • Viral PCR (CMV, parvovirus) • Complement panel: C3, C4, sC5b9, CH50, AH50, CFB, CFBp, CFH	• Complement gene mutations/ deletions • Complement antibody: Anti-CFH • Autoimmune workup: ANA, anti-Scl-70, APL antibodies, anti-ds DNA • Infection workup: *S. pneumonia* urinary antigen, HIV, CMV, EBV, parvovirus B19 PCR, stool culture, Shiga toxin stool PCR • ADAMTS13 mutation

BMP basic metabolic panel; *LFT* liver function test; *PT* prothrombin time; *PTT* partial thromboplastin time; *ADAMTS13* a disintegrin and metalloprotease with a thrombospondin type 1 motif member 13; *C3* complement factor 3; *C4* complement factor 4; *sC5b9* serum complement membrane attack complex; *CH50* functional assay for total hemolytic complement assay; *AH50* functional assay alternative complement pathway functional assay; *CFB* complement factor B; *CFBp* complement factor Bp; *CFH* complement factor H; *ANA* Antinuclear antibody; Anti-Scl-70 (also called anti-topoisomerase I), Antiphospholipid (APL) antibodies like lupus anticoagulant (LA) and anticardiolipin antibody (aCL), anti-beta 2 glycoprotein 1 (anti-ß2 GP); *anti-ds DNA* anti-double-stranded DNA antibody

pheresis can be initiated based on clinical judgment and a risk assessment using the PLASMIC score (platelets, lysis, active cancer, stem cell or solid organ transplant, MCV, INR, and creatinine), a score developed as a clinical predictor of severe ADAMTS13 deficiency. It identifies patients with TMA who are most likely to benefit from plasmapheresis while the workup is pending (Score > 5 has a high sensitivity for TTP). The distinction between TTP and HUS relies on the test of plasma ADAMTS13 activity. The activity of less than 10 IU/dL (often referred to as 10% of normal ADAMTS13 activity) is the hallmark of TTP. Treatment of TTP usually consists of plasmapheresis, glucocorticoids, and at times, the addition of rituximab and/or caplacizumab (a humanized monoclonal antibody that binds to von Willebrand factor). Eculizumab, a monoclonal antibody directed against C5, has no role in TTP but rather is a life-saving therapy for complement-mediated HUS [10, 11].

2. *Infection-associated TMA* is usually related to a bacterial infection from Shiga-toxin-producing *E. coli* (STEC) or *Streptococcus* pneumonia. Viruses have also been reported with cytomegalovirus (CMV) as the most frequently reported. Other viral causes include parvovirus B19, hepatitis C, and human immunodeficiency m virus. Fungal infections such as histoplasmosis have also been described [7–9]. The principal treatment for STEC-HUS infection is mainly supportive. Antibiotic therapy and plasmapheresis have not been proven to improve clinical outcomes. For pneumococcal-associated HUS, an antibiotic is indicated, but plasma infusions or plasmapheresis should be avoided because plasma containing natural IgM class antibodies to the T-antigen may aggravate hemolysis. CMV-associated TMA is treated with ganciclovir or valganciclovir, while parvovirus B19-associated TMA is treated with IVIG [7–12].

3. *Drug-induced TMA (DI-TMA)* can be immune-mediated or non-immune-mediated. Immune-mediated TMA is associated with drugs such as quinine, thienopyridines (ticlopidine, clopidogrel), trimethoprim-sulfamethoxazole, quetiapine, anti-tumor necrosis factor (TNF) monoclonal antibody adalimumab. The mainstay treatment of this group is the immediate withdrawal of the drug and complete avoidance for life. Plasmapheresis is controversial in this group, with some effectiveness in certain immune-mediated DI-TMAs. It is reasonable to consider in cases of uncertainty about the diagnosis of DI-TMA versus TTP. Non-immune mediated TMA is associated with drugs such as *proteasome inhibitors, gemcitabine, vascular endothelial growth factor (VEGF) inhibitors, and tyrosine kinase inhibitors*. Among immunosuppressants utilized for transplantation, calcineurin inhibitors (CNIs) are the main culprit, with a higher risk seen with cyclosporine than with tacrolimus, and some reported risk with mammalian target rapamycin inhibitors [mTORis]. The combination of CNI and mTORi has a higher risk of de novo TMA than either drug alone. The mainstay of treatment is withdrawal or dose reduction of the offending agent. Plasmapheresis is generally not effective in non-immune mediated DI-TMA [6, 7].

4. *Antibody-mediated rejection (ABMR)*, both acute and chronic, can activate the classical complement pathway and induce the development of TMA in renal allografts. Grafts with ABMR and TMA have a lower graft survival than those

Table 41.2 Defects in complement-mediated TMA

Defect in the alternate complement pathway	Known complement factor mutants
• Increased activity of complement factors	• C3 • CFB
• Decreased activity of inhibitory factors	• CFI • CFH • MCP
• Antibody formation to inhibitory factors	• Anti-FH
• Other mutants	• THBD • DGK-ε

C3 complement factor 3; *CFB* complement factor B; *CFI* complement factor I; *CFH* complement factor H; *MCP* membrane cofactor protein; *FH* factor H; *THBD* thrombomodulin; *DGK-ε* diacylglycerol kinase-epsilon

with AMR and no TMA. It is important to note that TMA may be present in other non-rejection conditions, such as recurrent aHUS or DI-TMA, so it is important to rule out other causes of TMA based on clinical history, degree of sensitization, and the presence of donor-specific antibodies. The Banff classification for diagnosis of ABMR requires the presence of morphologic, immunohistologic, and serologic evidence in distinguishing ABMR from other causes of TMA [6, 7, 12, 13].

5. *Complement-mediated TMA (aHUS)* is characterized by hyperactivity of the alternative complement pathway. Dysregulation of alternate complement pathways may result from increased activity of activating factors, decreased activity of inhibitory factors, or antibody formation with inhibitory factors (Table 41.2). The alternative complement pathway is activated in plasma by low-grade hydrolysis of complement factor C3 into C3a and C3b, a process accelerated by C3 convertase enzymes. Complement factor C3b propagates the C5 convertase enzyme that cleaves C5 to C5a and C5b. Complement factor C5b initiates the membrane attack complex. Innate immunity is subject to the balance between constitutive activation and adaptive inhibition. Hyperactivity of complement may cause endothelial damage, tissue factor release, fibrin activation, and microthrombi formation.

The majority of complement-mediated TMA cases are related to loss of function mutations in inhibitory factors complement factor H (~20–30%), complement factor I (2–12%), and membrane cofactor protein CD46 (10–15%). The minority are related to gain of function mutants of complement factor 3 (5–10%) or complement factor 3b (1–2%). Other mutations in thrombomodulin (THBD) and diacylglycerol kinase-epsilon (DGK-ε) have also been described. Antibody formation to complement factor H (anti-FH) is a unique disease entity that is more common in children and demonstrates a rapid progression to end-stage renal disease (ESRD). Genetic testing results should be interpreted cautiously because one-third of patients with complement-mediated TMA do not have an identifiable mutant [14–16].

Patients with complement-mediated TMA are at high risk for disease recurrence without anti-complement therapy after kidney transplantation. Therefore, it is crucial to screen for complement system abnormalities and perform a comprehensive evaluation for patients suspected to have aHUS as a cause of ESRD. It has been reported that in 80% of patients with pregnancy-associated TMA, TMA was complement-mediated [14].

In selecting the type of kidney donor for a patient with known aHUS, it is recommended that living-related donor kidney transplants be avoided due to the increased risk of recurrent disease in the recipient and de novo disease in the donor if the donor is a genetic mutation carrier. One can consider a living unrelated donor if genetic testing is negative or a deceased-donor kidney transplant [14–17].

Outcomes in kidney transplantation may vary by the underlying compliment abnormality [9]. CFH and CFI mutations are associated with high recurrence rates (~50–100%). MCP mutations are associated with low recurrence rates (10–15%). MCP regulates complement at the cell surface level, and thus recurrence should not occur in a kidney allograft expressing normal MCP.

Anti-complement therapy has improved treatment for patients with complement-mediated TMA and is an effective prophylactic therapy to prevent recurrence after kidney transplantation. It reduces the post-transplant recurrence rate from 49 to 12% in patients with aHUS [15–17]. Eculizumab and ravulizumab are humanized monoclonal antibodies directed against the terminal pathway protein complement factor C5. These drugs inhibit the formation of the membrane attack complex by preventing the cleavage of C5 into C5a and C5b. Other innate immune functions of C3 are preserved because these drugs operate downstream of C3 convertase. Eculizumab trough levels guide dosing, with a goal eculizumab trough level > 100 µg/mL. Total complement activity levels (CH50) measure the effectiveness of therapy, with a goal of CH50 < 10%. Therapeutic drug monitoring includes routine assessment of complete blood counts and markers of hemolysis. Patients receiving these drugs are at increased risk of infection with *Neisseria meningitides* and other encapsulated organisms and require meningitis and pneumonia vaccines two or more weeks prior to transplantation. Antimicrobial prophylaxis with penicillin or fluoroquinolone should also be considered [14–17]. Treatment of anti-FH disease targets the elimination of pathogenic autoantibodies [18]. Peri-transplant therapies may include therapeutic plasma exchange, rituximab, intravenous immunoglobulin therapy. In addition, eculizumab has been used in anti-FH disease as a means to tamper complement activity in the peri-transplant period. Anti-FH titers measure the effectiveness of therapy, with a higher risk of recurrence associated with anti-FH titer > 1000 AU/mL.

Summary

TMA is a histopathological diagnosis with many possible primary and secondary causes. Complement-mediated TMA results from overactivation of the alternate complement pathway. This may result from a loss of function in inhibitory complement factors, a gain of function in activating complement factors, or autoantibody formation to complement factor H. Kidney transplantation workup should include complement antigen levels and genetic variants in suspected cases of complement-mediated TMA. Eculizumab and ravulizumab are effective prophylactic and therapeutic agents in complement blockade to reduce the risk of recurrence of complement-mediated TMA.

Disclosures None.

Funding None.

References

1. Ruggenenti P, Noris M, Remuzzi G. Thrombotic microangiopathy, hemolytic uremic syndrome, and thrombotic thrombocytopenic purpura. Kidney Int. 2001;60(3):831–46. https://doi.org/10.1046/j.1523-1755.2001.060003831.x.
2. Salvadori M, Bertoni E. Complement related kidney diseases: recurrence after transplantation. World J Transplant 2016;6(4):632–645. https://doi.org/10.5500/wjt.v6.i4.632. PMID: 28058212; PMCID: PMC5175220.
3. George JN, Nester CM. Syndromes of thrombotic microangiopathy. N Engl J Med. 2014;371(7):654–66. https://doi.org/10.1056/NEJMra1312353.
4. Fakhouri F, Roumenina L, Provot F, Sallée M, Caillard S, Couzi L, Essig M, Ribes D, Dragon-Durey MA, Bridoux F, Rondeau E, Frémeaux-Bacchi V. Pregnancy-associated hemolytic uremic syndrome revisited in the era of complement gene mutations. J Am Soc Nephrol. 2010;21(5):859–67. https://doi.org/10.1681/ASN.2009070706. Epub 2010 Mar 4. PMID: 20203157; PMCID: PMC2865741
5. Palma LMP, Sridharan M, Sethi S. Complement in secondary thrombotic microangiopathy. Kidney Int Rep. 2021;6(1):11–23. https://doi.org/10.1016/j.ekir.2020.10.009. Epub 2020 Oct 21. PMID: 33102952; PMCID: PMC7575444
6. Go RS, Winters JL, Leung N, Murray DL, Willrich MA, Abraham RS, Amer H, Hogan WJ, Marshall AL, Sethi S, Tran CL, Chen D, Pruthi RK, Ashrani AA, Fervenza FC, Cramer CH 2nd, Rodriguez V, Wolanskyj AP, Thomé SD, Hook CC. Mayo clinic complement alternative pathway-thrombotic microangiopathy disease-oriented group. thrombotic microangiopathy care pathway: a consensus statement for the mayo clinic complement alternative pathway-thrombotic microangiopathy (cap-tma) disease-oriented group. Mayo Clin Proc. 2016;91(9):1189–211. https://doi.org/10.1016/j.mayocp.2016.05.015. Epub 2016 Aug 3
7. Ávila A, Gavela E, Sancho A. Thrombotic Microangiopathy after kidney transplantation: an underdiagnosed and potentially reversible entity. Front Med (Lausanne). 2021;8:642864. https://doi.org/10.3389/fmed.2021.642864. PMID: 33898482; PMCID: PMC8063690
8. Miller RB, Burke BA, Schmidt WJ, Gillingham KJ, Matas AJ, Mauer M, Kashtan CE. Recurrence of haemolytic-uraemic syndrome in renal transplants: a single-centre report. Nephrol Dial Transplant. 1997;12(7):1425–30. https://doi.org/10.1093/ndt/12.7.1425.
9. Lahlou A, Lang P, Charpentier B, Barrou B, Glotz D, Baron C, Hiesse C, Kreis H, Legendre C, Bedrossian J, Mougenot B, Sraer JD, Rondeau E. Hemolytic uremic syndrome. Recurrence after renal transplantation. Groupe Coopératif de l'Ile-de-France (GCIF). Medicine (Baltimore). 2000;79(2):90–102. https://doi.org/10.1097/00005792-200003000-00003.
10. Völker LA, Kaufeld J, Miesbach W, Brähler S, Reinhardt M, Kühne L, Mühlfeld A, Schreiber A, Gaedeke J, Tölle M, Jabs WJ, Özcan F, Markau S, Girndt M, Bauer F, Westhoff TH, Felten H, Hausberg M, Brand M, Gerth J, Bieringer M, Bommer M, Zschiedrich S, Schneider J, Elitok S, Gawlik A, Gäckler A, Kribben A, Schwenger V, Schoenermarck U, Roeder M, Radermacher

J, Bramstedt J, Morgner A, Herbst R, Harth A, Potthoff SA, von Auer C, Wendt R, Christ H, Brinkkoetter PT, Menne J. Real-world data confirm the effectiveness of caplacizumab in acquired thrombotic thrombocytopenic purpura. Blood Adv. 2020;4(13):3085–92. https://doi.org/10.1182/bloodadvances.2020001973. PMID: 32634236; PMCID: PMC7362370

11. Zheng XL, Vesely SK, Cataland SR, Coppo P, Geldziler B, Iorio A, Matsumoto M, Mustafa RA, Pai M, Rock G, Russell L, Tarawneh R, Valdes J, Peyvandi F. ISTH guidelines for treatment of thrombotic thrombocytopenic purpura. J Thromb Haemost. 2020;18(10):2496–502. https://doi.org/10.1111/jth.15010. Epub 2020 Sep 11. PMID: 32914526; PMCID: PMC8091490

12. Wu K, Budde K, Schmidt D, Neumayer HH, Lehner L, Bamoulid J, Rudolph B. The inferior impact of antibody-mediated rejection on on the clinical outcome of kidney allografts that develop de novo thrombotic microangiopathy. Clin Transpl. 2016;30(2):105–17. https://doi.org/10.1111/ctr.12645. Epub 2016 Jan 5

13. Jeong HJ. Diagnosis of renal transplant rejection: Banff classification and beyond. Kidney Res Clin Pract. 2020;39(1):17–31. https://doi.org/10.23876/j.krcp.20.003. PMID: 32164120; PMCID: PMC7105630

14. Java A. Peri- and post-operative evaluation and Management of Atypical Hemolytic Uremic Syndrome (aHUS) in kidney transplantation. Adv Chronic Kidney Dis. 2020;27(2):128–37. https://doi.org/10.1053/j.ackd.2019.11.003.

15. Pugh D, O'Sullivan ED, Duthie FA, Masson P, Kavanagh D. Interventions for atypical haemolytic uraemic syndrome. Cochrane Database Syst Rev. 2021;3(3):CD012862. https://doi.org/10.1002/14651858.CD012862.pub2. PMID: 33783815; PMCID: PMC8078160

16. Okumi M, Tanabe K. Prevention and treatment of atypical haemolytic uremic syndrome after kidney transplantation. Nephrology (Carlton). 2016;21(Suppl 1):9–13. https://doi.org/10.1111/nep.12776.

17. Zuber J, Frimat M, Caillard S, Kamar N, Gatault P, Petitprez F, Couzi L, Jourde-Chiche N, Chatelet V, Gaisne R, Bertrand D, Bamoulid J, Louis M, Sberro Soussan R, Navarro D, Westeel PF, Frimat L, Colosio C, Thierry A, Rivalan J, Albano L, Arzouk N, Cornec-Le Gall E, Claisse G, Elias M, El Karoui K, Chauvet S, Coindre JP, Rerolle JP, Tricot L, Sayegh J, Garrouste C, Charasse C, Delmas Y, Massy Z, Hourmant M, Servais A, Loirat C, Fakhouri F, Pouteil-Noble C, Peraldi MN, Legendre C, Rondeau E, Le Quintrec M, Frémeaux-Bacchi V. Use of highly individualized complement blockade has revolutionized clinical outcomes after kidney transplantation and renal epidemiology of atypical hemolytic uremic syndrome. J Am Soc Nephrol. 2019;30(12):2449–63. https://doi.org/10.1681/ASN.2019040331. Epub 2019 Oct 1. PMID: 31575699; PMCID: PMC6900783

18. Strobel S, Hoyer PF, Mache CJ, Sulyok E, Liu WS, Richter H, Oppermann M, Zipfel PF, Józsi M. Functional analyses indicate a pathogenic role of factor H autoantibodies in atypical haemolytic uraemic syndrome. Nephrol Dial Transplant. 2010;25(1):136–44. https://doi.org/10.1093/ndt/gfp388. Epub 2009 Aug 7

Chapter 42
IgA Nephropathy Post-Kidney Transplantation

Husain Hasan and Shaifali Sandal

Introduction

IgA nephropathy (IgAN) represents the leading cause of primary glomerulonephritis in the developed world. As such, a substantial portion of patients develop end-stage kidney disease and consequently undergo kidney transplantation (KT), and each of these patients faces the risk of recurrence in their allograft. In this clinical case-based discussion, we sought to review the epidemiology, immunopathogenesis, as well as diagnostic, therapeutic, and prognostic implications of IgAN recurrence to highlight and address the more challenging clinical aspects of this disease.

Case

A 66-year-old female with an end-stage kidney disease that was presumed to be due to diabetes underwent deceased-donor KT. At the time of transplantation, her calculated panel reactive antibody (cPRA) was 96%, and there were 5/6 HLA mismatches

H. Hasan
Department of Medicine, McGill University Health Centre, Canada Research Institute
of the McGill University Health Centre, Montreal, QC, Canada
e-mail: husain.hasan@mail.mcgill.ca

S. Sandal (✉)
Division of Nephrology, Department of Medicine, McGill University Health Centre,
Montreal, QC, Canada

Royal Victoria Hospital Glen Site, Montreal, QC, Canada

Research Institute of the McGill University Health Centre, Montreal, QC, Canada
e-mail: shaifali.sandal@mcgill.ca

© The Author(s), under exclusive license to Springer Nature
Switzerland AG 2022

F. Aziz, S. Parajuli (eds.), *Complications in Kidney Transplantation*,
https://doi.org/10.1007/978-3-031-13569-9_42

(HLA-A: 2/2, -B:2/2, and -DR: 1/2) with the donor. The flow crossmatch was negative, and the patient received induction therapy with alemtuzumab and methylprednisolone. Her maintenance immunosuppression included tacrolimus (target trough level 4–8 ng/mL), mycophenolate mofetil (720 mg twice a day), and prednisone that was tapered to 5 mg daily. Her other past medical history was also significant for coronary artery disease that was managed medically and hypertension, dyslipidemia, obesity, and microvascular complications from diabetes.

She had excellent graft function post-operatively with a baseline creatinine of 0.7–0.8 mg/dL and no significant albuminuria. However, a protocol test conducted at 3-months revealed three new donor-specific antibodies (DSAs); A3 with MFI 1248, A26 with MFI 3137, and Cw4 with MFI 1486. A for-indication biopsy thereafter revealed no features to suggest acute or chronic rejection or other pathology, and immunofluorescence was unremarkable. She was treated by maximizing the maintenance immunosuppression regimen. Her graft function remained stable, and she had no significant albuminuria. Follow-up measurements showed the absence of these DSAs up to 12 months post-KT.

However, 13 months post-KT, she developed new-onset mild albuminuria (80–100 mg/g). A history of an upper respiratory infection was reported 2–3 weeks prior. Laboratory investigations were otherwise unrevealing; no new DSAs, normal urinalysis, and stable creatinine. There was low suspicion of non-adherence to medications; thus, a kidney biopsy was performed. Light microscopy revealed no features to suggest T-cell mediated rejection. However, glomerular hypercellularity and mild mesangial expansion were noted in several glomeruli (Fig. 42.1a, b). The pathologist graded other findings as follows; c4d0, ptc0, and cg0. Immunofluorescence demonstrated strong positivity for IgA, and electron microscopy demonstrated the presence of mesangial, para-mesangial, and occasional subendothelial deposits (Fig. 42.1c, d).

Question 1

Based on this clinical history and pathology findings, what is the most likely diagnosis?

A. Acute antibody-mediated rejection.
B. Recurrent or de novo IgA nephropathy.
C. Donor-derived IgA deposits.
D. De novo membranous nephropathy.

The correct answer is B.

The patient's biopsy is diagnostic for IgAN. However, given the lack of a native kidney biopsy before KT, we could not distinguish whether this was a case of de novo or recurrent IgAN. There was very low suspicion for acute antibody-mediated rejection due to the absence of DSA, C4d peritubular capillary deposition, and peritubular capillaritis; thus, response A is incorrect. Response C is incorrect as the first biopsy performed 3-months post-KT did not demonstrate any evidence of IgA deposits; these changes are unlikely to be donor derived. The biopsy findings were not consistent with membranous nephropathy, rendering D incorrect.

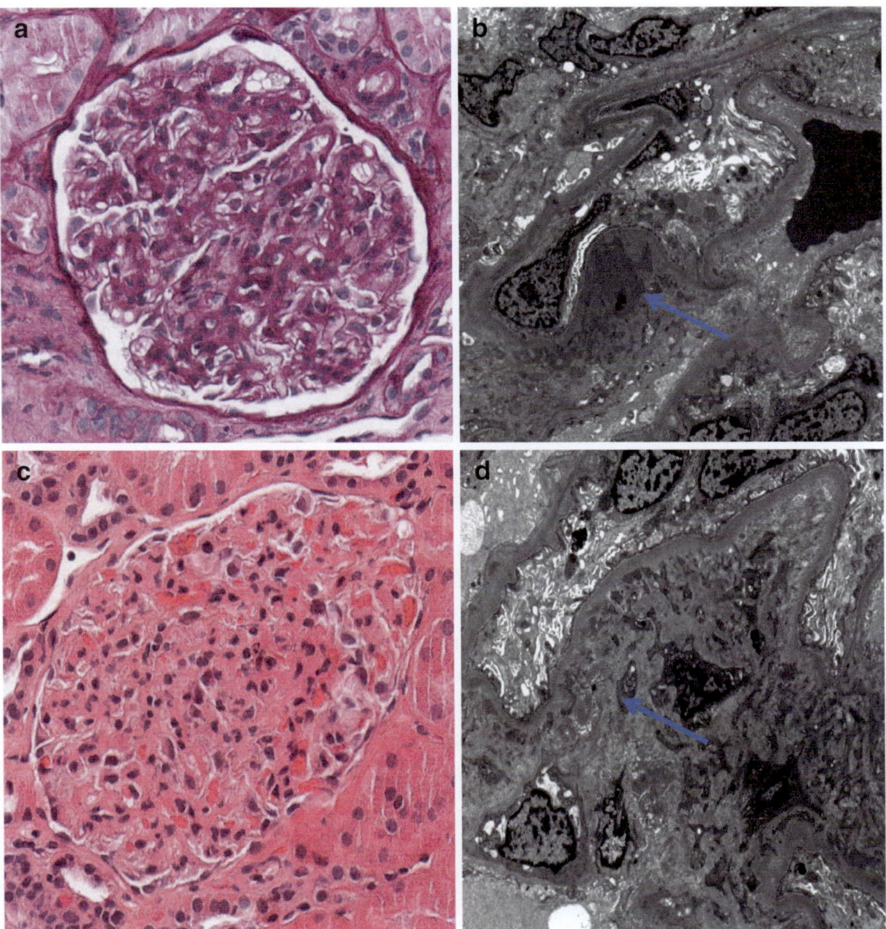

Fig. 42.1 A for-indication biopsy was performed for worsening proteinuria in a patient with kidney transplantation 13 months prior. On light microscopy, mesangial expansion and endocapillary hypercellularity were noted on PAS (**a**) and H&E (**b**) stains. Electron microscopy demonstrated mesangial expansion and deposits (starred in **c** and **d**)

Clinical Course

After diagnosing IgA nephropathy, the patient was seen in the clinic to discuss the management plan.

Question 2
Which of the following is the most appropriate next step in managing this patient?

A. Tonsillectomy.
B. Cyclophosphamide with glucocorticoids.

C. Blood pressure management and initiation of a RAASI.

D. B-cell depleting therapy, plasmapheresis, and glucocorticoids.

The correct response is C.

There are no proven therapies for IgAN in the post-KT setting that have demonstrated efficacy in large prospective studies. Overall, the primary focus in mild to moderate cases of IgAN is to target therapies to reduce proteinuria and optimize blood pressure. Patients who are deemed to be at high risk for progressive disease and those with crescents may require immunosuppressive therapy with glucocorticoids. Our patient was considered to be at low risk of progression and not to have antibody-mediated rejection; thus, responses B and D are incorrect. Tonsillectomy is not routinely recommended for treatment or prevention of IgAN post-KT, and response A is incorrect.

Follow-Up of the Case Presented

The patient was deemed to have IgAN and at low risk of progression, and thus management aimed at targeting proteinuria, blood pressure, and other lifestyle modifications. Candesartan was initiated and increased to a maximum tolerated dose of 32 mg daily. Her other blood pressure medications were optimized to target blood pressure of < 130/80 mmHg. She was referred to a dietician for weight control and dietary sodium restriction and an endocrinologist for optimal management of her diabetes. At 5-years post-KT, she continues to have mild albuminuria with stable graft function.

Discussion

Post-transplant glomerular diseases are a frequent complication after KT [1, 2]. They can be "recurrences" of the same original disease that affected the native kidney of the recipient or "de novo," in which the disease is unrelated to the original disease. When a post-KT biopsy reveals glomerular disease, it can be challenging to differentiate between the two. Most recipients have not had a biopsy before KT, and most of the time, pre-implantation biopsies to ascertain whether donor-derived changes are not performed [2]. In addition, in many cases, the recipient's pre-KT biopsy may reveal advanced changes, and the original disease may be difficult to ascertain. Regardless, glomerular disease post-KT affects graft function and portends a poor long-term graft survival [1, 2].

IgA nephropathy is the most prevalent primary glomerulonephritis worldwide, and the diagnostic hallmark is the predominance of IgA deposits in the glomerular mesangium on immunofluorescence [3, 4]. Generally, IgAN follows a slowly progressive course with approximately 25–30% of any cohort developing kidney failure within 20–25 years of presentation [4]. Treatment in most patients is supportive, with immunosuppressive management reserved for those at higher risk of progression [4]. In those who progress and develop kidney failure, KT is the best therapeutic option.

Pathogenesis

IgAN is an autoimmune disease mediated by circulating IgA-containing immune complexes [3–6]. This requires a critical interaction between an intrinsic antigen and circulating anti-glycan antibodies [5]. The intrinsic antigen is a circulatory IgA1 with a galactose deficiency in some carbohydrate side chains (O-glycans) attached to the hinge-region segment of the heavy chain [5]. Those affected have a genetic predisposition and experience a triggering event [5]. The trigger may occur after KT, leading to de novo disease. In those with a history of IgAN, the propensity to produce immune complex formation is not diminished after KT, thereby leading to recurrence. However, there is variability in whether the circulating immune complexes deposit in the mesangium and how immunosuppression modifies this [6]. The responses of mesangial cells and recruited inflammatory cells likely determine whether IgAN occurs or recurs [6]. It is of note that when grafts with IgA deposits are transplanted into recipients that are not predisposed to IgAN, the IgA deposits clear in follow-up biopsies [7]. Thus, IgAN is unlikely to be donor-derived unless the recipient is predisposed to developing this disease.

Risk of Recurrence

No large prospective study has quantified the risk of IgAN recurrence or development of de novo IgAN post-KT. In observational studies, recurrence rates are as high as 60% but vary widely across studies [6]. A few cases of de novo IgAN have been described. However, the overall incidence is unknown [2]. This is due to various reasons, such as the patient population being studied, donor type, immunosuppression protocols, differences in the indication for biopsies, and time from transplantation [6, 8]. The development of de novo DSA is associated with a 6.7 higher risk of IgAN recurrence [8].

Diagnosis

The diagnosis of IgAN requires histological evidence. In transplant recipients, clinical findings may or may not be present and are not very reliable [6]. When protocol biopsies are performed and demonstrate recurrence, many do not show clinical signs of the disease [6]. The features of IgAN on light microscopy vary significantly among patients and within the individual biopsy sample; however, an increase in mesangial matrix and hypercellularity is common [3, 5]. Other potential glomerular lesions include focal necrosis, segmental scarring, and crescents in Bowman's space [5]. An international panel of nephrologists and nephropathologists developed the Oxford classification of IgAN to identify specific pathological features that more accurately predict the risk of progression [3]. The "MEST" score comprises four histological features that are independent predictors of clinical outcome. These are the mesangial hypercellularity score, segmental glomerulosclerosis, endocapillary hypercellularity, and tubular atrophy/interstitial fibrosis. This classification has a prognostic role in the post-KT setting as well [9].

Treatments

There are no proven therapies to prevent IgAN recurrence. Over a short follow-up period, preoperative tonsillectomy did not impact the recurrence of IgAN [10]. In mild to moderate cases of IgAN, most recommend targeting therapies to reduce proteinuria, optimize blood pressure, and reduce the inflammatory state [6]. Angiotensin-converting enzyme inhibitors or angiotensin II receptor blockers should be used in those with proteinuria and may have a role in improving graft survival [11]. In those with the crescentic disease, a highly individualized approach with shared decision-making should be pursued. Some evidence suggests a role for immunosuppressive medications as therapeutic options. Steroid use was associated with a 50% reduced risk of recurrence post-KT [12]. Also, the use of anti-thymocyte globulin induction therapy was associated with an 80% reduction in the relative risk of IgAN recurrence [13]. More recently, immunosuppressive regimens were not associated with recurrent IgAN in multivariable analysis [8]. Overall, no large prospective studies demonstrate the efficacy of any of these approaches in transplant recipients.

Outcomes

There is a lack of prospective data with protocol biopsies to quantify the true risk of graft dysfunction and/or loss from de novo or recurrent disease. Those with mild to moderate mesangial cell proliferation generally have a favorable course, while those with crescents at biopsy have poor outcomes. Larger registry analyses report similar outcomes between patients with a history of IgAN and those with none; however, they lack granular data [14]. In a multicenter, international, retrospective study of 504 transplant recipients with IgA nephropathy, where 82 patients had recurrent IgA deposits, there was a 3.7 times higher risk of graft loss when compared with patients without IgA [8]. In another cohort of patients followed up for 15 years post-KT, death-censored graft survival was approximately 10% lower in patients who had IgAN than in controls [9]. Overall, the outcome of de novo or recurrent IgAN depends on pathology findings and duration post-KT.

Acknowledgments We would like to thank Dr. Chantal Bernard for providing the pathology images.

References

1. Chailimpamontree W, Dmitrienko S, Li G, Balshaw R, Magil A, Shapiro RJ, et al. Probability, predictors, and prognosis of posttransplantation glomerulonephritis. J Am Soc Nephrol. 2009;20(4):843–51.
2. Ponticelli C, Moroni G, Glassock RJ. De novo glomerular diseases after renal transplantation. Clin J Am Soc Nephrol. 2014;9(8):1479–87.
3. Cattran DC, Coppo R, Cook HT, Feehally J, Roberts IS, Troyanov S, et al. The Oxford classification of IgA nephropathy: rationale, clinicopathological correlations, and classification. Kidney Int. 2009;76(5):534–45.
4. KDIGO. 2021 clinical practice guideline for the Management of Glomerular Diseases. Kidney Int. 2021;100(4s):S1–s276.
5. Wyatt RJ, Julian BA. IgA nephropathy. N Engl J Med. 2013;368(25):2402–14.
6. Wyld ML, Chadban SJ. Recurrent IgA nephropathy after kidney transplantation. Transplantation. 2016;100(9):1827–32.
7. Silva FG, Chander P, Pirani CL, Hardy MA. Disappearance of glomerular mesangial IgA deposits after renal allograft transplantation. Transplantation. 1982;33(2):241–6.
8. Uffing A, Pérez-Saéz MJ, Jouve T, Bugnazet M, Malvezzi P, Muhsin SA, et al. Recurrence of IgA nephropathy after kidney transplantation in adults. Clin J Am Soc Nephrol. 2021;16(8):1247–55.
9. Moroni G, Longhi S, Quaglini S, Gallelli B, Banfi G, Montagnino G, et al. The long-term outcome of renal transplantation of IgA nephropathy and the impact of recurrence on graft survival. Nephrol Dial Transplant. 2013;28(5):1305–14.
10. Sato Y, Ishida H, Shimizu T, Tanabe K. Evaluation of tonsillectomy before kidney transplantation in patients with IgA nephropathy. Transpl Immunol. 2014;30(1):12–7.
11. Courtney AE, McNamee PT, Nelson WE, Maxwell AP. Does angiotensin blockade influence graft outcome in renal transplant recipients with IgA nephropathy? Nephrol Dial Transplant. 2006;21(12):3550–4.
12. Clayton P, McDonald S, Chadban S. Steroids and recurrent IgA nephropathy after kidney transplantation. American journal of transplantation. 2011;11(8):1645–9.
13. Berthoux F, El Deeb S, Mariat C, Diconne E, Laurent B, Thibaudin L. Antithymocyte globulin (ATG) induction therapy and disease recurrence in renal transplant recipients with primary IgA nephropathy. Transplantation. 2008;85(10):1505–7.
14. Ponticelli C, Traversi L, Feliciani A, Cesana BM, Banfi G, Tarantino A. Kidney transplantation in patients with IgA mesangial glomerulonephritis. Kidney Int. 2001;60(5):1948–54.

Chapter 43
C1q Nephropathy in Kidney Transplant Recipients

Kusum L. Sharma, Ravi B. Singh, and Weixiong Zhong

Introduction

C1q nephropathy (C1qN) is an uncommon, idiopathic glomerular disease characterized by dominant or codominant C1q deposition primarily in mesangium in patients without evidence of systemic lupus erythematosus, membranoproliferative glomerulonephritis, or infection. It generally presents as a nephrotic syndrome in older children and young adults but is also uncommonly discovered in renal allograft of the transplant patient. There is a wide range of variations in the clinical picture, and biopsy is often diagnostic. Management is conservative with variable outcomes depending on clinical and histological factors. The kidney transplant recipients usually have stable creatinine with no or stable proteinuria and no loss of graft function.

History

This 63-year-old female received a deceased donor kidney (DCD) transplant 2 years ago, which was complicated by delayed graft function. She had a history of end-stage kidney disease (ESKD) secondary to polycystic kidney disease (PCKD) and has hypertension and metabolic bone disease. Her immunosuppressive therapy

K. L. Sharma (✉) · W. Zhong
Department of Pathology and Laboratory Medicine, University of Wisconsin Hospital and Clinics, Madison, WI, USA
e-mail: ksharma@uwhealth.org; wzhongh3@wisc.edu

R. B. Singh
Department of Medicine, SUNY Upstate Medical University, Syracuse, NY, USA
e-mail: singhrav@upstate.edu

© The Author(s), under exclusive license to Springer Nature Switzerland AG 2022

F. Aziz, S. Parajuli (eds.), *Complications in Kidney Transplantation*,
https://doi.org/10.1007/978-3-031-13569-9_43

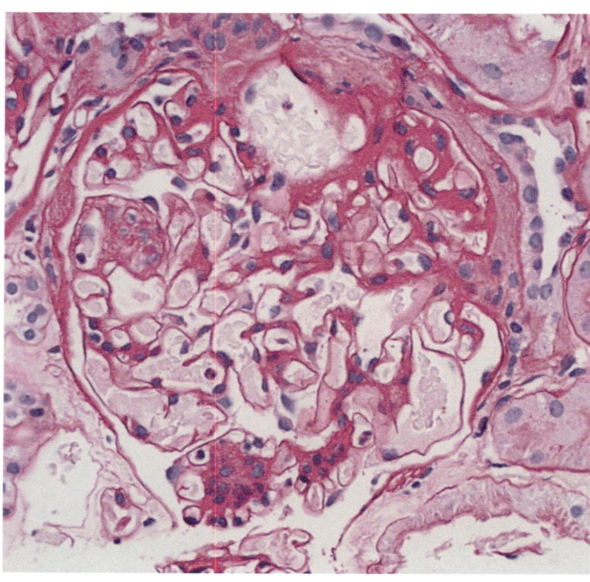

Fig. 43.1 PAS staining showing the glomerulus with segmental sclerosis and a segmental mild increase in mesangial cellularity and matrix

includes tacrolimus and is currently taking amlodipine 5 mg and metoprolol 50 mg daily as well as metformin. She does home blood pressure monitoring which averages between 120 and 130 mmHg for systolic and 60 and 80 mmHg for diastolic. She also monitors her blood sugar intermittently at home which averages at 120–130 mg/dL. She denies chest pain, shortness of breath (SOB), weight gain, edema, fever, chills, dysuria, or hematuria. Her baseline laboratory values include tacrolimus trough of 9.6 ng/mL, creatinine 1.6 mg/dL, eGFR 39 mL/min/1.73sqm, potassium 4.8 mmol/L, hematocrit 47.9%, white cell count 9.71 k/uL, urine creatinine 24 mg/dL, urine protein 2.5 mg/dL, and urine protein/creatinine ratio of 0.096. Today she underwent renal biopsy for enrollment into a study protocol.

Hematoxylin and eosin (H&E), periodic acid Schiff (PAS) (Fig. 43.1), periodic acid silver methenamine stain (PASM), and trichrome stained slides reveal sclerotic glomeruli, interstitial fibrosis, tubular atrophy, and dense chronic inflammation and no evidence of rejection.

Question 1

What is the most likely diagnosis based on the clinical findings and preliminary biopsy report?

A. Lupus nephritis.
B. Focal segmental glomerulosclerosis.
C. C1q nephropathy.
D. Membranous glomerulonephritis.
E. Accurate diagnosis cannot be assigned based on clinical picture or H&E alone and needs assessment with immunofluorescence findings.

The correct answer is E.

The light microscopic findings are nonspecific and nondiagnostic. To diagnose A, B, C, and D, immunofluorescence staining and ultrastructural study by electron microscopy are required.

Further study with electron microscopy (Fig. 43.2) reveals a mild mesangial matrix increase and segmental moderate amounts of electron-dense deposits in the mesangium but normal cellularity and no basement membrane double contours. There is segmental mild podocyte foot process effacement. Immunofluorescence staining shows glomeruli with mesangial staining for C1q (2+) in diffuse segmental distribution (Fig. 43.3).

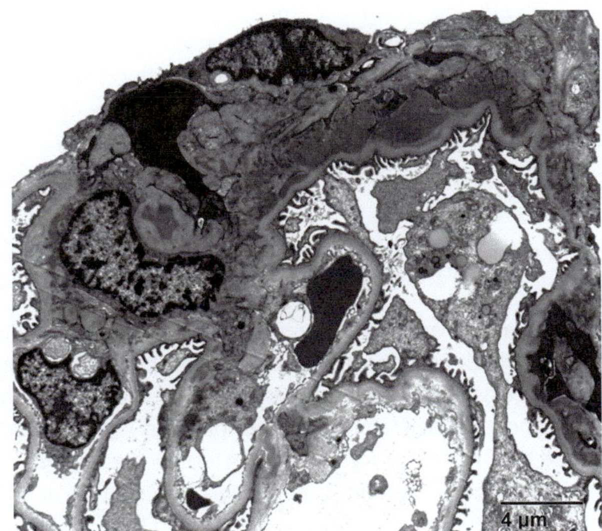

Fig. 43.2 Electron micrograph showing electron-dense deposits in the mycangium without significant podocyte foot process effacement

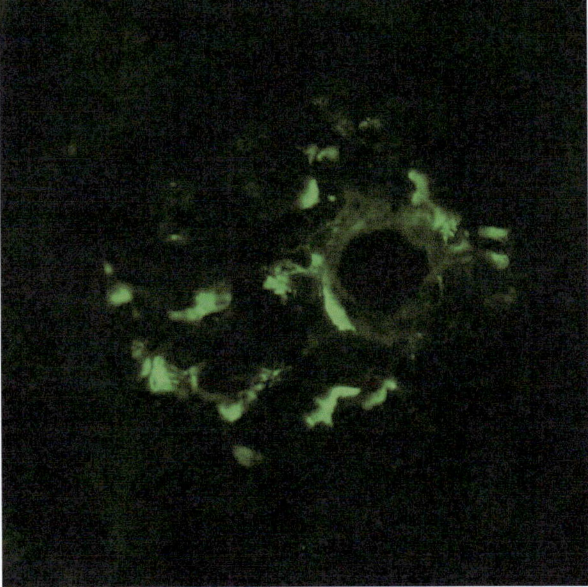

Fig. 43.3 Immuno-fluorescence staining showing C1q staining in the mesangium

Question 2

What is the most likely diagnosis?

A. Focal segmental glomerulosclerosis.
B. Lupus nephritis.
C. C1q nephropathy.
D. Membranous glomerulonephritis.

The correct answer is C.

Focal segmental glomerulosclerosis may have segmental nonspecific staining for IgM and C3 but should have severe podocyte foot process effacement, lupus nephritis typically has full-house immunofluorescence staining or IgG- or IgA-dominant plus C3 and C1q staining on kidney transplant biopsies, and membranous glomerulonephritis typically has positive immunofluorescence staining for IgG and C3 and subepithelial electron-dense deposits.

Further, the patient was managed conservatively.

Discussion

Complements are a heterogeneous group of 40 proteins circulating in the blood stream which get activated by specific molecules like autoantibodies, immune complexes (classical pathway), carbohydrate molecules (the MB lectin pathway), or spontaneously activated (alternate pathway) [1]. C1 molecule is a pentamer composed of C1q and two C1r and C1s molecules. The C1q is a glycoprotein produced in various cells including monocytes, microglial, dendritic, and endothelial cells, and the receptor for the C1q protein is also found in similar cells. It is the first member of the complement system in the classical pathway where it recognizes and binds to the immune complex and activates the other components of C1 [2].

First described as a distinct clinic-pathological entity by Jennette and Hipp in 1985, C1q nephropathy is a rare form of glomerulopathy [3]. The exact pathogenesis of C1q nephropathy is still not known. Within the mesangial cells of the kidneys, there are specialized C1q receptors that help in the binding of immune complexes [4]. C1q complement and immunoglobulin deposit detection in the glomeruli suggest an underlying immune complex mechanism. C1q molecule's affinity to various substances including DNA, RNA, viral proteins, immune cells suggests that a direct mechanism may exist, and immunoglobulins may just be bystanders in the process. Even though the role of podocyte injury has not been established, the detection of effacement of podocyte foot process raises the possibility of "podocytopathy" [5]. Some viruses such as Epstein–Barr virus [6] and BK virus [7] have been associated with C1q nephropathy, and there is histologic evidence of C1q dominant deposition in allograft kidneys in patient who did not have a prior diagnosis of C1q nephropathy [8].

C1q nephropathy is rare, and prevalence can vary from 0.2 to 16% of all renal biopsies, and in renal allograft transplant, patients can be seen after the first year of transplant [9, 10]. Generally, it is slightly more common in male (68%) patients and may present with a wide range of clinical presentations, ranging from no symptom and normal urine to asymptomatic proteinuria or hematuria to frank nephritic or nephrotic syndromes. The most common findings at the time of diagnosis are hypertension (35%) and renal insufficiency (5–46%) [5]. Rapidly progressive crescentic glomerulonephritis progressing to end-stage kidney disease (ESKD) [9] and acute renal failure requiring renal replacement therapy [11] have also been reported. Histologically, it is characterized by the deposition of C1q in the mesangium. Although there is no evidence of extrarenal disease, there are other histological features resembling lupus nephritis hence diagnosis is made in the absence of clinical or immunological features of systemic lupus erythematosus (SLE) [5, 12, 13].

Light microscopic examination with H&E, PAS, and PASM stains reveals heterogenous glomerular changes, ranging from no glomerular abnormalities resembling minimal change disease to mesangial proliferative glomerulonephritis to focal segmental glomerulosclerosis. Based on light microscopy, C1q nephropathy can be classified into two subtypes: a) MCD/FSGS group, with namely three variants of FSGS group: collapsing, cellular, and "not otherwise specified" variants and b) immune complex-mediated proliferative glomerulonephritis (GN) group. The latter may include focal or diffuse mesangial proliferative GN, membranous GN, and membranoproliferative GN [14].

Light microscopy is less specific than immunofluorescence microscopy. Moreover, staining of the C1q fragment of the complement component C1 by antiserum against C1q (prepared from goat) is more specific. Staining for C1q is evident in all cases of C1q nephropathy, and the staining pattern may be either dominant or codominant. Staining mainly highlights the deposits within the mesangium. IgM and IgG immunoglobulins are also identified, as these immunoglobulins provide ligands for C1q in the immune complex formation. In addition, C3 and C4 are also noted at 60% and 25%, respectively [12].

Histologic criteria require ≥ 2+ (on a scale of 0–4+) immunostaining for C1q with a predominantly mesangial distribution, frequently accompanied by IgG and IgM, which may be less intense, equally intense, or more intense [3, 15, 16]. An important fact to remember is that immunologic staining for C1q may be seen in many glomerular diseases. Jennette and Hipp [16] described high-intensity positivity in a high proportion of cases of proliferative lupus nephritis, membranous lupus nephritis, and type 1 membranoproliferative glomerulonephritis (MPGN). These findings formed the basis of their exclusion of SLE and type 1 MPGN in the diagnostic criteria of C1q nephropathy [16].

Finally, electron microscopy provides the diagnostic confirmation when amorphous electron-dense deposits are demonstrated in the mesangium, occasionally in the subendothelial space and rarely in the subepithelial space. These deposits are a consistent finding in all cases irrespective of their light microscopic subtype. Besides these deposits, podocyte injury characterized by foot process effacement and cytoskeleton condensation is seen to be expressed more commonly in the immune complex-mediated subtype. They occur more frequently in patients with nephrotic syndrome or nephrotic range proteinuria than in those with non-nephrotic proteinuria. Very rarely, tubuloreticular cytoplasmic inclusions may be seen on glomerular and peritubular capillary endothelial cells [12].

Many reports describe different symptoms, histopathologies, therapeutic responses, and prognoses suggesting that C1q nephropathy may be a combination of several disease groups rather than a single disease entity [17]. The therapy mainly involves treatment of the underlying light microscopic lesion, usually with corticosteroids. The disease is associated with a high proportion of steroid resistance, for which, multiple drugs have been tried either separately or in combination therapies, with good response. The most used drugs are methylprednisolone, cyclophosphamide, azathioprine, cyclosporine, mycophenolate, and tacrolimus. There is evidence of the use of rituximab, a monoclonal antibody to CD20, in a few patients who failed to respond to steroids, and they had a promising result in one of the cases, normalization of renal function was achieved avoiding hemodialysis [18].

Not only there is a wide range of variation in the clinical and microscopic picture, but even the outcomes are also variable, and outcomes are generally dependent on various clinical and histological factors [12].

Said et al. [10] performed a retrospective study in 24 patients with kidney transplants whose native kidney disease was not C1q nephropathy and none of these patients had any features of SLE. Histopathological evidence of de novo C1q glomerulonephritis was found by biopsy. The mean time from transplant to detection of mesangial C1q deposits was 37 months (>12 months in 71% of cases) and on follow-up (mean 1 year) of the 10 patients without rejection, most had stable creatinine with no or stable proteinuria, and none lost their graft function.

Among nearly 9000 kidney biopsies reviewed from 1994 to 2002 from Columbia University in New York, 19 were classified as C1q nephropathy [19]. Seventeen patients had FSGS (six with collapsing and two with cellular forms) on kidney biopsy, and two had MCD. At a mean follow-up period of 27 months, 12 of 16 available patients (75%) had stable kidney function, with 7 of 12 entering partial or complete remission (with or without immunosuppressive therapy). Two progressed to end-stage kidney disease (ESKD) (both of whom had FSGS) [19].

In a study of 4048 kidney biopsies from Slovenia, 82 revealed C1q nephropathy, with 11, 27, and 20 also revealing FSGS, no lesion by light microscopy, and proliferative glomerulonephritis, respectively [5]. Of patients who had no lesion by light microscopy, 22% had asymptomatic hematuria and/or mild to modest proteinuria; 63% had the nephrotic syndrome, and 7% had a normal urinalysis. All patients with FSGS presented with nephrotic syndrome. Of those with proliferative glomerulonephritis, 75% presented with chronic kidney disease. Thirty-three percent of those who presented with FSGS developed ESKD, whereas 77% of patients with a minimal change-like lesion had complete remission of nephrotic syndrome.

Similarly, in a study performed by Fukuma et al. [20], among 2221 children aged 3–15 years, 30 had biopsy-proven C1q nephropathy. Among them, 18 were asymptomatic but had hematuria and 12 had a nephrotic syndrome. Light microscopy revealed minimal change disease in 73% while others had immune-mediated glomerulonephritis or FSGS. All nephrotic children were treated with prednisolone with or without cyclosporine and only four of the asymptomatic children received glucocorticoid therapy, and the rest were treated with dipyridamole. Proteinuria decreased in both groups, and hematuria improved more in the asymptomatic group.

Conclusion

Originally described by Jennette and Hipp in 1985, C1 q nephropathy is a glomerulopathy that is subdivided into two groups, MCD/FSGS group and proliferative glomerulonephritis group. Controversy remains whether it is a distinct entity. To the best of our knowledge, there are no randomized trials that have evaluated the treatment of C1q nephropathy. Studies have shown a good clinical outcome for C1q nephropathy in renal transplant patients with a stable creatinine with no or stable proteinuria, and no loss in graft function. Generally, those with minimal proteinuria, nephritic syndrome, and the histologic variant of minimal change disease (MCD) generally have a favorable outcome while those with nephrotic range proteinuria and focal segmental glomerulosclerosis (FSGS) variant have unfavorable outcomes.

References

1. Walport MJ. Complement: first of two parts. N Engl J Med. 2001;344(14):1058–66.
2. Mueller W, Hanauske-Abel H, Loos M. Biosynthesis of the first component of complement by human and Guinea pig peritoneal macrophages: evidence for an independent production of the C1 subunits. J Immunol. 1978;121:1578–84.
3. Jennette JC, Hipp CG. C1q nephropathy: a distinct pathologic entity usually causing nephrotic syndrome. Am J Kidney Dis. 1985;6:103–10.
4. Berger SP, Roos A, Daha MR. Complement and the kidney: what the nephrologist needs to know in 2006? Nephrology Dialysis Transplantation. 2005;20:2613–9.
5. Vizjak A, Ferluga D, Rožič M, et al. Pathology, clinical presentations, and outcomes of C1q nephropathy. J Am Soc Nephrol. 2008;19:2237–44.
6. Lim IS, Yun KW, Moon KC, Cheong HI. Proteinuria in a boy with infectious mononucleosis, C1q nephropathy, and Dent's disease. Journal of Korean Medical Science. 2007;22(5):928–31. View at: Publisher Site|Google Scholar
7. Isaac J, Shihab FS. De novo C1q nephropathy in the renal allograft of a kidney pancreas transplant recipient: BK virus-induced nephropathy? Nephron. 2002;92:431–6.
8. Said SM, Cornell LD, Valeri AM, et al. C1q deposition in the renal allograft: a report of 24 cases. Mod Pathol. 2010;23(8):1080–8.
9. Srivastava T, Chadha V. C1q nephropathy presenting as rapidly progressive crescentic glomerulonephritis. Clinical and Experimental Nephrology. 2009;13(4):263–74.
10. Said SM, Cornell LD, Valeri AM, Sethi S, Fidler ME, Cosio FG, Nasr SH. C1q deposition in the renal allograft: a report of 24 cases. Mod Pathol. 2010;23(8):1080–8. https://doi.org/10.1038/modpathol.2010.92. Epub 2010 May 14
11. Malleshappa P, Ranganath R, Chaudhari AP, Ayiangar A, Lohitaksha S. C1q nephropathy presenting as acute renal failure. Saudi J Kidney Dis Transpl. 2011;22(2):324–6.
12. Joe Devasahayam, Gowrishankar Erode-Singaravelu, Zeenat Bhat, Tony Oliver, Arul Chandran, Xu Zeng, Paramesh Dakshinesh, and Unni Pillai. C1q nephropathy: the unique underrecognized pathological entity.

13. Sharman A, Furness P, Feehally J. Distinguishing C1q nephropathy from lupus nephritis. Nephrology Dialysis Transplantation. 2004;19(6):1420–6. https://doi.org/10.1093/ndt/gfh139.
14. Markowitz GS, Schwimmer JA, Stokes MB, et al. C1q nephropathy: a variant of focal segmental glomerulosclerosis. Kidney Int. 2003;64(4):1232–40.
15. Jennette JC, Falk RJ. C1q nephropathy. In: Massry SG, Glassock R, editors. Textbook of nephrology. 4th ed. Philadelphia: Lippincott-Williams & Wilkins; 2000. p. 730–3.
16. Jennette JC, Hipp CG. Immunohistopathologic evaluation of C1q in 800 renal biopsy specimens. Am J Clin Pathol. 1985;83:415–20.
17. Mii A, Shimizu A, Masuda Y, Fujita E, Aki K, Ishizaki M, Sato S, Griesemer A, Fukuda Y. Current status and issues of C1q nephropathy. Clin Exp Nephrol. 2009;13(4):263–74. https://doi.org/10.1007/s10157-009-0159-5. Epub 2009 Apr 17. PMID: 19373520
18. Sinha A, Nast CC, Hristea I, Vo AA, Jordan SC. Resolution of clinical and pathologic features of C1q nephropathy after rituximab therapy. Clin Exp Nephrol. 2011;15:164–70.
19. Markowitz GS, Schwimmer JA, Stokes MB, Nasr S, Seigle RL, Valeri AM, D'Agati VD. C1q nephropathy: a variant of focal segmental glomerulosclerosis. Kidney Int. 2003;64(4):1232–40. https://doi.org/10.1046/j.1523-1755.2003.00218.x.
20. Fukuma Y, Hisano S, Segawa Y, Niimi K, Tsuru N, Kaku Y, Hatae K, Kiyoshi Y, Mitsudome A, Iwasaki H. Clinicopathologic correlation of C1q nephropathy in children. Am J Kidney Dis. 2006;47(3):412–8. https://doi.org/10.1053/j.ajkd.2005.11.013.

Chapter 44
Vitamin-C Induced Oxalate Nephropathy in Kidney Transplant Recipient

Kusum L. Sharma, Ravi B. Singh, and Weixiong Zhong

Introduction

One of the most common types of crystalline nephropathy is oxalate nephropathy. It is characterized by the deposition of calcium oxalate crystals in the renal tubules, resulting in acute and chronic tubular injury, interstitial fibrosis, and progressive renal insufficiency. It remains a rare cause of renal failure in transplanted kidneys, and understanding the various etiologies of oxalate nephropathy and their prevention is of clinical importance.

Patient History

The patient is a 68-year-old female with a history of end-stage kidney disease secondary to long-standing diabetes mellitus with proliferative diabetic retinopathy, severe hypertension, and obesity. She received a living non-related kidney transplant 5 years ago and had recurrent post-coital urinary tract infections (UTI) with multidrug-resistant Klebsiella. She presented to the emergency department with 1 week of increasing fatigue, malaise, and anorexia. She had a few episodes of "explosive" diarrhea, which she related to taking Fosfomycin for her UTI. Besides,

K. L. Sharma (✉) · W. Zhong
Department of Pathology and Laboratory Medicine, University of Wisconsin Hospital and Clinics, Madison, WI, USA
e-mail: ksharma@uwhealth.org; wzhongh3@wisc.edu

R. B. Singh
Department of Medicine, SUNY Upstate Medical University, Syracuse, NY, USA
e-mail: singhrav@upstate.edu

© The Author(s), under exclusive license to Springer Nature Switzerland AG 2022

F. Aziz, S. Parajuli (eds.), *Complications in Kidney Transplantation*,
https://doi.org/10.1007/978-3-031-13569-9_44

her home glucose readings were between 100 and 200, with a recent HbA1c of 7.1. She had an approximate weight gain of 8 pounds over the last few weeks. She denied any lower extremity swelling, dyspnea, orthopnea, cough, or upper respiratory symptoms. She denied abdominal pain, vomiting, tenderness over her graft, dysuria/frequency, hematuria, or other lower urinary tract symptoms. She had been compliant with all her medications and immunosuppression. There were no recent medication changes. Laboratory investigations revealed significantly elevated serum Cr > 7.29 mg/dL (baseline of 1.2) and blood urea nitrogen (BUN) of 99 mg/dL, and mildly elevated potassium of 5.7 mEq/L. There was an elevated TSH with low fT4. Her Hb was 10.2 with a hematocrit of 32%, sodium was 145 mEq/L, chloride at 117 mEq/L, the glucose of 172 mg/dL, calcium at 8.2 gm/dL, and elevated parathyroid hormone at 417 mg/dL without proteinuria.

Question 1

What is the most likely diagnosis?

A. Acute interstitial nephritis.
B. Acute rejection.
C. Oxalate nephropathy.
D. Phosphate nephropathy.

The correct answer is C.

Diarrhea and excess consumption of Vit C are the risk factors for increasing intestinal absorption of calcium oxalate. Without recent antibiotic or NSAIDs use, acute interstitial nephritis is unlikely, without changes in immunosuppressive drugs, acute rejection is less likely, and phosphate nephropathy is unlikely with normal serum calcium levels.

She was diagnosed with acute kidney injury with acidosis and hyperkalemia on CKD stage 3 and was admitted to the hospital. At the time of admission, her X-ray, EKG, and transplant ultrasound were normal, she had an elevated blood pressure that was managed with nifedipine, and a biopsy of the allograft was performed. Hyperkalemia was treated with intravenous bicarbonate and diuretics. Nephrotoxic agents, losartan, hydrochlorothiazide, and tacrolimus were held. Urine output was adequate, and hemodialysis was not required. IV fluids and Lasix were given. The biopsy revealed diffuse rhomboid-shaped crystal deposits in tubules best seen on frozen section (Fig. 44.1). These crystals were birefringent under polarized light (Fig. 44.2). There was also moderate to severe acute tubular injury with focal mild interstitial mononuclear cell infiltrates. The glomeruli are unremarkable, tubulitis is not identified, and focal arteries show mild intimal fibrous thickening.

Question 2

What is the most likely etiology?

A. Calcium phosphate crystal accumulation.
B. Calcium oxalate crystal accumulation.
C. Drug-induced crystal accumulation.

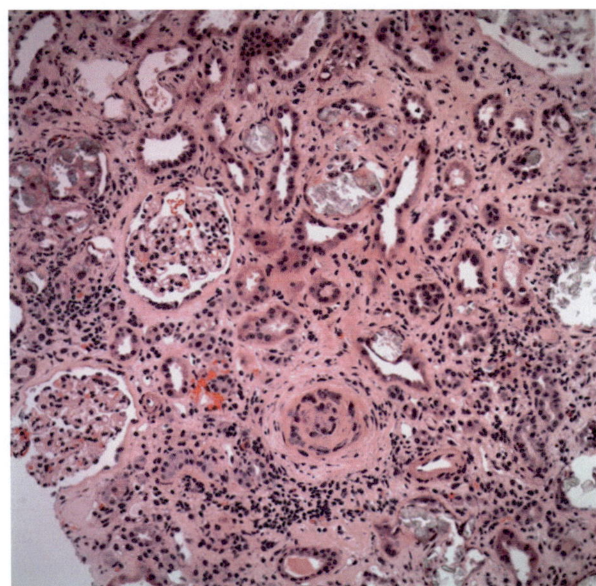

Fig. 44.1 H&E-stained slides showing birefringent calcium oxalate crystals

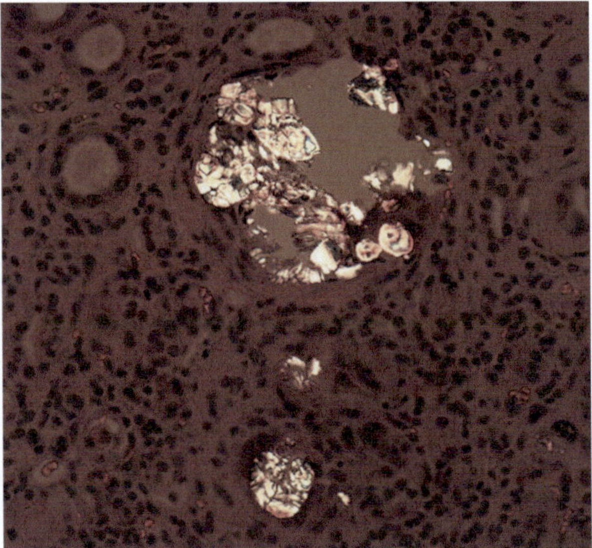

Fig. 44.2 Strongly birefringent calcium oxalate crystals viewed under polarized light (H&E, 100×)

D. Urate crystal accumulation.

E. Non-specific crystal accumulation.

The correct answer is B.

A diagnosis of oxalate crystal nephropathy with acute tubular necrosis was made, and there was no evidence of rejection. Hyperoxaluria could be related to her recent worsening of chronic diarrhea and impaired oxalate binding in the gut and increased absorption, dietary habits, and excess vitamin c intake, which she reported. She received dietary counseling to avoid worsening her condition. After 5 days of hospital stay, her creatinine improved to 5.85, and was discharged home with dietary recommendations including low oxalate, low sodium, and high calcium diet and with a plan to continue to follow-up with thrice-weekly labs and continued hold on losartan and hydrochlorothiazide. A calcium supplement was additionally added at discharge.

Discussion

Crystalline nephropathies are an important cause of kidney disease that are diagnosed with the histologic finding of intrarenal crystal deposition. Under favorable conditions, crystals of some molecules and ions precipitate and deposit within the tubular lumens [1]. The two most common crystalline nephropathies are calcium phosphate- and calcium oxalate-induced crystalline nephropathies. The most common cause is hypercalcemia/hypercalciuria, hyperphosphatemia/hyperphosphaturia, or hyperoxalemia/hyperoxaluria due to different etiologies. Generally, nephrocalcinosis is the term that applies to both of these situations based on crystalline nephropathies. However, in daily practice, calcium oxalate deposition is referred to as oxalate nephropathy or renal oxalosis [2].

The definitive diagnosis of oxalate nephropathy is histologic. In the established methodology, the kidney tissue obtained from the needle biopsy is cut into three pieces; two of them are small and processed for examination by immunofluorescent microscopy and by transmission electron microscopy (TEM). The large remainder portion is embedded in paraffin and finely sliced, a stained specimen for light microscopy (LM) is prepared, and the histological changes are examined. The information obtained from these three methodologies is consolidated for the pathological diagnosis of the renal biopsy specimen. For renal biopsy examination, the standard practice has become to observe specimens stained with HE, PAS, and Masson (or AZAN) stains plus silver impregnation stain periodic acid silver methenamine stain (PASM stain) [3]. Oxalate crystals are often partially or completely dissolved in tissue processing for paraffin sections, depending on the size of the crystals. The best method for evaluating oxalate crystals is viewing the H&E-stained frozen section under polarized light (Figs. 44.1 and 44.3).

Oxalic acid is a small decarboxylate ion (C_2O_4) and is the end-product of many metabolic pathways. Oxalic acid is eliminated through free glomerular filtration and secretion by the proximal tubule. The plasma concentration of oxalic acid is determined by the balance between dietary intake, intestinal absorption, endogenous production, and renal excretion. Normal plasma concentrations are below 5 μmol/L [4].

Hyperoxaluria, defined as excessive urinary excretion of oxalic acid, can be classified as primary or secondary hyperoxaluria. Primary hyperoxaluria is caused by

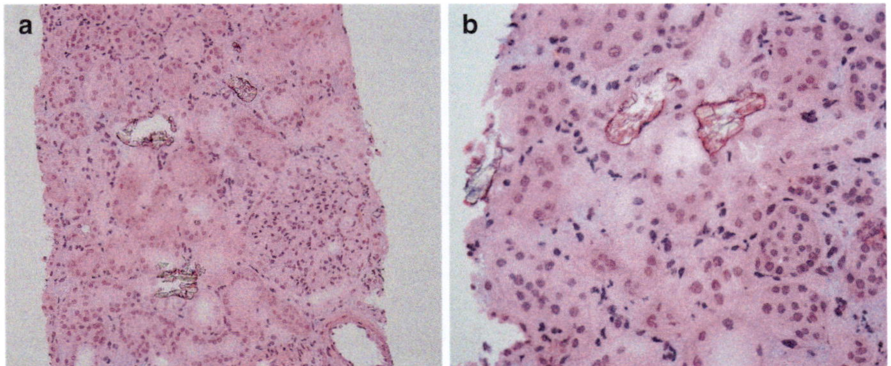

Fig. 44.3 Calcium oxalate crystal seen on frozen sections. (**a**) Strongly birefringent calcium oxalate crystals viewed under polarized light (H&E A) 200× and (**b**) 400×

rare autosomal recessive disorders which cause excessive production of oxalic acid. In primary hyperoxaluria, persistently elevated plasma oxalic acid concentrations cause CaOx deposition in the kidney, which leads to permanent loss of renal function [4].

Secondary hyperoxaluria is a more common disorder that results from increased dietary intake of oxalate, enteric conditions causing increased intestinal oxalate availability, decreased intestinal oxalate degradation, or increased colonic permeability to oxalate. Enteric hyperoxaluria occurs mostly in patients with malabsorption as a result of, e.g., small bowel resections, pancreatic insufficiency, or gastric bypass. A high intake of oxalic acid-containing food puts these patients at risk of renal stones or CaOx deposition in their kidneys [4]. When the GFR drops below 30–40 mL/min/1.73 m [2] oxalic acid elimination by the kidneys is impaired, and the plasma concentration rises [4]. The blood levels of oxalate can achieve supersaturation and precipitate mainly in kidneys, bones, joints, cardiac conductive system, blood vessels, and retina [4]. In our case, the patient had a new-onset diagnosis of hypothyroidism at the time of admission, requiring treatment with levothyroxine. One study suggested that primary hypothyroidism can result in the deposition of calcium oxalate in the thyroid tissue [5].

In a systematic review by Lumlertgul et al. [6], hyperoxaluria-enabling conditions were mainly divided into four categories: (1) increased dietary oxalate intake through excessive consumption; (2) increased oxalate availability in the colon caused by decreased intestinal calcium availability from fat malabsorption commonly resulting from Crohn's disease, celiac sprue, jejunoileal bypass, ileal resection, Roux-en-Y gastric bypass surgery, short bowel syndrome, chronic pancreatitis, pancreatic insufficiency, cystic fibrosis, and use of orlistat and a low calcium diet; (3) decreased intestinal oxalate degradation due to decreased intestinal colonization with oxalate-degrading bacteria (i.e., *Oxalobacter formigenes*); and (4) an increased colonic permeability to oxalate from injury to colonic mucosa in *Clostridium difficile* colitis, leading to a nonselective increase in oxalate absorption. Amongst these, fat malabsorption (75.0%) was the most attributed cause of secondary oxalate nephropathy, followed by excessive dietary oxalate consumption (30.6%) and decreased intestinal oxalate degradation (0.9%).

In our case, the patient had a history of chronic *Clostridium difficile* colitis with recent worsening. Cohen-Bucay et al. [7] described a case report of a 69-year-old man who presented with acute kidney injury in the setting of community-acquired *Clostridium difficile* colitis with biopsy-proven oxalate nephropathy. The potential mechanism was presumed to be increased colonic permeability to oxalate secondary due to infection.

Another important known cause of oxalate nephropathy is excessive consumption of vitamin C. In our case, the patient describes excessive consumption of vitamin C. Vitamin C should be replaced each day by a dietary intake of 70 –90 mg to maintain optimal health and ascorbic acid homeostasis. Urinary oxalate excretion begins to increase when amounts of ascorbic acid are above that required by the body are ingested [8]. Many reports of oxalate nephropathy are associated with moderate and large amounts of oral and intravenous administration of vitamin C in people with previously normal renal function [9–14]. In a short-term human experiment, Auer et al. [15] described a 25-year-old individual with no history of nephrolithiasis and normal renal function who ingested 8 g of ascorbic acid during an 8-day period time. After 8 days, he presented with hematuria after oxalate excretion had increased to 350%, showing crystalluria, and the protocol was immediately suspended. Although the authors highlighted the potential dangers of large dose ingestion of vitamin C in some individuals, they did not show alterations in renal function.

Some reports of patients with renal allografts developing oxalate nephropathy and worsening renal function with vitamin C ingestion have been reported [16, 17]. Getting JE et al. [16] described 65 patients with biopsy-proven calcium oxalate crystals. Five patients showed oxalate nephropathy associated with high intake of vitamin C, including two patients post kidney transplant and three patients with chronic kidney diseases. Suneja et al. [17] described three patients, two with a history of kidney transplant and one with a history of pancreas-kidney transplant. All three patients had a history of vitamin C ingestion. They presented with acute kidney allograft dysfunction and oxalate nephropathy on renal biopsies.

Conclusion

Oxalate nephropathy is more likely to develop in patients with more than one predisposing factor. In our case, the patient's oxalate nephropathy was attributed to her chronic worsening *Clostridium difficile* colitis, and due to excessive ingestion of vitamin C. Vitamin C is prescribed for a number of indications. Clinicians should be aware of the potential risks of high doses of vitamin C ingestion and the ingestion of large amounts of fruits rich in vitamin C, especially for patients with renal transplant or other nephropathies with concurrent enteric conditions.

References

1. Perazella MA, Herlitz LC. The crystalline nephropathies. Kidney Int Rep. 2021;6(12):2942–57. https://doi.org/10.1016/j.ekir.2021.09.003.
2. Nicholas Cossey L, Dvanajscak Z, Larsen CP. A diagnostician's field guide to crystalline nephropathies. Semin Diagn Pathol. 2020;37(3):135–42. https://doi.org/10.1053/j.semdp.2020.02.002. Epub 2020 Feb 21. PMID: 32178905
3. N.Yamanaka. Staining techniques. In: Japanese Renal Pathology Society and Japanese Society of Nephrology (Eds): Kidney Biopsy-Atlas and Text, 2nd Edition, Tokyo, Tokyo Igakusha 2017 pp. 32–43 (in Japanese).
4. Malou L. H. Snijders, Dennis A. Hesselink, Marian C. Clahsen-van Groningen, Joke I. Roodnat. Oxalate deposition in renal allograft biopsies within 3 months after transplantation is associated with allograft dysfunction.
5. Shatha M, Eisenberg I. Endocrine manifestations of primary hyperoxaluria. AACE Endocr Pract. 2017;23(12):1414–24. https://doi.org/10.4158/EP-2017-0029.
6. Lumlertgul N, Siribamrungwong M, Jaber BL, Susantitaphong P. Secondary oxalate nephropathy: a systematic review. Kidney Int Rep. 2018;3(6):1363–72. https://doi.org/10.1016/j.ekir.2018.07.020.
7. Cohen-Bucay A, Garimella P, Ezeokonkwo C. Acute oxalate nephropathy associated with *Clostridium difficile* colitis. Am J Kidney Dis. 2014;63:113–8.
8. Knight J, Madduma-Liyanage K, Mobley JA, Assimos DG, Holmes RP. Ascorbic acid intake and oxalate synthesis. Urolithiasis. 2016;44:289–97.
9. Mashour S, Turner JF, Merrel R. Acute renal failure, oxalosis, and vitamin C supplementation, a case report and review of the literature. Chest. 2000;118:561–3.
10. Nasr SH, Kashtanova Y, Levchuk V, Markowitz GS. Secondary oxalosis due to excess vitamin C intake. Kidney Int. 2006;70:1672.
11. Lamarche J, Nair R, Peguero A, Courville C. Vitamin C-induced oxalate nephropathy. Int J Nephrol. 2011;2011:146927. https://doi.org/10.4061/2011/146927.
12. Gurm H, Sheta MA, Nivera N, Tunkel A. Vitamin-C induced oxalate nephropathy. J Community HospInt Med Persp. 2012;2:17718. https://doi.org/10.3402/jchimp.v2i2.17718.
13. Cossey LN, Rahim F, Larsen CP. Oxalate nephropathy and intravenous vitamin C. Am J Kidney Dis. 2013;61:1032–5.
14. Moyses-Neto M, Brito BRS, de Araújo Brito DJ, et al. Vitamin C-induced oxalate nephropathy in a renal transplant patient related to excessive ingestion of cashew pseudofruit (Anacardium occidentale L.): a case report. BMC Nephrol. 2018;19:265. https://doi.org/10.1186/s12882-018-1060-9.
15. Auer BL, Auer D, Rodgers AL. Relative hyperoxaluria, crystalluria and haematuria after megadose ingestion of vitamin C. Eur J Clin Investig. 1998;28:695–700.
16. Getting JE, Gregoire JR, Phul A, Kasten MJ. Oxalate nephropathy due to "juicing": case report and review. Am J Med. 2013;126:768–72.
17. Suneja M, Kumar AB. Secondary oxalosis induced acute kidney injury in allograft kidneys. Clin Kidney J. 2013;1:84–6.

Chapter 45
Recurrent Heavy Proteinuria and Focal Segmental Glomerulosclerosis Post-Kidney Transplant

Rowena Delos Santos and Tarek Alhamad

Introduction

Proteinuric kidney diseases such as focal segmental glomerulosclerosis (FSGS) can recur after kidney transplantation. This case reviews the presentation and course of a patient with "minimal change disease" who had recurrence early after transplant. We later describe the patient's development of rejection, highlighting the need for ongoing vigilance with respect to suspicion of rejection in patients with recurrent native kidney disease. We discuss various treatments and long-term outcomes of patients with recurrent FSGS.

Case Presentation

A 48-year-old man with a history of end-stage kidney disease attributed to a biopsy-proven minimal change disease (vs. early or unsampled FSGS) underwent a deceased donor kidney transplant. His calculated panel reactive antibody (cPRA) was 0% with a 0A, 1B, 1DR mismatch, with cytomegalovirus (CMV) serology donor positive and recipient negative, with a kidney donor profile index (KDPI) of 17%. He made less than a cup of urine a day prior to the transplant. He had no pre-existing antibodies, and the pre-transplant cross matches were negative. He received induction with anti-thymocyte globulin and continued with maintenance immunosuppression, including tacrolimus (target trough 7–10 ng/mL), mycophenolate

R. D. Santos (✉) · T. Alhamad
Division of Nephrology, Department of Medicine, Washington University School of Medicine, St. Louis, MO, USA
e-mail: delossantos@wustl.edu; talhamad@wustl.edu

© The Author(s), under exclusive license to Springer Nature Switzerland AG 2022

F. Aziz, S. Parajuli (eds.), *Complications in Kidney Transplantation*,
https://doi.org/10.1007/978-3-031-13569-9_45

sodium starting at 720 mg bid, and prednisone. Prophylaxis with valganciclovir was planned for 9 months due to his CMV high-risk status.

The patient's kidney function and urine output improved until post-operation day (POD) 3, when he had a rise from Cr 5.9 to 6.8 mg/dL, and urine output decreased from 1.3 L down to only 500 cc with a urine protein/creatinine ratio of 10,489 mg/g. Evaluation including kidney ultrasound, CT abdomen/pelvis without contrast, and donor-specific testing were unremarkable. He underwent a biopsy on POD 5.

Question 1

What is the most likely cause of the patient's current presentation?

A. Acute cellular rejection, Banff 2A.
B. Active antibody-mediated rejection.
C. Recurrent FSGS.
D. Acute BK nephropathy.

The correct answer is C.

The patient had a cPRA 0%, no history of sensitization event, no evidence of pre-existing antibodies, and cross matches were negative. His history and timing of the transplant and biopsy would likely make rejection less likely. It would be unlikely that he would have BK nephropathy this early after kidney transplantation. With the high level of proteinuria found, a recurrent focal segmental glomerulosclerosis is a potential etiology for the current presentation. Assuming there was no pre-existing donor disease, the most likely cause for the current high-level proteinuria would be minimal change/recurrent FSGS.

Question 2

Which one of the following treatment regimens leads to more partial and complete remissions?

A. High dose IV corticosteroids with oral taper.
B. Cyclosporine.
C. Rituximab only.
D. Plasmapheresis with or without rituximab.

The correct answer is D.

The Post-Transplant Glomerular Disease (TANGO) project investigates glomerular disease recurrence post-transplant through an international cohort of over 11,000 patients worldwide. In this study, the treatment that appears to have the most partial and complete remissions compared with the other treatments listed above is plasmapheresis with or without rituximab.

Hospital Course

The patient underwent five sessions of plasmapheresis and received a dose of rituximab at the end of the plasmapheresis treatments, with an improvement of his urine output to 3 L and serum creatinine 3.83 mg/dL by the day of discharge

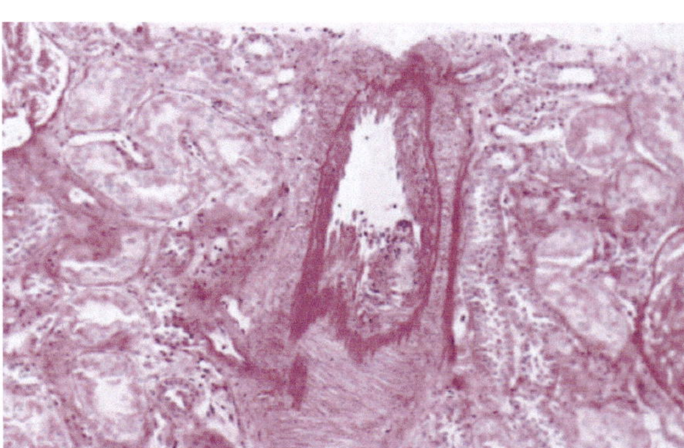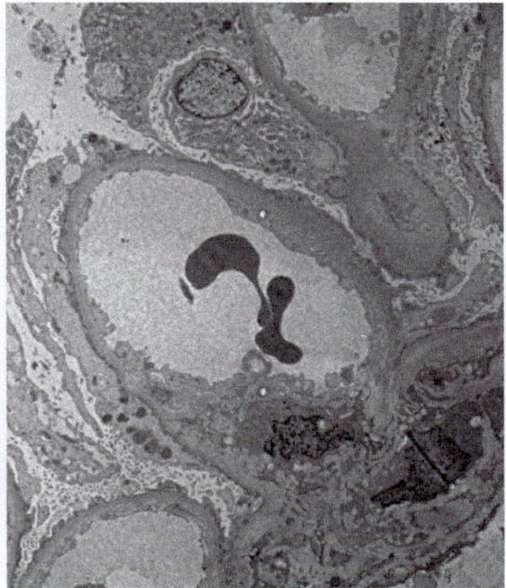

Fig. 45.1 Biopsy findings

on POD 11. The patient's serum creatinine decreased to a baseline between 1.3 and 1.5 mg/dL, but his proteinuria remained in the nephrotic range between 5000 and 7000 mg/g. Because of the persistent proteinuria, the patient was restarted on plasmapheresis treatments twice-weekly starting 4 months post-transplant. The kidney function remained stable for approximately 7 months post-transplant when it was noted that his serum creatinine increased to 1.9 mg/dL. His proteinuria remained elevated despite the plasmapheresis, and he underwent a second kidney transplant biopsy 7 months post-transplant, with biopsy results below.

Question 3

In addition to the podocyte foot process effacement seen on the electron microscopy picture (Fig. 45.1), what other prominent findings can be found in the slide?

A. C4d by immunofluorescence positivity consistent with an active antibody-mediated rejection.
B. Endothelialitis and endothelial injury of a small-sized artery consistent with Banff 2A or B acute cellular rejection.
C. Tip lesion on PAS stain consistent with recurrent FSGS.
D. SV40 staining consistent with BK nephropathy.

   The correct answer is B.

   Neither picture depicts immunofluorescence with C4d deposition present. Additionally, neither picture shows immunohistochemical staining for SV40 to indicate BK nephropathy. While the podocyte effacement of approximately 90% as seen on the electron microscopy may reveal the presence of recurrent FSGS, there is no tip lesion shown on either picture. The artery noted here is a small-sized artery with an inflammatory infiltrate and endothelialitis consistent with at least a Banff 2A or B acute cellular rejection. In this patient's case, the inflammatory infiltrate within the tubules was focal and mild.

Hospital Course and Follow-Up

The patient was diagnosed with a Banff 2A acute cellular rejection in addition to his already known recurrent FSGS. He was treated with anti-thymocyte globulin, IV corticosteroids with taper, as well as a repeated dose of rituximab. His plasmapheresis was continued as an outpatient after discharge. Over the course of the following 3 months (10 months post-transplant), the patient's serum creatinine decreased to his pre-rejection baseline of 1.3–1.5 mg/dL, with subnephrotic range proteinuria, prompting tapering of his plasmapheresis. The patient did undergo one more kidney transplant biopsy approximately 15 months post-transplant due to another increase in his serum creatinine to 2.0 mg/dL. There was no evidence of cellular or antibody-mediated rejection, and podocyte effacement decreased to 10%, and he was discharged to continue outpatient plasmapheresis. Over subsequent months, he improved to minimal proteinuria, and plasmapheresis was entirely discontinued by 22 months post-transplant. He maintains a serum creatinine between 1.3 and 1.5 mg/dL.

Discussion

Focal segmental glomerulosclerosis is one of the glomerular diseases that can recur in a kidney transplant. Typical signs and symptoms of FSGS recurrence include proteinuria, typically in the nephrotic range, an elevated serum creatinine, hyperlipidemia, and hypoalbuminemia, with associated edema. Generally, the rate of recurrence of FSGS in a first kidney transplant is approximately 30 and 80% in those requiring a second kidney transplant due to FSGS recurrence in a first transplant [1–3]. Recurrence of the disease carries an increased relative risk of allograft failure as well as decreased allograft survival compared with no recurrence [1, 2].

Data from the ANZDAT registry noted several risk factors associated with disease recurrence, including younger age, non-white ethnicity, and having a living donor [4]. Patients with disease recurrence experience lower 5-year allograft survival at 52% compared with those who did not experience disease recurrence, with 5-year allograft survival of 83% [4]. Though there was a higher association of recurrence in those with a living donor kidney transplant, they also had longer median allograft survival compared with deceased donor recipients [4].

Recent data from the international Post-Transplant glomerular Disease (TANGO) study has shown different findings. The risk of recurrence in a kidney transplant was similar, around 32%, with rather poor 5-year allograft survival of 61% [5]. In those who had the first transplant fail from FSGS recurrence, recurrence occurred in 45% (5 of 11) of those who had a second transplant, while disease recurrence was in 100% (5 of 5) of those who had a third transplant [5]. Contrasting with this was patients with a history of FSGS who lost their allograft due to other reasons, where only 15% (4 of 28) developed recurrence in a second transplant [5]. The group found that older age at diagnosis, Caucasian race, higher BMI, and patients with prior nephrectomy were at higher risk for FSGS recurrence in the allograft [5].

The development of nearly immediate recurrence of proteinuria in post-reperfusion allograft biopsies suggests a circulating factor affecting the glomeruli, leading to disease recurrence [6]. The first and perhaps most notable case report that illustrates this involved a living donor-recipient who underwent pre-transplant plasmapheresis before and after his surgery, with standard immunosuppressive therapy. By post-transplant day 2, the patient developed heavy proteinuria with a biopsy on POD6 showing diffuse podocyte foot process effacement consistent with recurrent disease [7]. Due to the massive proteinuria, hypoalbuminemia, and worsening kidney function, the decision was made to explant the allograft on POD14 and re-transplant it into another recipient on the waitlist [7]. The second recipient did well, with reversal of podocyte changes on two subsequent biopsies and on the last follow-up had an eGFR >90 mL/min/m2 BSA and mild proteinuria (0.27 g in 24 h) [7].

As mentioned above, a circulating factor in some patients may be the causative agent leading to recurrent FSGS. Several potential proteins have been evaluated, but the mechanisms of their pathophysiologic effects on the kidney are not yet elucidated. Due to its relatively poor allograft prognosis after recurrence, therapeutic interventions to prevent and/or treat the disease have been attempted, with varying responses. Gohh et al. described a cohort of 10 patients who were determined to be at high risk of FSGS recurrence and treated with eight sessions of perioperative plasmapheresis in addition to their center's induction and maintenance immunosuppression protocol [3]. Seven out of ten patients did not experience FSGS recurrence with treatment [3]. A multicenter study in France evaluated rituximab in 19 patients with recurrent FSGS and administered between one and four doses of 375 mg/m2 in instances of early recurrence, after treatment failure, or after titrating off plasmapheresis [8]. More patients who received rituximab achieved complete or partial remission of disease than those who did not receive the drug [8]. The TANGO study also showed that more patients had a full or partial response when treated with plasmapheresis with or without rituximab [5]. Other less commonly used medications include cyclosporine, cyclophosphamide in addition to plasmapheresis, immunoadsorption where available, and as reported, two retrospective series, ACTH gel [5, 9, 10].

At our center, we treat patients with recurrent FSGS or de novo FSGS with plasmapheresis and rituximab. We treat patients with ACTH gel who are refractory to plasmapheresis and rituximab, utilizing a strategy of at least 4–6 months of treatment and monitoring their proteinuria closely. Further studies to determine the pathophysiologic process of this disease are needed to guide our therapies better. LDL apheresis has shown promising results in the treatment of FSGS (in native and kidney transplantation). Additional studies with more significant numbers of patients, such as in the TANGO study, will provide more information on the most effective treatments. An additional learning point we wish to emphasize here is that though patients may have heavy proteinuria, a rise in serum creatinine should not be assumed to be related to worsening FSGS. Another biopsy may be warranted in some cases to evaluate for superimposed rejection, as seen in our patient.

References

1. Hariharan S, Adams MB, Brennan DC, et al. Recurrent and de novo glomerular disease after renal transplantation: a report from renal allograft disease registry (RADR). Transplantation. 1999;68(5):635–41.
2. Canaud G, Audard V, Kofman T, Lang P, Legendre C, Grimbert P. Recurrence from primary and secondary glomerulopathy after renal transplant. Transpl Int. 2012;25(8):812–24.
3. Gohh RY, Yango AF, Morrissey PE, et al. Preemptive plasmapheresis and recurrence of FSGS in high-risk renal transplant recipients. American journal of transplantation. 2005;5(12):2907–12.
4. Francis A, Trnka P, McTaggart SJ. Long-term outcome of kidney transplantation in recipients with focal segmental glomerulosclerosis. CJASN. 2016;11(11):2041–6.
5. Uffing A, Pérez-Sáez MJ, Mazzali M, et al. Recurrence of FSGS after kidney transplantation in adults. Clin J Am Soc Nephrol. 2020;15(2):247–56.
6. Chang JW, Pardo V, Sageshima J, et al. Podocyte foot process effacement in postreperfusion allograft biopsies correlates with early recurrence of proteinuria in focal segmental glomerulosclerosis. Transplantation. 2012;93(12):1238–44.
7. Gallon L, Leventhal J, Skaro A, Kanwar Y, Alvarado A. Resolution of recurrent focal segmental glomerulosclerosis after Retransplantation. N Engl J Med. 2012;366(17):1648–9.
8. Garrouste C, Canaud G, Büchler M, et al. Rituximab for recurrence of primary focal segmental glomerulosclerosis after kidney transplantation: clinical outcomes. Transplantation. 2017;101(3):649–56.
9. Alhamad T, Manllo Dieck J, Younus U, et al. ACTH gel in resistant focal segmental glomerulosclerosis after kidney transplantation. Transplantation. 2019;103(1):202–9.
10. Grafals M, Sharfuddin A. Adrenocorticotropic hormone in the treatment of focal segmental glomerulosclerosis following kidney transplantation. Transplant Proc. 2019;51(6):1831–7.

Chapter 46
Early Complications Following Kidney Allograft Biopsy

Shahul Valavoor and M. Yahya Jan

Introduction

Kidney allograft biopsy remains the gold standard for assessing graft function and diagnosis of rejection. It has been incorporated into graft surveillance as part of protocol biopsies by some transplant centers, while other centers utilize this when there is clinical suspicion for rejection. Ultrasound-guided allograft biopsy and pre-loaded biopsy needles have become the standard practice for this procedure. Bleeding and hematoma formation remain the most common complication. This chapter reviews some of the complications that can potentially be encountered during and after this procedure.

Case

A 19-year-old female with a history of kidney dysgenesis leading to ESKD status post LRKT from her mother 3 years ago was noted to have an elevated creatinine of 1.7 mg/dL compared to her baseline of 0.8 mg/dL on yearly follow-up. She has transitioned to adult transplant nephrology over the course of the past year. Her tacrolimus levels were noted to be sub-therapeutic. Over the past 3 months, the patient had missed routine surveillance lab testing. The patient had recently moved out of living with her parents, to start college and living with a roommate.

The patient was admitted for AKI. Given her presenting history, the index of suspicion was high for kidney allograft rejection, and a kidney allograft biopsy was

S. Valavoor · M. Y. Jan (✉)
Indiana University School of Medicine, Indianapolis, IN, USA
e-mail: myjan@iu.edu

© The Author(s), under exclusive license to Springer Nature Switzerland AG 2022

F. Aziz, S. Parajuli (eds.), *Complications in Kidney Transplantation*,
https://doi.org/10.1007/978-3-031-13569-9_46

planned the next day. Appropriate consent for the procedure was obtained, explaining the risks and benefits. Pre-transplant labs showed a hemoglobin of 11.2 g/dL, platelets of 167k/microL, and an INR of 1.1 with normal PT and APTT. BP on the morning of the biopsy was 138/78. Blood pressure overnight and the day prior were in the 120/70 range. The patient had been NPO overnight. The patient's BMI was 22.3 kg/m^2.

A pre-biopsy allograft ultrasound was performed and showed a kidney allograft with the longest dimension of 10.5 cm, no cysts, hydronephrosis, and no perinephric fluid collection. The allograft was at a 3–4 cm depth from the skin.

A 16-gauge pre-loaded biopsy needle was used to obtain samples, and 3 cores of tissue were planned. The first and second biopsy cores were obtained and examined at the bedside microscope.

During the pass for the third biopsy core, the patient reported feeling dizzy and lightheaded. The needle was withdrawn, and vital signs showed a BP of 104/72. 500 mL of normal saline bolus was given immediately to improve BP to 122/76. A scanning ultrasound of the allograft was performed. The third core was deferred, and the patient was returned to their room in supine position. Stat labs were drawn for hemoglobin and hematocrit. Vital signs were obtained q 15 min as per protocol.

During this time, the patient continued to feel lightheaded and reported feeling nauseous. This was accompanied by reported discomfort at the site of needle insertion for the biopsy. She voided once since the biopsy and urine color was light yellow. She was moved to a progressive care unit for higher acuity of monitoring.

Question 1

Which of the following is the most common complication of an allograft kidney biopsy?

A. Injury to surrounding abdominal viscera.
B. Perinephric hematoma.
C. Subcapsular hematoma.
D. Infection.
E. Graft loss.

The correct answer is B.

Ultrasound-guided percutaneous kidney allograft biopsy is the gold standard in monitoring the status of kidney allografts and investigating the cause of kidney allograft dysfunction. Depending on specific transplant center practices, these are performed as "protocol biopsies," i.e., performed at set intervals regardless of kidney allograft functional status or as "by indication," i.e., if a clinical or laboratory concern arises for allograft dysfunction. In either case, the relative risk of complications from the procedure must be weighed against the possible benefits, and informed consent of the patient is a key step in this process. Generally, the risks of performing kidney allograft biopsies have decreased over recent years, with practices such as the use of larger gauge biopsy needles and the use of ultrasound guidance [1].

Transplant kidney biopsy carries a lower complication rate than native kidney biopsy. The rate of complication secondary to transplant kidney biopsy has been variously reported between 6 and 13% [2, 3]. The transplanted kidney is much more superficial than the native kidney, separated from the skin only by a thin layer of muscle, fascia, and subcutaneous tissue of the anterior abdominal wall. It is, therefore, much better visualized because of less acoustic impedance from these structures. Furthermore, because the biopsy needle has to travel through a thinner layer of tissue, the operator has better directional control. The safety and efficacy of the smaller 18-gauge automated biopsy needle compared with the conventional Tru-Cut biopsy needles have been documented by various authors [3, 4].

The variation in the frequency of the reported complications depends on multiple factors. These include the operator's experience, utilization of imaging guidance, the gauge of the biopsy needle, and a proactive effort on the part of the operator to pursue subclinical complications by follow-up imaging [1]. Bleeding is the predominant complication related to transplant biopsy and may occur acutely as microscopic or gross hematuria or subcapsular hematoma. The rate of frank and occult hematuria secondary to kidney biopsy has been reported to be between 5 and 40% [2]. Clinical findings that should raise suspicion for a significant bleed after the biopsy include the development of abdominal pain or flank pain or both, especially if sudden, as well as passing blood clots in the urine. Tachycardia and down trending blood pressure or frank hypotension are other signs of a potentially significant bleed.

Clinical Course

The patient's BP remained below her norm in the 110/60s range. The patient's lightheadedness improved. Her CBC was reported with a hemoglobin of 8.9 g/dL, and a type and screen were sent to the lab.

Question 2

What is the next best step in the management of this patient?

A. Wait for blood products to arrive and re-assess after transfusion.
B. Given that the patient's symptoms have resolved, she should be closely monitored without any further interventions.
C. Repeat ultrasound of the kidney.
D. CT Angiogram (CTA) of the abdomen and pelvis.
E. Surgical consultation for exploration.
F. Interventional radiology consultation for embolization of bleeding vessel.

The correct answer is D.

The patient has had a bleeding complication during an allograft biopsy. Though the immediate post-biopsy ultrasound and doppler did not show any significant hematoma or active bleed, the concern remains supported by a drop in hemoglobin. While it is prudent to transfuse promptly, the patient is stable enough to undergo an urgent CT scan of the abdomen and pelvis to evaluate for hematoma or an active bleed. The location and size of the hematoma on CT scan will determine the next best approach, and the patient can be transfused in the meantime. It would also make the radiological intervention more timely if required.

Further Clinical Course

CTA of the abdomen showed a large perinephric hematoma without mass effect on the kidney allograft parenchyma and the absence of an active bleeding vessel. The patient returned to the progressive care unit and was transfused with packed red cells resulting in stabilization of hemoglobin levels around 10 g/dL. CBC was trended every 6 h and remained stable. The patient remained asymptomatic and was discharged on the third post-biopsy day. No radiological or surgical intervention was required.

Discussion

Prior to a percutaneous kidney biopsy, a history, a physical examination, and selected laboratory tests should be obtained to determine patient-specific risks for complications. The skin overlying the biopsy site should be free from signs of infection, and the patient's blood pressure should be well controlled. In certain cases, this may require admission to the hospital a day prior for better BP control. It is suggested that the blood pressure before and after the biopsy should be controlled to a goal of less than 140/90 mmHg. Hypertension is a risk factor for bleeding complications; performing elective kidney biopsy should be avoided if the patient has a systolic blood pressure of > 170 mmHg [1, 8–10].

Recommended laboratory tests include a complete metabolic profile, complete blood count, platelet count, prothrombin time and international normalized ratio (INR), and activated partial thromboplastin time. A bleeding diathesis and qualitative or quantitative platelet dysfunction, if discovered, should be appropriately evaluated and treated prior to undertaking an elective kidney biopsy [11]. Patients taking antiplatelet or antithrombotic agents should ideally discontinue these medications for *at least one to 2 weeks* prior to a scheduled elective biopsy and remain off of them for 1–2 weeks after the biopsy if possible. The management of patients on chronic anticoagulation must be individualized. Cardiology and hematology consultation is often necessary to decide on holding anticoagulation for the procedure [11]. In cases of acute kidney injury or worsening CKD with elevated blood urea nitrogen, administration of desmopressin can be considered on a *case-by-case* basis, and the risks of desmopressin administration such as thrombosis and hyponatremia should be weighed against the risk of bleeding [3].

Given the higher complication rate of previous kidney biopsy techniques, patients were traditionally admitted to the hospital overnight after the procedure for observation. With the emergence of safer biopsy devices, combined with improvements in kidney localization and real-time visualization of the process of tissue acquisition, the complication rates have decreased. In addition to this, increasing health care costs have prompted many physicians to perform a kidney biopsy as an outpatient procedure. Following the kidney biopsy procedure, the patient should be supine for

4–6 h. To help detect bleeding and other complications, vital signs are closely monitored. One such protocol is to check vital signs every 15 min for the first hour, then every 30 min for the next 4 h, then per routine if the patient remains stable. A complete blood count is obtained at various time points after the biopsy, the first generally within 6 h after the procedure. To minimize the risk of bleeding, blood pressure should be well controlled to a goal of <140/90 mmHg [1, 8, 10, 12]. Voided urine samples should be obtained and observed at the bedside for the presence of worsening hematuria.

In patients with suspected bleeding, a complete blood count should be obtained, and abdominal imaging with either ultrasound or computed tomography should be performed. If the patient is hemodynamically unstable, urgent referral for angiography or surgery without imaging may be warranted. An arterial injury may also result in arteriovenous fistulae or a pseudoaneurysm formation. A subcapsular fluid collection/hematoma is generally managed conservatively but may require percutaneous or surgical intervention if there is evidence of compromised kidney function. A small percentage of patients with decreased hemoglobin levels or hemodynamic instability may require blood product transfusion. Other complications include pain lasting more than 12 h, peri-kidney soft tissue infection, and rarely puncture of the liver, pancreas, spleen, or even aorta may occur, as well as urinoma formation from puncture of the urinary tract. Another rare complication from a sub-acute or chronic development and persistence of subcapsular hematoma is chronic hypertension due to "Page kidney" (Fig. 46.1). In this scenario, pressure-induced ischemia from a large subcapsular hematoma can lead to hypertension due to persistent activation of the renin–angiotensin system. Surgical intervention is often required to salvage the transplanted kidney. These are summarized in Table 46.1. Loss of a kidney allograft as a complication of biopsy is rare [8, 12].

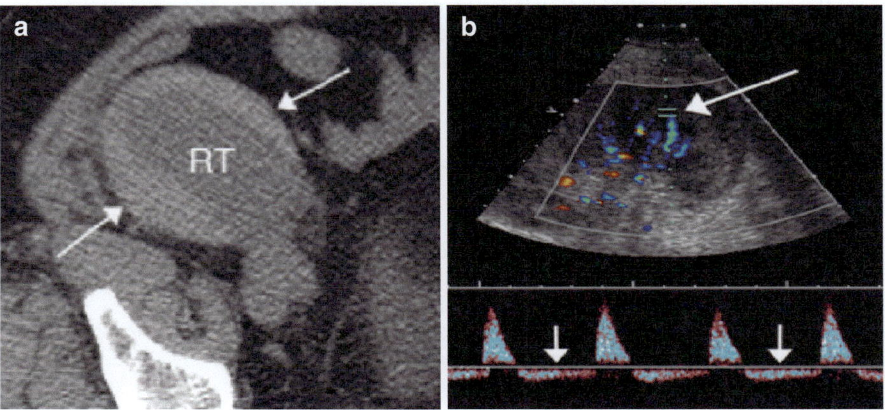

Fig. 46.1 (a) Non-contrast computed tomography scan with hyperdense areas between arrows showing "page kidney." (b) Ultrasound Doppler shows a diastolic flow reversal consistent with "page kidney" [7]

Table 46.1 Complications of transplant kidney biopsy [5, 6]

Complication type	Percentage (%)
Gross hematuria	3.5
Peri-kidney hematomas	2.5
Arteriovenous fistulas	7.3
Vasovagal reactions	0.5
Hospitalization	1.9

Other potential complications of a kidney allograft biopsy include the inability to obtain adequate samples and sampling of the kidney medulla, which does not allow assessment of glomeruli. Both these situations may prompt a need to re-biopsy. Clinical and lab monitoring, along with physician awareness for potential complications, remains paramount to patient care following allograft kidney biopsy.

References

1. Ahmad I. Biopsy of the transplanted kidney. Semin Intervent Radiol. 2004;21(4):275–81.
2. Kersnik Levart T, Kenig A, Buturović Ponikvar J, Ferluga D, Avgustin Cavić M, Kenda RB. Real-time ultrasound-guided kidney biopsy with a biopsy gun in children: safety and efficacy. Acta Paediatr. 2001;90(12):1394–7.
3. Riehl J, Maigatter S, Kierdorf H, Schmitt H, Maurin N, Sieberth HG. Percutaneous kidney biopsy: comparison of manual and automated puncture techniques with native and transplanted kidneys. Nephrol Dial Transplant. 1994;9(11):1568–74.
4. Nyman RS, Cappelen-Smith J, Al Suhaibani H, Alfurayh O, Shakweer W, Akhtar M. Yield and complications in percutaneous kidney biopsy:A comparison between ultrasound-guided gun-biopsy and manual techniques in native and transplant kidneys. Acta Radiol. 1997;38(3):431–6.
5. Peters B, Andersson Y, Stegmayr B, et al. A study of clinical complications and risk factors in 1,001 native and transplant kidney biopsies in Sweden. Acta Radiol. 2014;55(7):890–6.
6. Schwarz A, Gwinner W, Hiss M, Radermacher J, Mengel M, Haller H. Safety and adequacy of kidney transplant protocol biopsies. Am J Transplant. 2005;5(8):1992–6.
7. Morgan TA, Chandran S, Burger IM, Zhang CA, Goldstein RB. Complications of ultrasound-guided kidney transplant biopsies. Am J Transplant. 2016;16(4):1298–305.
8. Chesney DS, Brouhard BH, Cunningham RJ. Safety and cost effectiveness of pediatric percutaneous kidney biopsy. Pediatr Nephrol. 1996;10(4):493–5.
9. Murphy BF, MacIsaac A. Percutaneous kidney biopsy as a day-patient procedure. Am J Kidney Dis. 1989;14(1):77.
10. Plattner BW, Chen P, Cross R, Leavitt MA, Killen PD, Heung M. Complications and adequacy of transplant kidney biopsies: a comparison of techniques. J Vasc Access. 2018;19(3):291–6.
11. Korbet SM. Percutaneous kidney biopsy. Semin Nephrol. 2002;22(3):254–67.
12. Rosenbaum R, Hoffsten PE, Stanley RJ, Klahr S. Use of computerized tomography to diagnose complications of percutaneous kidney biopsy. Kidney Int. 1978;14(1):87–92.

Chapter 47
Post-Transplant Lymphoproliferative Disorder: Overview

M. Yahya Jan and Asif A. Sharfuddin

Introduction

Post-Transplant Lymphoproliferative Disorder (PTLD) is a life-limiting transplant complication with serious implications. It is most commonly encountered in the first year after transplant and is related to the degree of immunosuppressive therapy and donor/recipient EBV serostatus. Diagnostic workup involves a clinical review of symptoms, as well as laboratory and radiological testing. Diagnosis is confirmed by obtaining tissue biopsy and histopathological evaluation. A cornerstone of treatment involves reducing immunosuppression and PTLD directed therapy in consultation with hematological oncology. No EBV directed anti-viral treatment is currently the standard of care for prophylaxis or treatment of EBV viremia.

Case

A 57-year-old male with the past medical history of ESKD secondary to HTN nephrosclerosis status post deceased donor kidney transplantation presents with abdominal pain, fatigue, and reduced appetite. He underwent a kidney transplant 9 months ago, with an induction regimen of anti-thymocyte globulin (ATG) and methylprednisolone with rapid taper off and transition to maintenance immunosuppression (IS) with tacrolimus and mycophenolate. He did well with improved functional status and overall health and returned to his job as a warehouse worker. His creatinine stabilized to a baseline of 1.4–1.5 mg/dL. At the 7 months post-transplant

M. Y. Jan (✉) · A. A. Sharfuddin
Indiana University School of Medicine, Indianapolis, IN, USA
e-mail: myjan@iu.edu; asharfud@iu.edu

© The Author(s), under exclusive license to Springer Nature Switzerland AG 2022

F. Aziz, S. Parajuli (eds.), *Complications in Kidney Transplantation*,
https://doi.org/10.1007/978-3-031-13569-9_47

follow-up, his creatinine was elevated to 1.9 mg/dL, and an allograft biopsy showed acute cellular rejection IIA treated with Anti-thymocyte Globulin (ATG). His donor-specific antibody levels (DSA) remained + but low. Donor and recipient serological status for CMV IgG and EBV IgG was positive. He received CMV prophylaxis with valganciclovir for 6 months and was re-instituted at the time of repeat ATG treatment.

He reports deep dull abdominal pain over the RLQ, not related to eating or drinking. This is accompanied by intermittent diarrhea for the last 2–3 weeks, without blood. He has lost 8 lbs. over this course and has a low energy level, unable to get through his entire shift, leading him to stay off work. He was admitted to the hospital for a workup of abdominal pain. Labs were notable for creatinine of 1.7 mg/dL, improved with administration of IV fluids. CT scan of the abdomen and pelvis showed enlarged lymph nodes around the superior mesenteric vessels. No masses were identified. GI medicine was consulted, and an EGD and colonoscopy were done with biopsies. Biopsies from the terminal ileum were reported as Diffuse Large B Cell Lymphoma (DLBCL), and stains were positive for EBV and CD 20 marker.

Question 1

Which one of the following is a significant risk factor for post-transplant lymphoproliferative disorder in this patient?

A. EBV positive donor to EBV negative recipient transplant.
B. Anti-thymocyte globulin induction treatment.
C. An episode of rejection requiring intensification of immunosuppression regimen.
D. All of the above.

The correct answer is D.

Overall, up to two-thirds of PTLD cases are seen in the presence of Epstein–Barr virus (EBV) mediated B cell proliferative process in immunosuppression. Previous exposure or infection with EBV results from latent B cells that are kept in check by T cytotoxic cell immune response to these infected B cells. After transplant with suppression of T cell function, those B cells with EBV are allowed to proliferate, leading to PTLD.

The main risk factors for PTLD include the degree of immunosuppression in general and T cell-directed immunosuppression in particular. This has been shown by a study of more than 50,000 kidney and heart transplant recipients showing the incidence of PTLD to be highest in the first year after transplantation [1]. Similarly, the intensity of maintenance therapy has also been noted to impact the development of PTLD due to a more pronounced T cell inhibition being highest in intestinal transplants and lowest in liver transplant recipients [1]. Multiple studies have shown the absence of a pre-transplant exposure to EBV as a risk factor for subsequent PTLD among solid organ transplant recipients [2, 3]. Treatment with anti-thymocyte globulin has been shown to have a higher risk of developing PTLD than IL-2 inhibitor-based induction therapy [4].

Clinical Course

The biopsy findings were discussed with the patient, and he opted to pursue treatment for this diagnosis. Hematological oncology was consulted, and a PET CT was obtained, which showed extensive lymphadenopathy in the pelvis and abdomen along with the terminal ileum. Immunosuppression was reduced by stopping mycophenolate and continuing low-dose tacrolimus with a trough goal of 4–6 ng/mL. Subsequently, he was started on Rituximab, Cyclophosphamide, Vincristine, Doxorubicin, Prednisone (R-CHOP) chemotherapy.

Question 2

Which of the following is the most important initial step in treating PTLD in kidney transplant recipients?

A. Radiation therapy to affected organs.
B. Reduction of immunosuppression therapy and avoidance of agents likely to worsen PTLD.
C. Surgical oncology evaluation.
D. Early institution of immunochemotherapy with CHOP based chemotherapy with or without rituximab.

The correct answer is B.

Reduction in immunosuppression is the cornerstone of all forms of PTLD management with acceptance of higher risk for allograft rejection. PTLD is a spectrum of disease and has been classified into four different categories [5] (Table 47.1):

After reducing immunosuppression, chemoimmunotherapy may be pursued depending on the type of PTLD. In selected cases of CD 20 + Polymorphic PTLD and most cases of monomorphic PTLD, reduction in immunosuppression is not enough to control the disease [6]. Similar to CD 20+ Polymorphic PTLD, rituximab is used as part of initial therapy in all cases along with chemotherapy with CHOP regimen. For those who are frail or have poor functional status precluding chemotherapy, the recommendation is for single-agent rituximab, along with a reduction in immunosuppression. For a disease that has a mass effect or causes the visceral

Table 47.1 Categories of PTLD based on 2008 WHO classification [5]

Category of PTLD	Immunosuppression	Treatment
Early lesion	Reduce	Reduction of IS
Polymorphic PTLD	Reduce	+/− rituximab for CD 20 +
Monomorphic PTLD	Reduce	Rituximab for CD 20+ disease, CHOP
Hodgkin lymphoma like PTLD	Reduce	Treat as per Hodgkin lymphoma regimens

IS Immunosuppression, *CD* Cluster of Differentiation.

mass effect, e.g., small bowel obstruction, surgical resection is appropriate. In certain cases, localized radiation therapy may be pursued.

Discussion

PTLD is the second most commonly encountered cancer following kidney transplantation, with high mortality and morbidity after non-melanoma skin cancer [7]. In most cases, it is associated with EBV virus exposure or re-activation following transplant. The most common risk factors include T cell-directed therapies at induction and maintenance immunosuppression and its intensity.

It is important to be aware of individual risk factors heading into transplant, including EBV serostatus, previous history of malignancy, especially hematological malignancy with previous chemo/immune therapy received, and co-existing auto-immune condition requiring immunosuppressive treatment. However, there are various risks factors that cannot be anticipated, including donor EBV seropositivity and episodes of rejection, which may require intensification of immunosuppressive regimens. Given these, a high index of suspicion is required to evaluate any new patient symptoms and lab abnormalities. This is important as it is often a time of significant transition for patients changing from life on dialysis to life after transplant, adjusting to new medications, and dealing with potential complications of transplant. Although presenting symptoms can vary, some of the symptoms may mimic symptoms that are commonly encountered after a transplant, such as weight loss, poor appetite, nausea or vomiting, or those related to side effects of immunosuppressive medications. Certain symptoms may be related to viremia, such as fever, lymphadenopathy, or those related to effects on involved organ systems.

The diagnostic and treatment algorithm is summarized in Fig. 47.1.

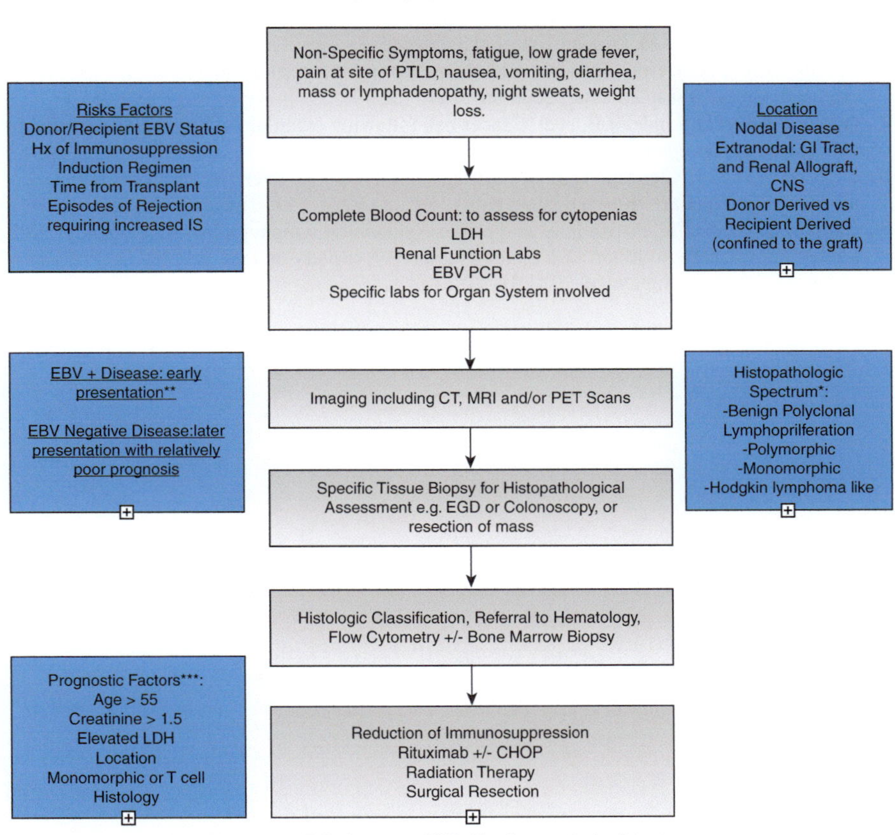

Fig. 47.1 Post transplant lymphoprofilerative disorder (PTLD) * [5], ** [8], *** [9]

References

1. Walker RC, Paya CV, Marshall WF, et al. Pretransplantation seronegative Epstein-Barr virus status is the primary risk factor for posttransplantation lymphoproliferative disorder in adult heart, lung, and other solid organ transplantations. J Heart Lung Transplant. 1995;14(2):214–21.
2. McDonald RA, Smith JM, Ho M, et al. Incidence of PTLD in pediatric renal transplant recipients receiving basiliximab, calcineurin inhibitor, sirolimus and steroids. Am J Transplant. 2008;8(5):984–9.
3. Caillard S, Lelong C, Pessione F, Moulin B. Post-transplant lymphoproliferative disorders occurring after renal transplantation in adults: report of 230 cases from the French registry. Am J Transplant. 2006;6(11):2735–42.
4. Ali H, Soliman K, Daoud A, et al. Relationship between rabbit anti-thymocyte globulin and development of PTLD and its aggressive form in renal transplant population. Ren Fail. 2020;42(1):489–94.

5. Swerdlow SH, Campo E, Harris NL, et al. WHO classification of tumours of haematopoietic and lymphoid tissues, vol. 2. France: International agency for research on cancer Lyon; 2008.
6. Swinnen LJ, LeBlanc M, Grogan TM, et al. Prospective study of sequential reduction in immunosuppression, interferon alpha-2B, and chemotherapy for posttransplantation lymphoproliferative disorder. Transplantation. 2008;86(2):215–22.
7. Adami J, Gäbel H, Lindelöf B, et al. Cancer risk following organ transplantation: a nationwide cohort study in Sweden. Br J Cancer. 2003;89(7):1221–7.
8. Leblond V, Davi F, Charlotte F, et al. Posttransplant lymphoproliferative disorders not associated with Epstein-Barr virus: a distinct entity? J Clin Oncol. 1998;16(6):2052–9.
9. Caillard S, Porcher R, Provot F, et al. Post-transplantation lymphoproliferative disorder after kidney transplantation: report of a nationwide French registry and the development of a new prognostic score. J Clin Oncol. 2013;31(10):1302–9.

Chapter 48
Post-Transplant Lymphoproliferative Disorders: Management

Sambhavi Krishnamoorthy and Tarek Alhamad

Introduction

Post-transplant lymphoproliferative disorders (PTLD) are a heterogeneous group of disorders that could present as indolent hyperplasia or aggressive lymphomas with distinct pathological subtypes and variable clinical presentations (Table 48.1). Increased incidence of late-onset EBV negative monomorphic PTLD associated with therapeutic immunosuppression has been observed with solid organ transplant recipients [1]. Advances in chemotherapeutic agents and cell therapy in the management of PTLD have made a significant impact on patient outcomes, given the significant morbidity and mortality related to this complication. In this chapter, we review a case of PTLD to understand the risks and benefits of treating this challenging disease and the serious impact it has in solid organ transplantation.

The patient is a 57-year-old woman with a history of end-stage kidney disease (ESKD) due to IgA nephropathy who received a deceased donor kidney transplant in 2005. The induction agent was anti-thymocyte globulin, and maintenance immunosuppression consisted of mycophenolic acid, tacrolimus, and prednisone. Fifteen years after kidney transplantation patient developed persistent nausea, satiety, and weight loss. She underwent a CT scan of her abdomen/pelvis that showed a large infiltrative mass in the left pelvis 10 × 15 cm continuous with retroperitoneal

S. Krishnamoorthy (✉)
Division of Nephrology, University of Chicago, Chicago, IL, USA
e-mail: samk@medicine.bsd.uchicago.edu

T. Alhamad
Division of Nephrology, Department of Medicine, Washington University School of Medicine, St. Louis, MO, USA
e-mail: talhamad@wustl.edu

© The Author(s), under exclusive license to Springer Nature Switzerland AG 2022

F. Aziz, S. Parajuli (eds.), *Complications in Kidney Transplantation*,
https://doi.org/10.1007/978-3-031-13569-9_48

Table 48.1 WHO classification of PTLD

Benign polyclonal lymphoproliferation
Florid follicular hyperplasia
Polymorphic PTLD
Monomorphic PTLD
Diffuse large B cell lymphoma
Burkitt lymphoma
Plasma cell neoplasm
Peripheral T cell lymphoma, not otherwise specified
Classic Hodgkin lymphoma type PTLD

WHO Classification of Tumours of Haematopoietic and Lymphoid Tissues, revised fourth edition, Swerdlow SH, Campo E, Harris NL, et al. (Eds), International Agency for Research on Cancer (IARC), Lyon 2017

lymphadenopathy. A biopsy of the mass was consistent with EBV (Epstein–Barr virus) negative, non-germinal center B-cell-like (non-GCB), diffuse large B cell lymphoma (DLBCL).

Question 1

What is the best treatment strategy for this patient?

A. Reduction in immunosuppression as first-line therapy.
B. Reduction in immunosuppression with rituximab.
C. Reduction in immunosuppression with rituximab with or without sequential or concomitant chemotherapy.
D. Chimeric antigen receptor T cell (CAR-T) therapy.

The correct answer is C.

Reducing immunosuppression with or without rituximab is usually the first-line therapy for early or minimally symptomatic PTLD. But for monomorphic PTLD, with significant symptoms, a combination of rituximab with or without sequential R- CHOP (rituximab, cyclophosphamide, doxorubicin, vincristine, and prednisone) therapy with a reduction in immunosuppression is recommended based on PTLD-1 trial [2]. CAR-T therapy is usually considered after the failure of first- and second-line salvage therapy.

Clinical Course

The patient's antimetabolite and tacrolimus were stopped as she received 4 cycles of R-CHOP chemotherapy with incomplete response noted on follow-up PET scan done 3 months later. Subsequently, the patient received 3 cycles of R-ICE (rituximab, ifosfamide, carboplatin, and etoposide) salvage therapy, with continued failure to reach clinical remission. A decision was made to proceed with CAR-T therapy. The patient underwent leukapheresis followed by lymphodepletion therapy and CAR-T infusion. On day 2 of CAR-T infusion, the patient developed a high-grade fever of 102.5 F and developed hypotension with a BP of 80/50.

Question 2

What is the most likely cause of the patient's fever and hypotension?

A. Sepsis, likely bacteremia due to immunosuppression from chemotherapy.
B. Serum sickness from CAR-T infusion.
C. Acute pyelonephritis of allograft.
D. Cytokine release syndrome.

The correct answer is D.

In autologous CAR-T therapy, T cells are separated from a patient's blood using apheresis. These cells are then genetically modified to express chimeric surface antigen receptors. In the currently approved CARs, these receptors allow the T cells to recognize and bind a tumor targeting the pan B-cell marker CD19. Though sepsis and pyelonephritis would be considered in the differential, cytokine release syndrome (CRS) is the most common adverse reaction noted after CAR-T therapy, with an incidence ranging from 35 to 93% [3]. CAR-T does not cause serum sickness.

Additional Clinical Course

The patient received tocilizumab for severe cytokine release syndrome. Her post-CAR-T course was also complicated by ICANS (immune effector cell-associated neurotoxicity syndrome), for which she received steroids and seizure prophylaxis. She ultimately developed aspiration pneumonia with pseudomonas aeruginosa requiring intubation and mechanical ventilation due to hypoxia. She required vaso-pressors for a septic shock as well. She developed acute kidney injury requiring kidney replacement therapy. The patient developed refractory shock despite treatment with broad-spectrum antibiotics and vasopressors. The family decided to pursue comfort care.

Discussion

PTLD is a devastating and potentially fatal long-term complication associated with immunosuppression and/or EBV infection in solid organ transplant patients. The overall incidence of PTLD is about 20% in SOT recipients, and the incidence varies by organs, with intestinal and multiorgan transplants having the highest risk and kidney transplants having the lowest risk. Early-onset PTLD is usually EBV associated and polymorphic, whereas late-onset PTLD is usually EBV negative and monomorphic. Though about 90% PTLDs originate from B cells, in the minority, they could be of T cell or null cell origin as well [1]. Reduction in immunosuppression remains the cornerstone of therapy, especially for early PTLD. Outcomes for PTLD of B cell origin have substantially improved with the introduction of rituximab [4], and the subsequent PTLD trials show better survival with the combination of rituximab and chemotherapy [2]. Radiation therapy may be considered for CNS involvement. The reduction in immunosuppression must be balanced with the risk of allograft rejection and allograft loss. This decision is especially difficult in life-sustaining organs such as heart transplants.

Additionally, refractory PTLD continues to have inferior outcomes. Various strategies include salvage regimens such as R-ICE (rituximab, ifosfamide, carboplatin, and etoposide), R-GemOx (rituximab, gemcitabine, and oxaliplatin), and R-DHAX (rituximab, dexamethasone, cytarabine, and oxaliplatin) are usually employed as second-line therapy [1]. CAR-T therapy is an adoptive T cell therapy that was first studied in pediatric ALL and showed improved outcomes. It has shown a disease-free survival of 35–40% in 1–2 years after therapy with a complete response rate of 50% in DLBCL [5, 6]. CRS and ICANS are well observed common adverse reactions to CAR-T therapy [3, 7]. Dexamethasone, seizure prophylaxis with/without IL-6 antibody or IL-6 receptor antibody may be used to manage these adverse effects. Gupta et al. reported that CAR-T therapy is associated with AKI. The 60-day mortality in patients with acute tubular necrosis after CAR-T therapy was 67% [8]. A recent case series of 3 solid organ recipients who underwent CAR-T therapy for PTLD showed poor response to therapy and significant adverse effects [9]. Further research is needed to increase CAR-T efficacy with better strategies to manage their adverse effects and improve outcomes in refractory PTLD without affecting allograft outcomes in solid organ transplant recipients.

References

1. Dharnidharka VR, Webster AC, Martinez OM, Preiksaitis JK, Leblond V, Choquet S. Post-transplant lymphoproliferative disorders. Nat Rev Dis Primers. 2016;2:15088.
2. Trappe R, Oertel S, Leblond V, Mollee P, Sender M, Reinke P, et al. Sequential treatment with rituximab followed by CHOP chemotherapy in adult B-cell post-transplant lymphoproliferative disorder (PTLD): the prospective international multicentre phase 2 PTLD-1 trial. Lancet Oncol. 2012;13(2):196–206.
3. Hirayama AV, Turtle CJ. Toxicities of CD19 CAR-T cell immunotherapy. Am J Hematol. 2019;94(S1):S42–S9.
4. Choquet S, Leblond V, Herbrecht R, Socié G, Stoppa AM, Vandenberghe P, et al. Efficacy and safety of rituximab in B-cell post-transplantation lymphoproliferative disorders: results of a prospective multicenter phase 2 study. Blood. 2006;107(8):3053–7.
5. Neelapu SS, Locke FL, Bartlett NL, Lekakis LJ, Miklos DB, Jacobson CA, et al. Axicabtagene Ciloleucel CAR T-cell therapy in refractory large B-cell lymphoma. N Engl J Med. 2017;377(26):2531–44.
6. Locke FL, Ghobadi A, Jacobson CA, Miklos DB, Lekakis LJ, Oluwole OO, et al. Long-term safety and activity of axicabtagene ciloleucel in refractory large B-cell lymphoma (ZUMA-1): a single-arm, multicentre, phase 1-2 trial. Lancet Oncol. 2019;20(1):31–42.

7. Gust J, Hay KA, Hanafi LA, Li D, Myerson D, Gonzalez-Cuyar LF, et al. Endothelial activation and blood-brain barrier disruption in neurotoxicity after adoptive immunotherapy with CD19 CAR-T cells. Cancer Discov. 2017;7(12):1404–19.
8. Gupta S, Seethapathy H, Strohbehn IA, Frigault MJ, O'Donnell EK, Jacobson CA, et al. Acute kidney injury and electrolyte abnormalities after chimeric antigen receptor T-cell (CAR-T) therapy for diffuse large B-cell lymphoma. Am J Kidney Dis. 2020;76(1):63–71.
9. Krishnamoorthy S, Ghobadi A, Santos RD, Schilling JD, Malone AF, Murad H, et al. CAR-T therapy in solid organ transplant recipients with treatment refractory posttransplant lymphoproliferative disorder. Am J Transplant. 2021;21(2):809–14.

Chapter 49
Central Nervous System Post-Transplant Lymphoproliferative Disorder after Kidney Transplantation

Elie Fadel and Shaifali Sandal

Introduction

Post-transplant lymphoproliferative disorder (PTLD) is a well-known complication following kidney transplantation (KT) that entails the uncontrolled proliferation of lymphoid cells. Extra-nodal involvement, including the central nervous system (CNS), can occur and is associated with poor survival, although outcomes may be improving over time. We present a fatal case of a recipient who developed CNS-PTLD. We then provide a brief overview of the disease incidence, the clinical presentation, risk factors, diagnostic and therapeutic approaches, outcomes, and prognosis.

E. Fadel
Division of Nephrology, Department of Medicine, McGill University Health Centre, Montreal, QC, Canada
e-mail: elie.fadel2@mail.mcgill.ca

S. Sandal (✉)
Division of Nephrology, Department of Medicine, McGill University Health Centre, Montreal, QC, Canada

Research Institute of the McGill University Health Centre, Montreal, QC, Canada

Royal Victoria Hospital Glen Site, Montreal, QC, Canada
e-mail: shaifali.sandal@mcgill.ca

© The Author(s), under exclusive license to Springer Nature Switzerland AG 2022

F. Aziz, S. Parajuli (eds.), *Complications in Kidney Transplantation*,
https://doi.org/10.1007/978-3-031-13569-9_49

Case

A 66-year-old lady of Asian background received a flow crossmatch negative deceased donor kidney transplantation. She had a past medical history of end-stage kidney disease due to IgM nephropathy and was on peritoneal dialysis. Her other medical problems included a history of hypertension, hypothyroidism, and pulmonary tuberculosis treated 40 years prior. She had a cPRA of 98, and thus she received alemtuzumab and steroid induction. She had a good postoperative course, and her creatinine stabilized in the 0.6–0.7 mg/dL range. The maintenance immunosuppression regimen consisted of long-acting tacrolimus (target trough 6–8 ng/mL), mycophenolate sodium (720 mg twice a day), and prednisone (5 mg daily).

Six months after transplant, the patient presented with a 3-week history of deterioration in cognitive function, weakness, memory problems, and difficulty with ambulation. On presentation to the emergency room, she was afebrile, her vital signs were normal, but she had some new neurological deficits. She was noted to have ataxia in both arms and mild pronator drift on the right side. Her muscle strength was good, and no other abnormalities were noted in her physical exam. Her blood work was unremarkable except for elevated lactate dehydrogenase. A CT scan of the head revealed multiple intraparenchymal enhancing lesions (Fig. 49.1).

Question 1
Which of the following can explain the patient's presentation?

A. Primary CNS malignancy.
B. Infection.

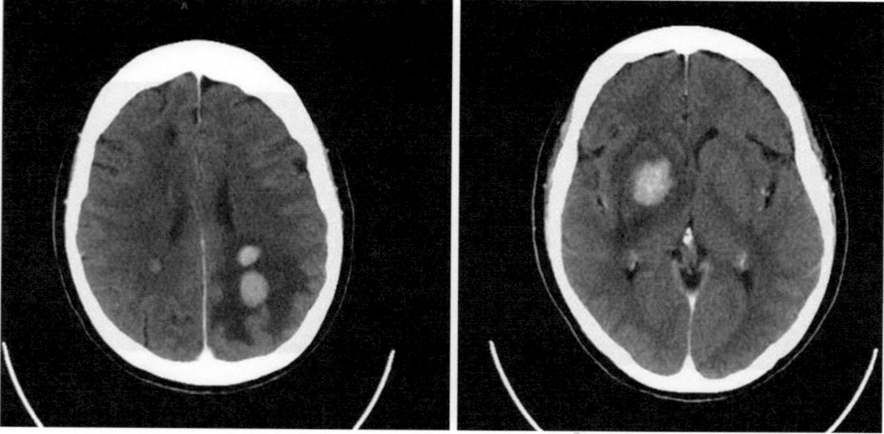

Fig. 49.1 The initial CT scan head of a kidney transplant recipient demonstrating multiple intra-parenchymal enhancing lesions who was diagnosed to have primary CNS-PTLD

C. Metastases.
D. All of the above.

The correct response is D.

The differential of brain lesion/s in an immunocompromised host is broad and includes primary CNS lymphoma, glioblastoma, metastatic disease, abscess, or other infections. Further imaging and a biopsy are needed to establish the diagnosis in this patient.

Clinical Course

CT thorax and abdomen did not reveal any other lesions. MRI of the head was pursued to define the brain lesions better, and they were described as heterogeneous, mainly low signal intensity in the T2-weighted images with a central hyperintensity. The diffusion images documented a very minimal restriction. A neurosurgical consultation was pursued, and the patient underwent a left parietal stereotactic biopsy. Pathology evidence demonstrated that the brain was infiltrated by a population of large, dis-cohesive cells with irregular nuclear morphology that had a prominent angiocentric distribution. By immunohistochemistry, the cells were positive for CD45, and the majority were positive for CD20. Toxoplasmosis stains were negative. The patient did not have Epstein–Barr viremia, and Epstein–Barr virus (EBV) encoded small RNAs in situ hybridization of the tissue sample was negative. Overall, this was diagnostic of diffuse large B-cell lymphoma. After a complete workup, this case was discussed at the tumor board, and she was diagnosed with CNS-PTLD.

Chemotherapy was initiated (cytarabine, high-dose methotrexate, and rituximab), and tacrolimus and mycophenolate were stopped. Following two cycles of chemotherapy, she developed neutropenic fever, and before the initiation of the third cycle of chemotherapy, the patient had an acute change in her mental status. A new CT head demonstrated a marked increase in the size of her CNS lesions with a severe increase in the associated vasogenic edema. Following this, the patient's family and the primary team of physicians pursued comfort approaches only, and the patient passed away 9-months after transplantation.

Question 2

Which of the following statements about the management of CNS-PTLD in this patient are correct?

A. Progression of disease and infection is the most common cause of death.
B. Bone marrow should have been pursued.
C. Immunosuppression reduction alone should have been the primary first-line treatment.
D. PTLD-1 trial approach of sequential immunochemotherapy would have been ideal in this patient.

The correct response is A.

In most case series, disease progression or infection during treatment or after complete/partial remission was the most common cause of death. Bone marrow biopsy is not essential if the systemic disease is excluded, and there is no evidence to suggest a concurrent low-grade lymphoma. The ideal treatment option in CNS-PTLD is not known, and the PTLD-1 trial that supported the use of sequential immunochemotherapy with rituximab and CHOP excluded patients with meningeal and CNS involvement. A minority of PTLD cases in the literature have responded to a reduction in immunosuppressive medications alone; however, this strategy has not been extensively studied in patients with primary CNS-PTLD. Thus, responses C and D are incorrect. Generally, given the poor prognosis of patients with CNS-PTLD, aggressive approaches are recommended unless a palliative approach is sought.

Discussion

Extra-nodal PTLD is frequently described in transplant recipients and far more common than nodal PTLD [1]. CNS involvement can occur as primary CNS lymphoma or systemic PTLD with secondary CNS disease. Here-in we present a brief discussion on CNS-PTLD.

For adult recipients of KT, standardized incidence ratios for PTLD are 8.4, and this is much higher in younger patients who have standardized incidence ratio as high as 86.6 [1]. CNS-PTLD is reported to occur in approximately 7–15% cases of PTLD [2]. Among CNS disorders presenting after transplantation, CNS-PTLD is reported to be the third most common in frequency after cerebrovascular disease and infection [3].

Patients with CNS-PTLD can only present with solid intracranial tumor masses, intraspinal masses, or leptomeningeal disease with cytomorphological CSF involvement [4]. A range of symptoms and signs have been reported; behavioral change, memory and language impairment, focal motor deficits, seizures, raised intracranial pressure, and neuropsychiatric symptoms [5]. Up to 20% of patients may have intra-ocular involvement, resembling chronic uveitis [5]. Also, systemic symptoms may be present such as fever, weight loss, night sweats, and mood disturbances [3]. Time to diagnosis ranges from 11 months to 12.5 years post-KT [1, 4, 6, 7].

EBV is a key pathogenic driver in many cases of PTLD, particularly the early-onset cases, and recipient EBV seronegativity is a risk factor [3, 8]. Most patients of CNS-PTLD reported in the literature were EBV-associated [6, 7]. Other risk factors are the intensity of immunosuppression, mycophenolate mofetil use, and hypogammaglobulinemia [2, 6, 8].

Contrast-enhanced brain MRI is the neuroimaging modality of choice for both diagnosis and response assessment [5]. Cranial MRI scans demonstrate contrast-enhancing lesions with perifocal edema and central necrosis [6]. Diagnosis, however, requires histopathology obtained either by stereotactic biopsy or resection [6]. Cerebrospinal fluid cytology and flow cytometry may be used in cases where a biopsy is not possible or to investigate leptomeningeal involvement [5]. Bone marrow biopsy is not essential if the systemic disease is excluded, there is no evidence of a concurrent low-grade lymphoma, and in the context of typical histology from tissue samples [5].

CNS-PTLD classification follows the 2016 WHO classification of hematopoietic and lymphoid tumors [9]. Six distinctive subsets are plasmacytic hyperplasia PTLD, infectious mononucleosis PTLD, florid follicular hyperplasia PTLD, polymorphic PTLD, monomorphic PTLD (B-cell types and T-cell types/NK-cell types), and Hodgkin PTLD. Most cases are monomorphic, and the most common histological subtype is diffuse large B-cell lymphoma [2–4, 6].

In general, the management of PTLD centers around balancing the competing risks of preserving the graft and delivering effective therapy. The ideal treatment option in CNS-PTLD is not known, and the PTLD-1 trial that supported the use of sequential immunochemotherapy with rituximab and CHOP in PTLD excluded patients with CNS involvement [10]. Treatment options for CNS-PTLD include a combination of systemic chemotherapy, surgery, antiviral therapy, use of EBV-specific T-cells, radiation therapy, and immunosuppression reduction [2, 4, 6, 7, 11, 12]. While this has not been investigated in KT, based on the patient's fitness level, four cycles of MATRix (high-dose methotrexate, cytarabine, thiotepa, rituximab) immunochemotherapy are recommended [5]. Antiviral approach may improve survival [12], and intrathecal rituximab may be an option for some patients with isolated CNS-PTLD [13].

CNS involvement is generally considered a poor prognostic factor in patients with PTLD and is associated with inferior survival. The median survival ranges from 17 to 47 months, but treatments used are heterogeneous, and the extent of the disease varies [2, 6, 11]. For example, a 2013 multicenter retrospective review by Evens and colleagues analyzed first-line treatment after reduction of immunosuppression in 84 patients with primary CNS-PTLD [2]. In this cohort, the following were given alone or in combination: high-dose methotrexate (48%), high-dose cytarabine (33%), and rituximab (45%) of patients. Also, 8% received all three therapies. The overall response rate was 60%, and complete response was observed in 38% of the patients. Although not significant, complete response rates appeared highest with high-dose methotrexate and/or high-dose cytarabine-based therapy. In another pediatric cohort of 25 patients, 48% were alive after first complete remission [4].

Outcomes of patients with CNS-PTLD may be improving over time due to better therapeutic options, early diagnosis, and improved supportive care measures [2, 4, 7]. In a recent report of 91 patients with monomorphic diffuse large B-cell lymphoma PTLD that included 21 patients with primary CNS-PTLD and two with systemic disease plus CNS involvement, there was no difference in overall survival for patients with systemic PTLD versus patients with CNS involvement [7]. Most patients received rituximab monotherapy with radiation or rituximab-based chemotherapy.

Progressive disease and infection are the most common causes of death [2, 6]. Predictors of poor survival are poor performance status, hypoalbuminemia, female sex, poor response to initial therapy, and elevated lactate dehydrogenase levels [2].

The most prominent prognostic factor identified in one case series was a response to first-line treatment [2]. Sporadic cases of a second KT after successful treatment of PCNS-PTLD have been reported [12].

Preventative strategies for CNS-PTLD are not known. Pre-emptive intervention with monitoring EBV levels is a potential strategy for PTLD prevention and early detection [8]. Beyond the first year of KT, there are no clear guidelines recommending monitoring EBV in peripheral blood [3].

Acknowledgments None.

References

1. Francis A, Johnson DW, Teixeira-Pinto A, Craig JC, Wong G. Incidence and predictors of post-transplant lymphoproliferative disease after kidney transplantation during adulthood and childhood: a registry study. Nephrol Dial Transplant. 2018;33(5):881–9.
2. Evens AM, Choquet S, Kroll-Desrosiers AR, et al. Primary CNS posttransplant lymphoproliferative disease (PTLD): an international report of 84 cases in the modern era. Am J Transplant. 2013;13(6):1512–22.
3. Velvet AJJ, Bhutani S, Papachristos S, et al. A single-center experience of post-transplant lymphomas involving the central nervous system with a review of current literature. Oncotarget. 2019;10(4):437–48.
4. Taj MM, Maecker-Kolhoff B, Ling R, et al. Primary post-transplant lymphoproliferative disorder of the central nervous system: characteristics, management, and outcome in 25 paediatric patients. Br J Haematol. 2021;193(6):1178–84.
5. Fox CP, Phillips EH, Smith J, et al. Guidelines for the diagnosis and management of primary central nervous system diffuse large B-cell lymphoma. Br J Haematol. 2019;184(3):348–63.
6. Zimmermann H, Nitsche M, Pott C, et al. Reduction of immunosuppression combined with whole-brain radiotherapy and concurrent systemic rituximab is an effective yet toxic treatment of primary central nervous system post-transplant lymphoproliferative disorder (pCNS-PTLD): 14 cases from the prospective German PTLD registry. Ann Hematol. 2021;100(8):2043–50.
7. Boyle S, Tobin JWD, Perram J, et al. Management and outcomes of diffuse large B-cell lymphoma post-transplant lymphoproliferative disorder in the era of PET and rituximab: a multi-center study from the Australasian lymphoma Alliance. Hema. 2021;5(11):e648.
8. Dharnidharka VR, Webster AC, Martinez OM, Preiksaitis JK, Leblond V, Choquet S. Post-transplant lymphoproliferative disorders. Nat Rev Dis Primers. 2016;2:15088.
9. Swerdlow SH, Campo E, Pileri SA, et al. The 2016 revision of the World Health Organization classification of lymphoid neoplasms. Blood. 2016;127(20):2375–90.
10. Trappe R, Oertel S, Leblond V, et al. Sequential treatment with rituximab followed by CHOP chemotherapy in adult B-cell post-transplant lymphoproliferative disorder (PTLD): the prospective international multicentre phase 2 PTLD-1 trial. Lancet Oncol. 2012;13(2):196–206.
11. Cavaliere R, Petroni G, Lopes MB, Schiff D. Primary central nervous system post-transplantation lymphoproliferative disorder: an international primary central nervous system lymphoma collaborative group report. Cancer. 2010;116(4):863–70.
12. Dugan JP, Haverkos BM, Villagomez L, et al. Complete and durable responses in primary central nervous system Posttransplant lymphoproliferative disorder with zidovudine, ganciclovir, rituximab, and dexamethasone. Clin Cancer Res. 2018;24(14):3273–81.
13. Anastasiou M, Mamez AC, Masouridi S, et al. Successful treatment of central nervous system lymphoproliferative disorder in a kidney-pancreas and stem cell transplanted patient using intrathecal rituximab. BMJ Case Rep. 2021;14(8)

Chapter 50
A Case of Early EBV-Negative Kidney Allograft-Limited Post-Transplant Lymphoproliferative Disorder

Estefania Abasolo and Fahad Aziz

Introduction

A large majority of post-transplant lymphoproliferative disorders (PTLD) occurring within the first year after transplant are associated with Epstein–Barr virus (EBV). EBV-negative PTLD is mainly late-onset. Here, we describe a case of a kidney and pancreas transplant recipient presenting with acute kidney injury diagnosed with EBV-negative PTLD at 6 weeks post-transplant.

Patient History

A 38-year-old male with a history of chronic kidney disease stage 5 secondary to insulin-dependent diabetes underwent a deceased donor simultaneous pancreas and kidney transplant (SPK). At the time of transplant, his panel reactive antibody (PRA) was 0%, and he had no preformed donor-specific antibodies (DSA). He received induction with anti-thymocyte globulin. His maintenance immunosuppression included tacrolimus (target trough 6–8 ng/mL), mycophenolate sodium 720 mg twice a day, and prednisone 5 mg daily. He achieved a baseline creatinine of 1.4 mg/dL with eGFR of 50 mL/min/1.73m^2. He developed CMV viremia at 3 weeks post-transplant and was treated with Valcyte, with the subsequent decrease in CMV viral load. Acute kidney injury with a creatinine of 3 mg/dL was noted at his routine

E. Abasolo (✉) · F. Aziz
Department of Medicine, University of Wisconsin—Madison School of Medicine and Public Health, University of Wisconsin Hospital and Clinics, Madison, WI, USA
e-mail: EAbasoloLopez@uwhealth.org; faziz@wisc.edu

© The Author(s), under exclusive license to Springer Nature Switzerland AG 2022

F. Aziz, S. Parajuli (eds.), *Complications in Kidney Transplantation*,
https://doi.org/10.1007/978-3-031-13569-9_50

6-week post-transplant visit. He had normal pancreas allograft function. He denies any fever, nausea, vomiting, or diarrhea. Ultrasound doppler of the kidney allograft showed good blood flow to the allograft.

Question 1

What should be the next step in the management?

A. Intravenous fluids.
B. Antibiotics.
C. Kidney biopsy.
D. CT abdomen.

The correct answer is C.

There can be multiple reasons for acute kidney injury in kidney transplant recipients, including acute allograft rejection, calcineurin inhibitor toxicity, thrombotic microangiopathy, transplant renal artery stenosis, urinary obstruction, and viral infections. This patient's tacrolimus level was within the therapeutic range; his renal ultrasound was negative for any abnormality that could identify a creatinine elevation; hence an allograft kidney biopsy should be obtained to evaluate the etiology further.

Hospital Course

Due to unexplained elevated creatinine, the patient underwent a kidney biopsy that showed diffuse dense lymphoplasmacytic infiltrates with predominantly CD138-positive polyclonal plasma cells interspersed with CD20-positive B cells and fewer numbers of CD3-positive T cells scattered throughout (Figs. 50.1, 50.2 and 50.3).

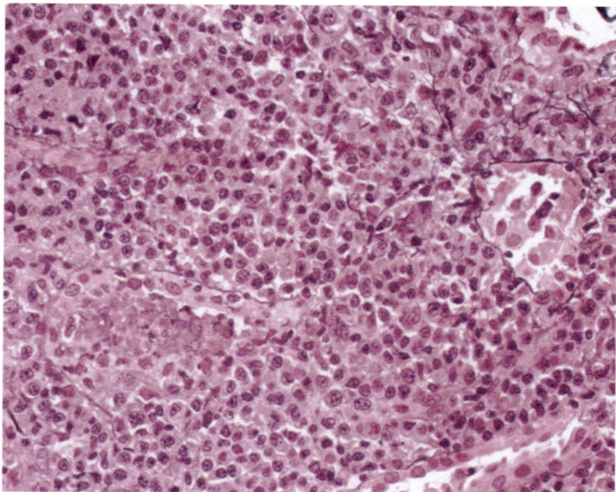

Fig. 50.1 E stain showing plasma cell-enriched infiltrates

Fig. 50.2 CD 20 stain

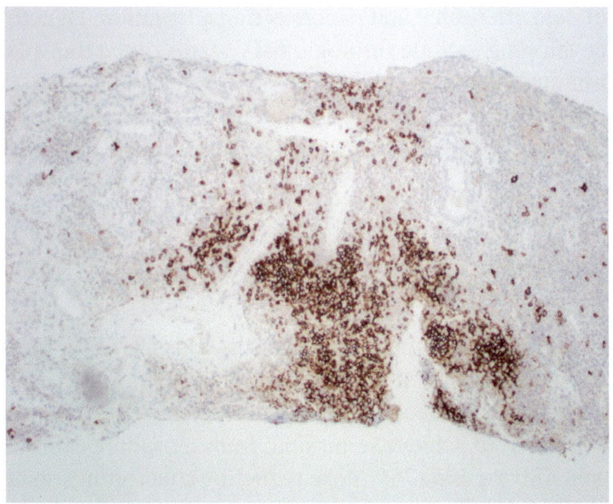

Fig. 50.3 CD30 stain

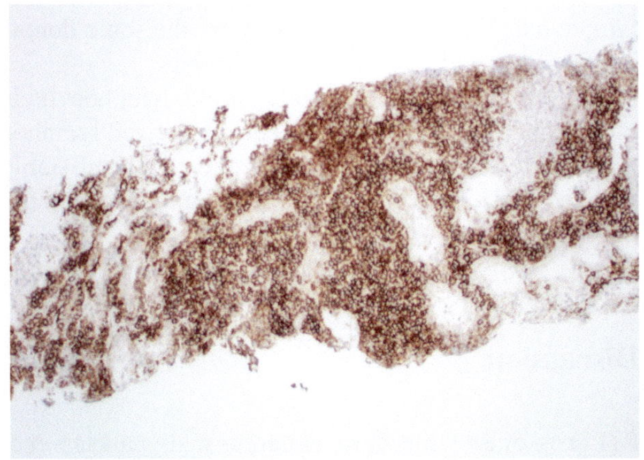

PET-CT demonstrated intense focal uptake limited to the upper and lower poles of the transplanted kidney. PET-CT did not show any pancreas involvement. These findings suggest PTLD of the kidney allograft.

Question 2
Which viral infection is the most associated with PTLD?

A. Cytomegalovirus.
B. HIV.
C. Adenovirus.
D. Epstein–Barr virus.

The answer is D.
Epstein–Barr Virus (EBV). The pathogenesis of PTLD is related to EBV-infected B-cell expansion in the setting of T cell immune suppression, which is the standard

of care after renal and pancreas transplantation. Hence, considerable risk factors for developing include serologic EBV status of the transplant receiver and the degree of immunosuppression [1]. Immunosuppression in an EBV-infected patient is a strong risk factor for PTLD development since patients lack the specific cytotoxic T cell response to control the growth of EBV-infected B cells [2].

Further Course

Interestingly, the patient's serum and tissue EBV were negative. The diagnosis of EBV-negative renal allograft-limited polymorphic PTLD was made. Oncology was consulted and recommended immunosuppression reduction with four doses of rituximab to achieve remission. Immunosuppression was reduced to mycophenolic acid 180 mg bid (75% dose reduction), tacrolimus with trough levels of 4–6 ng/mL (50% reduction), prednisone 5 mg daily, and rituximab (700 mg × 4) was administered. Looking retrospectively, his donor was 5 years old with no history concerning lymphoma. Two other recipients from the same donor were doing well when last inquired. Donor EBV status was negative.

Further, the presence of polymorphic lymphocytic infiltrates in the transplanted kidney makes it less likely to be donor-derived lymphoma. At 4 months after transplant, serum creatinine improved and remained stable 8 months post-transplant, with reduced uptake on PET-CT scan. Pancreatic function remained normal throughout his course.

Discussion

PTLD is one of the most common malignancies encountered in post-transplant patients. Solid-organ transplant increases the risk of de novo malignancy by two- to fourfold [2], and is a higher risk with more intense and more prolonged immunosuppression. The spectrum of disease presentation is broad, and the World Health Organization (WHO) classifies it based on histology. Non-Hodgkin's lymphoma comprises the majority of PTLD cases, and about 80–90% of cases are associated with an EBV infection [2]. Lymphoma accounts for 4–5% of cancer in the general immunocompetent population compared with 21% in solid transplant recipients [3]. The median presentation time is 18–18.5 months after transplantation, with EBV-negative PTLD cases often five or more years later [2].

The highest incidence of PTLD is seen with small bowel and multiple visceral transplantations. In patients with simultaneous kidney and pancreas transplantation, the incidence is 2–3% [2]. Age is an important determinant as well, with PTLD being the most common post-transplant malignancy in children, whereas, in adults, it is second to non-melanoma skin cancers.

Clinical manifestations are broad and include constitutional symptoms such as fevers, night sweats, and weight loss. The presentation can range from an incidental finding in a clinically asymptomatic patient to a more fulminant course with organ dysfunction [4]. Differential diagnoses to consider include graft rejection and sepsis. Evaluation is done with imaging studies, including CT, MRI, and PET scans. Tissue biopsy is the gold standard for a definitive diagnosis and to characterize PTLD type.

Treatment is a combination of reduction or discontinuation of immunosuppressive therapy, particularly tacrolimus, cyclosporine, and mycophenolate. Despite immunosuppression reduction, patients with the persistent disease can benefit from rituximab with positive predictive factors for success, including an EBV-positive PTLD, fewer sites involved, a shorter period of presentation from transplantation time, and a normal LDH [2]. Overall response is 49–77% in patients receiving immunosuppression reduction combined with rituximab, with complete remission rates between 20 and 55% [4]. If the above treatment has failed, chemotherapy can be used, and a CHOP regimen (cyclophosphamide, adriamycin, vincristine, and prednisone) with or without rituximab is usually the choice. One of the indications to start chemotherapy is histologic findings on biopsy, including Burkitt's lymphoma, Hodgkin's lymphoma, peripheral T cell lymphoma, primary central nervous system lymphoma [4]. Adoptive immunotherapy consists of EBV-specific cytotoxic lymphocytes infused either from the recipient, donor, or partially matched HLA donor [4]. Steroids are generally safe to use.

The previously mentioned therapeutic strategies have improved outcomes of PTLD in transplanted patients, which historically has had a poor prognosis. In the PTLD-1 trial, 70% had a complete remission with an overall median survival of 6.6 years [4]. New therapies such as BTK inhibition, proteasome inhibition, radio-immunotherapy, checkpoint inhibitors, and anti-CD-30 therapy are still experimental but may provide further therapeutic advances in the future.

References

1. Kotton CN, Fishman JA. Viral infection in the renal transplant recipient. J Am Soc Nephrol. 2005;16(6):1758–74.
2. Pham PT, Danovitch GM, Pham PC. Medical Management of the Kidney Transplant Recipient - Infections and Malignant Neoplasms. Comprehensive Clinical Nephrology. 2010:1177–88.
3. Siegel RL, Miller KD, Jemal A. Cancer statistics, 2016. CA Cancer J Clin. 2016;66(1):7–30.
4. Dierickx D, Habermann TM. Post-transplantation lymphoproliferative disorders in adults. N Engl J Med. 2018;378(6):549–62.

Chapter 51
Renal Cell Carcinoma in Kidney Transplant Recipients

Vignesh Viswanathan, Aisha Fatima, and Sami Alasfar

Introduction

Kidney transplant recipients suffer substantial complications, including cardiovascular disease and cancer, which constitute the major causes of kidney-transplant-associated morbidity and mortality. Patients with End-Stage Kidney Disease (ESKD) and kidney transplants carry multiple risk factors for Renal Cell Carcinoma (RCC). There is currently no consensus on screening for RCC before or after transplant, though treatment and follow-up strategies have significantly improved over the past several years.

Patient History

A 55-year-old man with ESKD secondary to diabetes underwent a deceased donor kidney transplant 3 years after initiating dialysis. One year after transplantation, he developed microscopic hematuria. CT of the abdomen and pelvis revealed a 5.6 cm solid mass in the left native kidney. He had no evidence of metastatic disease.

V. Viswanathan (✉) · S. Alasfar
Division of Nephrology, Department of Medicine, The Johns Hopkins University School of Medicine, Baltimore, MD, USA
e-mail: vviswan5@jhmi.edu; salasfa1@jhu.edu

A. Fatima
Department of Pathology, the Johns Hopkins University School of Medicine, Baltimore, MD, USA
e-mail: afatima2@jhmi.edu

© The Author(s), under exclusive license to Springer Nature Switzerland AG 2022

F. Aziz, S. Parajuli (eds.), *Complications in Kidney Transplantation*,
https://doi.org/10.1007/978-3-031-13569-9_51

What is the best next step in managing this condition?

A. Active surveillance.
B. Kidney mass biopsy.
C. Reduction of immunosuppression.
D. Radical nephrectomy and reduction of immunosuppression.

The correct answer is D.

Active surveillance is an option for the initial management of kidney masses suspicious for cancer, especially if they are small (<2 cm) or when the risk of intervention outweighs the potential benefits of treatment. A kidney mass biopsy can be considered for additional risk stratification. It is pursued if the mass is suspected to be hematologic, metastatic, inflammatory, or infectious. Partial nephrectomy should be considered for managing kidney masses less than 4 cm, as it is associated with favorable outcomes. Radical nephrectomy is preferred if the patient has a high tumor size, complexity, and normal contralateral kidney. Thermal ablation can be considered as an alternative approach for the management of a T1a renal mass less than 3 cm in size [1]. In patients with kidney transplantation, careful reduction of immunosuppression should always be considered in addition to the standard cancer treatment.

Clinical Course

The patient underwent a radical left nephrectomy which confirmed stage I papillary renal cell carcinoma (RCC) (Fig. 51.1). His 1-year follow-up CT surveillance showed no evidence of recurrence or metastatic disease. He was supposed to get routine CT screening 1 year later, but he was lost to follow-up. He remained asymptomatic for 3 years after his nephrectomy until he presented with complaints of dyspnea. A chest CT demonstrated a large anterior mediastinal mass and pulmonary

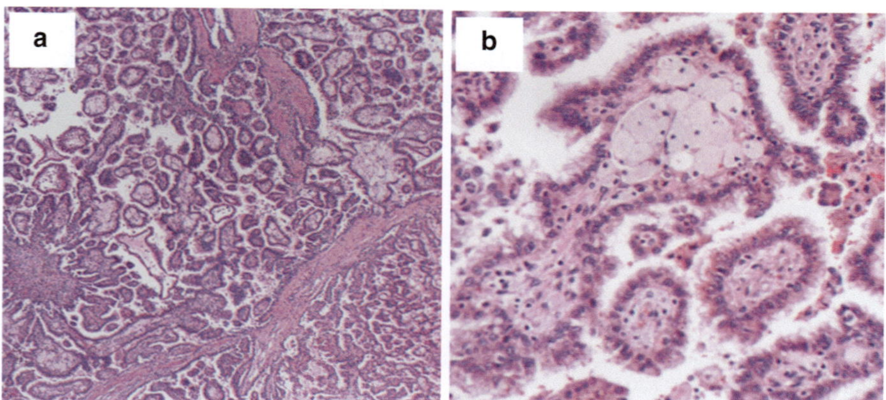

Fig. 51.1 (**a**) Papillary renal cell carcinoma with multiple papillary structures (40×). (**b**) Higher magnification shows papillae with fibrovascular cores and foamy macrophages. (200×)

nodules consistent with metastatic disease. At the presentation, he was in septic shock and developed acute kidney injury. He passed away a few days after admission due to hypoxic respiratory failure.

Question 1

What is the risk of recurrence after surgical excision of RCC?

A. 10–20%
B. 20–30%
C. 30–40%
D. >50%.

The correct answer is B.

The risk of recurrence after surgical excision of RCC is 20–30%. There is limited data on the risk of recurrence in patients with a history of kidney transplantation. For follow-up of radical or partial nephrectomy in localized disease, the National Comprehensive Cancer Network panel recommends yearly history and physical with laboratory testing. A baseline CT and MRI between months 3 and 12 after surgery followed by yearly imaging for 3 years or longer are also recommended. For RCC stages II and III, follow-up imaging is recommended every 6 months for 3 years, annually up to year 5, and longer if indicated [2].

Discussion

By 2018, an estimated 582,727 people were living with kidney and renal pelvis cancer in the United States. The estimated new cases for 2021 are around 76,000, with estimated deaths expected to be around 14,000 due to renal cell carcinoma. The 5-year survival has been reported at 75.6% [3]. Patients with ESKD carry risk factors for RCC, such as acquired cystic disease of the kidney. RCC develops in approximately 2% of individuals with acquired cysts and given the low incidence and high mortality of patients with ESKD, RCC screening is not routinely done in this population. However, some transplant programs have adopted variable screening processes for ESKD patients on the transplant waiting list [4].

The Kidney Disease Improving Global Outcomes (KDIGO) guidelines for kidney transplant recipients recommend screening for RCC with ultrasonography for patients at increased risk (>3 years of dialysis, family history of renal cancer, acquired cystic disease, analgesic nephropathy). After surgical removal of early RCC and before transplantation, a 2-year wait time is recommended. For invasive disease, a 5-year wait time is recommended by both the KDIGO and the Canadian Society of Transplantation [5, 6].

The incidence of RCC in kidney transplant recipients is four- to fivefold higher than matched controls in the general population. The increased risk has been attributed to long-term immunosuppression and other characteristics such as race, cause of kidney disease, and immunological factors [5]. Immunosuppressive medications can cause deprivation of tumor surveillance. Reduction of dendritic cells, NK cells activity, and increased immunosenescent T cells and regulatory T cells may contribute to tumor progression [5]. The standardized incidence ratio (SIR) for RCC posttransplant from the Australian and New Zealand registry was 5.0 (3.4–7.1) [6]. A similar SIR has been reported in other registries and multicenter studies [7, 8].

The subtypes of RCC are clear cell, papillary, and chromophobe. In cases where a tumor does not fit any subtype, it is designated as unclassified RCC. Approximately 75% of renal cell carcinomas (RCCs) are clear cell RCC. The risk factors for RCC include obesity, hypertension, and smoking [9]. Genetic factors must be evaluated in patients who develop RCC before the age of 46 [2]. Patients can present with symptoms of flank pain, gross hematuria, a palpable abdominal mass, though most diagnoses are incidental findings. Some unusual presentations from paraneoplastic syndromes due to hormones or cytokines released by the tumor include hypercalcemia, fever, erythrocytosis [10].

The staging of RCC is based on size, metastasis, and lymph node involvement. Stage I and stage II tumors are enclosed in the kidney. Stage III tumors are within the Gerota's fascia but can extend to the adrenal gland and major vein. Stage IV tumors have distant metastases or invade beyond the fascia.

Treatment of RCC in transplant recipients includes standard of care for RCC and reduction of immunosuppression. The standard treatment is dependent on the initial cancer stage. For T1a tumors, partial nephrectomy can be considered, especially if the tumor is in a favorable position. Radical nephrectomy is the curative treatment for stage II, III and those tumors that invade the IVC. Kidney mass biopsy is recommended before undertaking ablative therapies in non-surgical candidates and before chemotherapy in patients with metastatic disease. Post-surgical surveillance after obtaining a baseline CT usually includes yearly imaging for 5 years in stage I. For stage II and III, CT can be done every 6 months for 3 years and annually until year 5. A follow-up plan should be individualized to the patient and based on clinical judgment [2, 9]. Active surveillance can be considered for patients with tumor size < 2 cm and with other co-morbidities. These patients should undergo annual chest and abdominal imaging. Intervention is usually considered for growth to greater than 3–4 cm or by >0.4–0.5 cm/year [11]. Medical management is considered for advanced cancers. There is no role for adjuvant chemotherapy in patients with localized RCC except for patients with stage III clear cell histology due to the high risk of recurrence. Systemic treatment for relapsed or stage IV disease includes therapies such as tyrosine kinase inhibitors targeting the VEGF signaling axis [2, 9]. With recent advancements in the medical management of advanced malignancies, there has been a rise in the use of checkpoint inhibitors in advanced RCC. It is worth noting that several studies showed a high rate of acute allograft rejection in kidney transplantation patients who are treated with immune checkpoint inhibitors, and these patients must be closely monitored for rejection once cancer treatment has commenced [5].

Given the potential role of immunosuppression in promoting cancer growth, the consensus is to reduce immunosuppression doses in kidney transplant recipients after a cancer diagnosis. This, however, must carefully be balanced against the potential risks of allograft rejection, and treatment must be prescribed on a case-by-case basis, especially since limited evidence supports the efficacy of reducing immunosuppression in the treatment of most cancers. Using mTOR inhibitors instead of calcineurin inhibitors as a management strategy is controversial in RCC.

Regarding the prognosis of RCC in kidney transplant recipients, a meta-analysis showed that the pooled estimated mortality rate of kidney transplant patients with RCC is 15% at a mean follow-up of 42 months after diagnosis [12]. A large nationwide study from Korea showed that RCC after kidney transplantation is associated with a standardized mortality ratio of 5.8 (2.6–10.7) [13].

In conclusion, kidney transplant recipients have up to a fourfold to a fivefold higher risk of RCC and RCC-related death than matched individuals in the general population. The above literature review and clinical vignette suggest the importance of close surveillance in kidney transplant recipients who develop RCC. A tailored approach to the management of RCC in this patient population may result in improved outcomes.

Disclosures V. Viswanathan reports employment with Johns Hopkins University.

Sami Alasfar reports employment with the Johns Hopkins University; receiving research funding from CareDx and the World Health Organization (WHO).

Funding None.

References

1. Campbell S, et al. Renal mass and localized renal cancer: AUA guideline. J Urol. 2017;198(3):520–9.
2. Motzer RJ, et al. NCCN guidelines insights: kidney cancer, version 1.2021: featured updates to the NCCN guidelines. J Natl Compr Cancer Netw. 2020;18(9):1160–70.
3. SEER. Stat fact sheets: kidney and renal pelvis cancer. National Cancer Institute. 2016; http://seer.cancer.gov/statfacts/html/kidrp.html
4. Holley JL. Screening, diagnosis, and treatment of cancer in long-term dialysis patients. Clin J Am Soc Nephrol. 2007;2(3):604–10.
5. Chadban SJ, et al. KDIGO clinical practice guideline on the evaluation and management of candidates for kidney transplantation. Transplantation. 2020;104(4S1):S11–S103.
6. Knoll G, et al. Canadian society of transplantation: consensus guidelines on eligibility for kidney transplantation. CMAJ. 2005;173(10):S1–S25.
7. Au E, Wong G, Chapman JR. Cancer in kidney transplant recipients. Nat Rev Nephrol. 2018;14(8):508–20.
8. Vajdic CM, et al. Cancer incidence before and after kidney transplantation. JAMA. 2006;296(23):2823–31.
9. Hsieh JJ, et al. Renal cell carcinoma. Nat Rev Dis Primers. 2017;3(1):1–19.
10. Palapattu GS, Kristo B, Rajfer J. Paraneoplastic syndromes in urologic malignancy: the many faces of renal cell carcinoma. Reviews in urology. 2002;4(4):163.
11. Lane BR, Tobert CM, Riedinger CB. Growth kinetics and active surveillance for small renal masses. Curr Opin Urol. 2012;22(5):353–9.
12. Chewcharat A, et al. Incidence and mortality of renal cell carcinoma after kidney transplantation: a meta-analysis. J Clin Med. 2019;8(4):530.
13. Jeong S, et al. Incidence of malignancy and related mortality after kidney transplantation: a nationwide, population-based cohort study in Korea. Sci Rep. 2020;10(1):1–10.

Chapter 52
Posttransplant Erythrocytosis in Kidney Transplant Recipients

Karla Carias Martinez and Sami Alasfar

Introduction

Although kidney transplantation remains the treatment of choice for patients with end-stage kidney disease (ESKD), many patients develop posttransplant complications. Hematological complications are prevalent in this population and require close follow-up and proper management. Posttransplant erythrocytosis (PTE) is a hematological phenomenon that develops in up to 8–20% of kidney transplant recipients and is associated with potentially life-threatening complications.

Patient History

A 44-year-old African American non-smoker male with a history of ESKD secondary to diabetic nephropathy underwent kidney transplantation from a deceased donor with a Kidney Donor Profile Index (KDPI) score of 38%. His induction immunosuppression consisted of anti-thymocyte globulin (5 mg/kg), and his maintenance immunosuppression consisted of tacrolimus, mycophenolate mofetil, and prednisone. At the time of transplantation, the recipient's hematocrit and hemoglobin were 42.8% and 15.5 g/dL, respectively. Seven months after transplantation, he was noted to have an increase in hemoglobin to 16.5–17.3 g/dL range and hematocrit to 52.2–58.6% range on routine laboratory tests over 3 months. On review of systems, he did not endorse any headaches, blurry vision, itching, or dizziness.

K. Carias Martinez (✉) · S. Alasfar
Division of Nephrology, Department of Medicine, The Johns Hopkins University School of Medicine, Baltimore, MD, USA
e-mail: kcarias1@jhmi.edu; salasfa1@jhu.edu

© The Author(s), under exclusive license to Springer Nature Switzerland AG 2022

F. Aziz, S. Parajuli (eds.), *Complications in Kidney Transplantation*,
https://doi.org/10.1007/978-3-031-13569-9_52

Physical exam revealed a blood pressure of 131/84, stable weight over the last 3 months, moist mucous membranes, normal skin turgor, and the presence of plethora. The rest of his laboratory testing was unremarkable, and there was no associated leukocytosis or thrombocytosis. In addition to his maintenance immunosuppression regimen, his medications include amlodipine 5 mg daily, omeprazole 20 mg daily, and furosemide 20 mg daily.

Question 1

What is the most likely cause of the patient's elevated hematocrit and hemoglobin?

A. Posttransplant Erythrocytosis (PTE).
B. Polycythemia Vera (PCV).
C. Erythrocytosis due to renal artery stenosis.
D. Dehydration.
E. Erythrocytosis due to furosemide use.

The correct answer is A.

The only identifiable etiology in a patient's presentation is posttransplant erythrocytosis (PTE), usually present within the first year after kidney transplantation. PCV can present similarly, but the timeline and age of the patient are more consistent with PTE. Well-controlled hypertension and stable kidney function make renal artery stenosis less likely. Dehydration and diuretic use can also lead to a high hemoglobin/hematocrit, but there is no mention in the clinical vignette of poor oral intake, gastrointestinal losses, or physical signs of dehydration.

Clinical Course

Erythrocytosis resolved after 3 months without any intervention. One year later, he had a recurrence of erythrocytosis with hemoglobin ranging between 19.7 and 20.8 g/dL and hematocrit between 64.2 and 64.8%.

Question 2

What is the first line of treatment for PTE?

A. Therapeutic phlebotomy.
B. Renin Angiotensin Aldosterone System Inhibition (RAASi) with angiotensin-converting enzyme inhibitors (ACEi) or angiotensin receptor blockers (ARB).
C. Theophylline.
D. Change tacrolimus to sirolimus.
E. Observation.

The correct answer is B.

The mainstay pharmacologic therapy in patients with PTE consists of blocking the renin—angiotensin—aldosterone system if tolerated and no contraindication to their use. It is also essential to rule out and correct reversible causes of erythrocytosis, such as dehydration leading to hemoconcentration. The mechanism of action of RAASi in PTE is decreased production of erythropoietin and altering sensitivity of the erythroid progenitors in the bone marrow to erythropoietin. Therapeutic phlebotomy is reserved for patients who do not tolerate or respond to RAASi. It is also reserved for patients with HCT above 55% despite a maximally tolerated dose of RAASi.

Clinical Course

The patient's past medical history was again reviewed, and no other contributing factors for his erythrocytosis were found. He was a non-smoker and did not have underlying pulmonary disease or malignancy. To evaluate for renal cell carcinoma, he underwent the transplant and native kidney ultrasounds, with no suspicious masses found. There was no evidence of renal artery stenosis on the kidney transplant doppler.

He was started on therapeutic phlebotomy every 2 weeks, aspirin 81 mg daily, and losartan which was titrated to 50 mg daily but had to be discontinued due to hyperkalemia. The patient has not had any episode of thromboembolic disease.

Discussion

PTE is an often recognized, but poorly understood, a complication of kidney transplantation defined as a persistently elevated hematocrit level greater than 51% or hemoglobin greater than 17 g/dL following kidney transplantation [1–3] per Kidney Disease Improving Global Outcomes (KDIGO) 2009 guidelines [4], in the absence of other potential causes like malignancy, COPD, OSA, and renal artery stenosis. The criteria do not specify the duration of erythrocytosis or take the normal physiologic differences between sexes in erythropoiesis into account. In 2017, the WHO revised the cutoff to define erythrocytosis to include hemoglobin > 16.5 g/dL in men and > 16 g/dL in women, hematocrit > 49% in men, and > 48% in women.

PTE has a reported incidence between 8 and 20% of kidney transplant recipients usually presenting after 8–24 months [1, 3, 5] with recent reports showing a declining incidence (4–8%) [3, 6]. This broad range is explained by the lack of standardized definitions in most studies [6]. The pathogenesis of PTE was traditionally thought to be solely related to excess erythropoietin (EPO); however, various studies showed it is a multifactorial process that results from the combined effect of several hormonal systems and growth factors, including the renin—angiotensin—aldosterone system (RAAS), insulin-like growth factors, endogenous androgens, and local renal hypoxia (Fig. 52.1) [3].

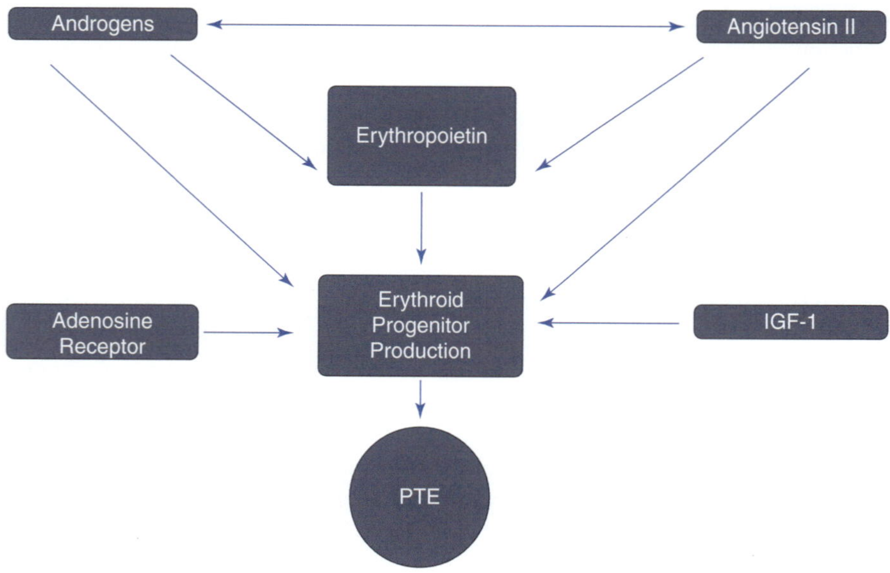

Fig. 52.1 Pathogenesis of PTE

Predisposing clinical factors include male sex, young age, smoking, good kidney quality, well-preserved kidney allograft function, and rejection-free course [6, 7]. Patients with ESKD due to polycystic kidney disease have a higher incidence of PTE due to excess production of erythropoietin from the native kidneys [6, 7].

Most patients with PTE experience mild symptoms like malaise, headache, plethora, lethargy, dizziness [1, 3]. Venous and arterial thromboembolic events occur in 10–30% of the cases, and 1–2% of patients die due to complications [1]. However, recent reports showed that the incidence of such events in PTE patients is similar to those without PTE, likely reflective of the appropriate recognition and management [3].

Spontaneous remission is observed in one-fourth of patients within 2 years from onset, whereas in the remaining patients, PTE persists for several years [1]. The primary goal of treatment in patients with persistent PTE is to control symptoms and reduce the risk of thromboembolic events. Several clinical trials in the late 1990s and early 2000s showed that the inactivation of the RAAS is very effective and safe (4). RAASi effectiveness is dose and time-dependent, with most patients reaching a plateau effect after 8 weeks of therapy. In patients with a contraindication or intolerance to RAASi, therapeutic phlebotomy should be used. Other treatments include theophylline—which also inhibits erythropoietin production but has an unpredictable response and several side effects, mTOR inhibitors which are associated with increased risk of rejection, and a now less commonly performed practice of bilateral native nephrectomy. Nephrectomy should be considered in patients with cystic kidney disease.

In conclusion, the incidence of PTE has declined over the last few decades. PTE is usually associated with a benign course if it is recognized and treated. RAASi is very effective in managing PTE and remains the mainstay of treatment after excluding reversible causes.

Disclosures K. Carias Martinez reports employment with the Johns Hopkins University.

Sami Alasfar reports employment with the Johns Hopkins University; receiving research funding from CareDx and the World Health Organization (WHO).

Funding None.

References

1. Vlahakos DV, Marathias KP, Agroyannis B, Madias NE. Posttransplant erythrocytosis. Kidney Int. 2003;63(4):1187–94. https://doi.org/10.1046/j.1523-1755.2003.00850.x.
2. Kiberd BA. Post-transplant erythrocytosis: a disappearing phenomenon? Clin Transpl. 2009;23(6):800–6. https://doi.org/10.1111/j.1399-0012.2008.00947.x.
3. Alzoubi B, Kharel A, Machhi R, Aziz F, Swanson KJ, Parajuli S. Post-transplant erythrocytosis after kidney transplantation: a review. World J Transplant. 2021;11(6):220–30. https://doi.org/10.5500/wjt.v11.i6.220.
4. Kidney disease: improving global outcomes (KDIGO) transplant work group. KDIGO clinical practice guideline for the care of kidney transplant recipients. Am J Transplant. 2009;9(Suppl 3):S1–S155. https://doi.org/10.1111/j.1600-6143.2009.02834.x.
5. Perazella MA, Bia MJ. Posttransplant erythrocytosis: case report and review of newer treatment modalities. J Am Soc Nephrol. 1993;3(10):1653–9. https://doi.org/10.1681/ASN.V3101653.
6. Alasfar S, Hall IE, Mansour SG, et al. Contemporary incidence and risk factors of post transplant erythrocytosis in deceased donor kidney transplantation. BMC Nephrol. 2021;22(1):26. https://doi.org/10.1186/s12882-021-02231-2.
7. Einollahi B, Lessan-Pezeshki M, Nafar M, et al. Erythrocytosis after renal transplantation: review of 101 cases. Transplant Proc. 2005;37(7):3101–2. https://doi.org/10.1016/j.transproceed.2005.08.023.

Chapter 53
Tacrolimus-Induced Serositis

Kurtis J. Swanson and Margaret R. Jorgenson

Introduction

Tacrolimus is an integral component of the maintenance immunosuppression in preventing allograft rejection. As has been well described in the literature, tacrolimus has been associated with favorable outcomes compared to its predecessor, cyclosporine. Despite these documented benefits, tacrolimus has a narrow therapeutic window and, as such, has a plethora of known adverse effects, including both serious (acute nephrotoxicity, posterior reversible encephalopathy syndrome, thrombotic microangiopathy) and common (neurotoxicity, alopecia, hyperglycemia) ones.

Serositis is a non-specific inflammatory process of serous membranes, such as the pericardium, peritoneum, or pleura. While serositis is a cardinal sign of several autoimmune/connective tissue diseases, it can arise from many causes, including medications.

In this chapter, we describe a case of a kidney transplant recipient who developed recurrent systemic serositis, which, after multiple thorough investigations, the process of elimination, and discontinuation of tacrolimus, was found to be secondary to tacrolimus.

Tacrolimus-induced serositis is an underappreciated cause of this disease in kidney transplant recipients that ought to be part of the differential for recurrent, otherwise unexplained ascites, pleural and pericardial effusions.

K. J. Swanson (✉)
Division of Nephrology and Hypertension, University of Minnesota, Minneapolis, MN, USA

M. R. Jorgenson
Department of Pharmacy, UW Health, Madison, WI, USA
e-mail: MJorgenson@uwhealth.org

© The Author(s), under exclusive license to Springer Nature Switzerland AG 2022
F. Aziz, S. Parajuli (eds.), *Complications in Kidney Transplantation*,
https://doi.org/10.1007/978-3-031-13569-9_53

Patient History

A 51-year-old woman with a history of end-stage kidney disease secondary to polycystic kidney disease underwent a deceased donor kidney transplantation. From the time of transplant, she was maintained on a triple-drug immunosuppressive regimen of tacrolimus, mycophenolate, and prednisone. Two years after the transplant, she began to experience recurrent serositis, including ascites, pleural, and pericardial effusions.

Ascites was first noted on a CT scan 2 years post-transplant. She underwent diagnostic paracentesis, where the fluid was sterile and exudative. She was then evaluated by hepatology and underwent MRI/MR elastogram inconsistent with portal hypertension or non-alcoholic fatty liver disease. Nine months later, she had recurrent ascites, prompting transjugular liver biopsy, which was negative for portal hypertension. On biopsy, she had grade 1 hemosiderosis, a minimal fatty change consistent with secondary iron overload, but no evidence of fibrosis or cirrhosis. At that time, her hepatologist thought she had presinusoidal portal hypertension from nodular regenerative hyperplasia, noting this is a diagnosis of exclusion. She was placed on spironolactone and furosemide, and at her follow-up appointment 4 months later, her ascites was well controlled on this regimen.

Pericardial effusion was also first diagnosed 2 years after transplant and was later redemonstrated on a transthoracic echocardiogram as part of pre-operative testing. The effusion had grown and was moderate to large at 1.4–1.7 cm. Repeat transthoracic echocardiogram showed no improvement. She was later referred to an outside hospital for progressive pleuritic chest pain and admitted for an elective pericardiocentesis and pericardial drain placement. She underwent pericardiocentesis with 360 mL of straw-colored fluid removed along with a drain placement. She was also placed on colchicine. Due to high drain output, she eventually underwent pericardial window and thoracic drain placement. Her pericardial effusion was transudative.

Pleural effusion was first noted on the same CT scan as her ascites 2 years post-transplant, where it was described as moderate in size. Later this was demonstrated on a CT scan to evaluate a perinephric fluid collection. She underwent diagnostic and therapeutic pleurocentesis with the resolution of her shortness of breath, which was consistent with a transudative effusion. On most recent imaging, no pleural effusion was appreciated.

Question 1

What is the incidence of pleural effusion and ascites related to tacrolimus based on an open-label, randomized multicentered trial evaluating 1-year outcomes?

A. 0–10%
B. 5–15%

C. 10–20%

D. 20–30%.

The correct answer is D.

According to the U.S Multicenter FK506 Liver Study comparing tacrolimus and cyclosporine for immunosuppression in liver transplantation, the incidence of pleural effusion and ascites in the first year after liver transplant ranged from 20% to 30% [1]. As aforementioned, from the time of transplantation, the patient was on tacrolimus as part of her maintenance immunosuppression regimen. This was maintained during the time of her new ascites and pleural effusion. However, after her pericardial effusion, tacrolimus was discontinued.

Question 2

Which immunosuppressant is more highly associated with late (defined as >4 years post-transplant) pericardial effusion in kidney transplant recipients?

A. Tacrolimus.

B. Mycophenolate.

C. Sirolimus.

D. Prednisone.

The correct answer is C.

In their single-center retrospective study from June 2021, Wang et al. showed that after multivariate analysis, adjusting for eGFR, sirolimus use was associated with late pericardial effusion development with an adjusted odds ratio of 3.58 (95% CI: 1.25–10.20, $p = 0.017$). This is demonstrated in the above Fig. 53.1.

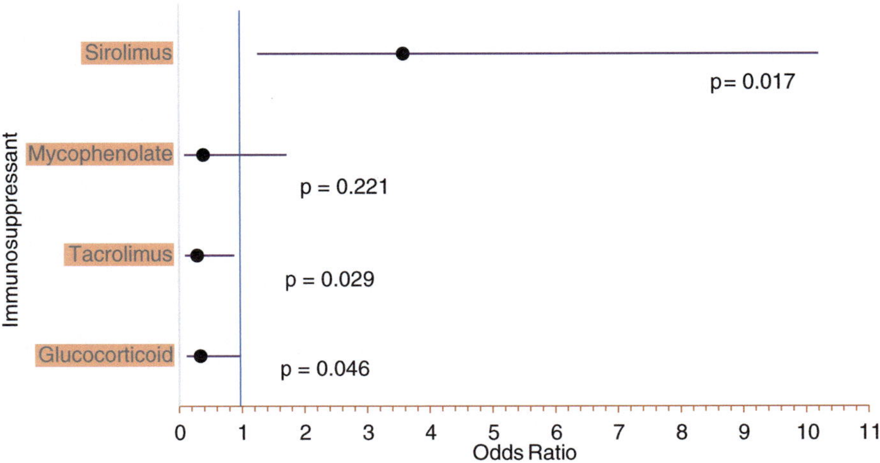

Fig. 53.1 Risk of pericardial effusion based on various immunosuppression

While unable to demonstrate correlation, the authors noted that KTRs with early-onset effusion had significantly higher tacrolimus levels (5.39 ± 2.72 ng/mL and 3.36 ± 1.86 ng/mL [$p < 0.001$]) [2].

Additional Clinical Course

Since pericardial effusion requiring invasive thoracotomy and pericardial window resulted in discontinuation of tacrolimus, the patient did not have recurrent serositis as seen on physical exam serial imaging, nor has she required any para-, pericardio-, or pleurocenteses.

Discussion

Here we describe a case of a middle-aged female kidney transplant recipient who developed recurrent serositis after 2 years post-kidney transplant. While her poly-cystic liver disease, evidence of iron overload, female sex, history of kidney trans-plantation, and induction/maintenance immunosuppression put her at risk for myriad causes of serositis, repeated non-revealing workups of these fluid collec-tions assessing broadly for vascular, infectious/inflammatory, traumatic, autoim-mune, metabolic, and neoplastic causes, in addition to disease recurrence and resolution after the discontinuation of tacrolimus strongly suggest a drug-induced phenomenon.

In the literature to date, 5 case reports exist describing tacrolimus-induced sero-sitis: 2 episodes of pericardial effusion with one leading to cardiac tamponade, 1 case report describing massive pleural effusion, and 2 cases of tacrolimus-induced ascites: 1 after kidney transplantation and the other after liver transplantation [3–7].

How tacrolimus leads to serositis has not been completely elucidated. Broadly speaking, fluid and salt retention are known adverse effects of tacrolimus described in the literature [5, 6]. While mechanistic studies pertaining to tacrolimus-mediated fluid retention are lacking, theoretically, processes similar to those described by Naesens et al. in their seminal work on calcineurin inhibitor nephrotoxicity are involved, i.e., TGF-beta and angiotensin II lead to the generation of reactive oxygen species and a proinflammatory state driving serosal inflammation and fluid genera-tion [8].

When specifically considering ascites, it has been postulated that this could be secondary to the development of sinusoidal obstruction syndrome and hepatic medi-ated alterations in tacrolimus pharmacodynamics [4]. Indeed, fluid retention/altera-tions appear to be quite common in the liver transplant population, with the incidence of peripheral edema, ascites, and pleural effusion reported to be 15–35% of patients on tacrolimus for maintenance immunosuppression [1, 6]. Notably, as Prashar et al. mention, the US Food and Drug Administration (FDA) has reported pericardial effusion in Phase IV studies as a post-marketing side effect [5]. As of September 2020, the FDA noted in their less frequently reported adverse reactions (>3–<15% in liver, kidney, and heart transplant patients) the following: pulmonary edema and generalized edema. In their post-marketing adverse reactions, the following were described: pericardial effusion and pancreatitis [9].

In summary, tacrolimus-induced serositis is an infrequently described but important adverse drug reaction that requires consideration in the differential of ascites, pleural effusion, pericardial effusion in kidney transplant recipients.

References

1. European FK506 multicentre liver study group. Randomised trial comparing tacrolimus (FK506) and cyclosporin in prevention of liver allograft rejection. Lancet. 1994;344(8920):423–8.
2. Wang SC, Pashkovetsky E, Conti D, Ata A, Torosoff M, Fein S, et al. Pericardial effusion after renal transplantation: timing and clinical characteristics. Transplant Proc. 2021;53(5):1606–10.
3. Doobay R, Gambhir HS. Cardiac tamponade induced by tacrolimus toxicity. Am J Ther. 2018;25(6):e683–4.
4. Hosseini M, Aliakbarian M, Akhavan-Rezayat K, Shadkam O, Milani S. Tacrolimus-induced ascites after liver transplant. Int J Organ Transplant Med. 2018;9(2):102–4.
5. Prashar R, Stewart D, Moza A. Tacrolimus as a rare cause of pericardial effusion in a renal transplant recipient. Heart Views. 2017;18(4):145–8.
6. Nayagam LS, Vijayanand B, Balasubramanian S. Massive pleural effusion in a renal transplant recipient on tacrolimus. Indian J Nephrol. 2014;24(5):318–20.
7. Mese M, Parmaksiz E. Tacrolimus induced ascites after 10 years renal transplantation. Prog Transplant. 2021;31(1):281–2.
8. Naesens M, Kuypers DR, Sarwal M. Calcineurin inhibitor nephrotoxicity. Clin J Am Soc Nephrol. 2009;4(2):481–508.
9. Tacrolimus human prescription drug label. National Institute of health U.S. National Library of Medicine. 2020.

Chapter 54
Arteriovenous Fistula Associated High-Output Heart Failure After Kidney Transplantation: Initial Workup

Vidya A. Fleetwood and Fadee Abualrub

Introduction

High-output heart failure is an uncommon but highly morbid complication of high-flow brachial fistulas. Early identification and treatment of this syndrome are key to a successful cardiac outcome. We present a case of arteriovenous fistula-related high-output heart failure after kidney transplantation and discuss diagnosis, management, and treatment considerations.

Case Presentation

A 55-year-old white male with a history of a kidney transplant 5 years ago presented to the emergency room with gradual weight gain, increasing shortness of breath, and lower extremity edema. He endorsed a history of end-stage kidney (ESKD) disease secondary to diabetes mellitus type II and had received a deceased donor kidney transplant with an uncomplicated postoperative course and no history of rejection. His serum creatinine had nadired at 1.2 mg/dL, and he was maintained on tacrolimus and mycophenolic acid.

His vital signs were significant for hypertension (159/95), a heart rate of 95 bpm, and an oxygen saturation of 80% on room air. On physical examination, he had fine crackles in bilateral lung bases and a distinct systolic ejection murmur, as well as bilateral 3+ pitting edema. His graft was non-tender with no bruit. His brachiocephalic fistula was large and tortuous with an intact thrill. Laboratory investigations

V. A. Fleetwood (✉) · F. Abualrub
Center for Abdominal Transplantation, Saint Louis University, St. Louis, MO, USA
e-mail: Vidyaratna.fleetwood@health.slu.edu; Fadee.Abualrub@health.slu.edu

© The Author(s), under exclusive license to Springer Nature Switzerland AG 2022
F. Aziz, S. Parajuli (eds.), *Complications in Kidney Transplantation*,
https://doi.org/10.1007/978-3-031-13569-9_54

showed serum creatinine of 1.9 mg/dL and a tacrolimus level of 5 ng/mL. Beta natriuretic peptide (BNP) was 890 pg/uL; troponins were normal. A chest X-ray showed bilateral infiltrates in the bases. An EKG showed left ventricular hypertrophy.

Question 1

Due to his elevated BNP, echocardiography was performed, which showed an ejection fraction of 40%, diastolic dysfunction with increased left ventricle thickness, mild mitral regurgitation, sclerosis of the aortic valve, and systolic pulmonary pressure of 50 mmHg.

What is the next step in management?

A. Intravenous loop diuretics.
B. Left heart catheterization.
C. Pulmonary function tests.
D. Ultrasound of the kidney allograft.
E. Check urine for protein and donor-specific antibodies.

The correct answer is A.

The patient presents with symptoms of acute congestive heart failure, and diuresis would be the first step in management, then diagnostic procedures can follow. Decreasing the preload will improve the patient's symptoms and lower both the systemic and pulmonary blood pressure, as well as decrease the oxygen requirement.

The patient responded well to diuresis, with weight decreasing and oxygenation improving. He continued to complain of orthopnea, however, and a repeat exam showed a heart rate of 95 bpm with an oxygen saturation of 90% at rest. His lower extremity edema improved only mildly.

Question 2

What is the next step in diagnosis and management?

A. Coronary angiography by left heart catheterization.
B. Start an angiotensin convertase enzyme inhibitor.
C. Start an angiotensin receptor blocker.
D. Start a sodium-glucose co-transporter-2 (SGLT-2) inhibitor.
E. Repeat the echocardiogram while compressing the fistula by blood pressure cuff.

The correct answer is E.

The patient's symptoms are not suggestive of an acute coronary syndrome, and there are no acute indications for coronary angiography. Although he may have had a silent myocardial infarction given his history of diabetes, angiography is invasive and uses contrast, worsening his AKI. All of the medications listed (b, c, d) may have long-term benefits but are not expected to improve the patient's symptoms in the short term and may not benefit him if the underlying cause of heart failure is not addressed. Echocardiography (E) is noninvasive and may elucidate whether fistula-related high-output heart failure is the cause of his symptoms.

Most of the time, repeating the echo while compressing the fistula by a blood pressure cough can show an immediate improvement in the hemodynamics, in which case the fistula needs to be ligated or revised.

Additional Clinical Course

Transthoracic echocardiography with and without fistula compression was performed. With compression, the heart rate improved to 79, the systolic pulmonary pressure improved to 40, and the ejection fraction improved to 48%. The patient was referred to a vascular surgeon for fistula ligation, which improved his heart failure symptoms.

Discussion

Cardiac death is the most common cause of mortality in the first year after kidney transplantation [1]. Diabetes and hypertension, common etiologies of kidney failure, are significant contributors to the development of cardiac disease; furthermore, the inflammatory effects of hemodialysis may hasten the development of atherosclerosis [2]. After transplant, steroid and calcineurin inhibitor use may further contribute to heart disease [2].

Although necessary in many patients for adequate dialysis, arteriovenous fistulas may also worsen cardiac disease and lead to heart failure [3]. Formation of an arteriovenous fistula requires increased blood flow through the brachial or femoral artery (depending on fistula location) and is associated with a significant increase in left ventricular (LV) and right ventricular end-systolic volume [4]. In most patients, these changes, while clinically significant, are not symptomatic. However, in a small subset, a high-flow fistula can lead to the development of high-output heart failure.

High-output heart failure (HOHF) is characterized by eccentric left ventricular remodeling, natriuretic peptide activation, high filling pressures, pulmonary hypertension, and increased cardiac output, despite similar ejection fraction (Table 54.1) [3] The pathophysiology is thought to be related to decreased systemic vascular resistance [3]. Multiple etiologies have been described, most prominently obesity and liver disease, but iatrogenic arteriovenous fistulas were seen to account for 14% of cases in one study [3].

HOHF can be seen most commonly with brachial artery fistulas, although it has been documented with femoral fistulas [5]. The syndrome typically develops when flow through the access is >2000 mL/min. Clinical symptoms may be similar with low- and high-output heart failure, manifesting with dyspnea on exertion, fatigue, and weight gain; high-output heart failure tends to be accompanied by a widened pulse pressure and an S3 gallop. HOHF may present with steal syndrome—neuropathy and possible weakness of the ipsilateral hand—but this is not a sensitive marker for the presence of HOHF. A transthoracic echocardiogram (TTE) may be obtained to assess for the previously mentioned derangements in cardiac remodeling and to assess cardiac output; the normal range is 2.5–4.2 L/min/m^2, but HOHF may present with flows of greater than 9 L/min/m^2 [4]. Notably, contractility may be

Table 54.1 Diagnosis and management of arteriovenous fistula-related high-output heart failure

Suggestive findings
    Physical exam
        Hypervolemia
        S3 gallop
        Widened pulse pressure
    Imaging findings
        Chest X-ray
            Pulmonary edema
        Transthoracic echocardiogram
            Pulmonary hypertension
            Eccentric LVH
            Increased cardiac output
            Normal EF
        Fistula duplex
            Qa >2 L/min

Alternate etiologies
    Beri-beri
    Thyrotoxicosis
    Liver cirrhosis
    Pregnancy

Confirmation
    Nicoladoni-Branham sign

Treatment
    Supportive care and heart failure management
    If stable renal function:
        Fistula ligation
    If poor renal function:
        Fistula banding
        Distalization of access

either hyperdynamic or decreased, depending on the degree of heart failure; however, pulmonary hypertension and left ventricular hypertrophy are expected [6]. If the diagnosis remains in question, right heart catheterization will definitively prove the presence or absence of a high-output state but may be unnecessary if TTE is revealing.

If echocardiography findings are consistent with HOHF, further investigation is needed to determine if the fistula is the culprit. Other common etiologies—anemia, thyrotoxicosis, cirrhosis, pregnancy—should be excluded or addressed. Doppler ultrasound of the fistula should reveal a flow (Qa) of >2 L/min, with an 89% sensitivity and a 100% specificity for HOHF [7]. Additionally, the Nicoladoni–Branham sign [8] can be elicited with manual compression of the fistula: the maneuver causes an immediate decrease in pulse and increase in blood pressure driven by the drop in SVR with compression of the fistula. Performing this sign during TTE can provide direct visualization of the effect on some cardiac derangements, particularly high pulmonary artery systolic pressure. Correction of HOHF due to a high-output fistula may be accomplished with surgical banding or ligation and can commonly be done under local anesthesia with monitored anesthesia care.

Due to the deleterious effects of high-flow fistulas on cardiac remodeling, elective and prophylactic ligation of the arteriovenous fistula in renal transplant recipients with stable renal function has been proposed. Ligation of the fistula even in patients without clinical signs of heart failure has been shown to result in a reduction of left ventricular end-diastolic diameter and mass index [9]. However, the transplant nephrologist must weigh the benefit of ligation in patients *without* heart failure symptoms against the possibility of losing access in patients who may return to dialysis in the future. Distalization of the access using a non-autogenous jump graft to the radial artery [10] has been suggested and would preserve dialysis access while decreasing flow. However, few patients are likely to be acceptable candidates for this treatment due to calcification or the small size of the radial artery.

Patients displaying signs of heart failure should undergo surveillance imaging of their hemodialysis access and consult with vascular surgery regarding the need for ligation and the ease of future access. No recommendations can currently be made regarding prophylactic AVF ligation, but it may be considered in patients with stable renal function.

References

1. Saran R, Robinson B, Abbott KC, et al. US renal data system 2017 annual data report: epidemiology of kidney disease in the United States. Am J Kidney Dis. 2018;71(3 Suppl 1):A7.
2. Devine PA, Courtney AE, Maxwell AP. Cardiovascular risk in renal transplant recipients. J Nephrol. 2019;32(3):389–99.
3. Reddy YNV, Melenovsky V, Redfield MM, Nishimura RA, Borlaug BA. High-output heart failure: a 15-year experience. J Am Coll Cardiol. 2016;68(5):473–82.
4. Dundon BK, Torpey K, Nelson AJ, et al. The deleterious effects of arteriovenous fistula-creation on the cardiovascular system: a longitudinal magnetic resonance imaging study. Int J Nephrol Renovasc Dis. 2014;7:337–45.
5. Bertrand D, Desbuissons G, Pallet N, et al. Acute renal failure and volume overload syndrome secondary to a femorofemoral arteriovenous fistula angioplasty in a kidney transplant recipient. Case Rep Transplant. 2013;2013:197524.
6. Stern AB, Klemmer PJ. High-output heart failure secondary to arteriovenous fistula. Hemodial Int. 2011;15(1):104–7.
7. Basile C, Lomonte C, Vernaglione L, Casucci F, Antonelli M, Losurdo N. The relationship between the flow of arteriovenous fistula and cardiac output in haemodialysis patients. Nephrol Dial Transplant. 2008;23(1):282–7.
8. Reis GJ, Hirsch AT, Come PC. Detection and treatment of high-output cardiac failure resulting from a large hemodialysis fistula. Catheter Cardiovasc Diagn. 1988;14(4):263–5.
9. van Duijnhoven EC, Cheriex EC, Tordoir JH, Kooman JP, van Hooff JP. Effect of closure of the arteriovenous fistula on left ventricular dimensions in renal transplant patients. Nephrol Dial Transplant. 2001;16(2):368–72.
10. Chemla ES, Morsy M, Anderson L, Whitemore A. Inflow reduction by distalization of anastomosis treats efficiently high-inflow high-cardiac output vascular access for hemodialysis. Semin Dial. 2007;20(1):68–72.

Chapter 55
High Output Heart Failure
Due to Arteriovenous Fistula in a Kidney
Transplant Patient: Management

Ravi V. Patel and Ali Ibrahim Gardezi

Introduction

Cardiovascular deaths remain the number one cause of mortality in post-kidney transplant patients [1]. Despite a downward trend, cardiovascular death accounts for nearly one-fourth of all deaths in patients with a functioning kidney graft [1]. Heart failure (HF) is a leading cause of hospitalization in kidney transplant recipients. Normal cardiac output ranges from 2.5 to 4.2 L/min. Patients with higher cardiac output are at risk of developing high output heart failure. High output heart failure secondary to arteriovenous (AV) fistula in the hemodialysis (HD) population was first described in the 1970s [2]. Yet, it remains an under-recognized condition in this population. This is partly due to high rates of pre-existing heart failure and multiple co-morbidities with similar presentation.

Here, we present a case of high output heart failure due to a high flow AV fistula and discuss our approach in managing such patients.

Case

A 58-year-old Caucasian male with a history of coronary artery disease s/p coronary artery bypass graft, end-stage kidney disease due to idiopathic focal segmental glomerulosclerosis received a deceased donor kidney transplant with alemtuzumab induction. For 9 years before the kidney transplant, he was undergoing

R. V. Patel (✉) · A. I. Gardezi
Division of Nephrology, Department of Medicine, University of Wisconsin—Madison School of Medicine and Public Health, Madison, WI, USA
e-mail: rvpatel7@wisc.edu; agardezi@uwhealth.org

© The Author(s), under exclusive license to Springer Nature Switzerland AG 2022

F. Aziz, S. Parajuli (eds.), *Complications in Kidney Transplantation*, https://doi.org/10.1007/978-3-031-13569-9_55

hemodialysis three times a week using the right brachiobasilic AV fistula. His post-transplant course was complicated by delayed graft function and multiple hospitalizations due to HF exacerbation. Two years after his transplant, his creatinine had stabilized around 2 mg/dL with eGFR of ~30 mL/min/m^2. He presented to the Emergency Department with shortness of breath on minimal exertion, early satiety, abdominal bloating, nausea, fatigue, and increasing weight gain despite an escalating dose of diuretics at home.

In the Emergency Department, the patient's vitals were as follows: blood pressure of 105/66 mmHg, pulse rate of 94 bpm, respiratory rate of 20/min, BMI 23 kg/m^2. The patient was noted to have bilateral crackles on lung auscultation, jugular venous pulse 5 cm above the clavicle in sitting position, and 2+ pedal edema. B-type Natriuretic Peptide (BNP) level was 1136 pg/mL. An echocardiogram showed a left ventricular ejection fraction (LVEF) of 60%, dilated right ventricle with severely reduced systolic function, and elevated right atrial pressure. The patient was started on intravenous diuretics and admitted to the hospital for further management.

Question 1

Which of the following echocardiogram findings is least likely associated with high output heart failure?

A. Dilation of the inferior vena cava.
B. Right ventricular enlargement or dysfunction.
C. Reduced left ventricular ejection fraction.
D. Elevation in estimated pulmonary artery pressures.
E. Left ventricular enlargement.

The correct answer is C.

With the increased venous return, there is increased preload, leading to elevated left ventricular end-diastolic pressure and volume, which causes increased pressure on the pulmonary vasculature and right side of the heart. Left ventricular systolic function is usually preserved in the beginning.

Case Follow-Up

On day 3 of hospitalization, the patient underwent right heart catheterization that showed high cardiac output (Fick CO: 5.7 L/min) with low normal systemic vascular resistance (749 dynes/s/cm^{-5}). It also showed elevated right atrial pressure and pulmonary hypertension (64/2 mmHg). Upon occlusion of the fistula, cardiac output decreased (Fick CO: 4.0 L/min) along with the reduction in right atrial pressure.

Question 2

Based on the above information, what would be the best management option for the patient?

A. Angioplasty.
B. Banding of the inflow to reduce the flow.

C. Ligation of the fistula.
D. B or C.

The correct answer is D.

Angioplasty is used to treat the stenosis in the fistula, which in case of a high output failure may result in worsening due to improvement in the flow after angioplasty. Patients with a confirmed diagnosis of high output heart failure due to AV fistula will require either fistula ligation or inflow reduction to reduce fistula flow to help improve HF.

Case Follow-Up

Based on the right heart catheterization findings and his suboptimal renal function, a decision was made to revise the fistula. The patient underwent a minimally invasive limited ligation endoluminal-assisted revision (MILLER) banding procedure to reduce fistula flow. Immediately following the procedure, the patient reported improved shortness of breath. At the month 3 follow-up, the patient reported increased exercise tolerance and good appetite. Over the last 3 years since his fistula banding, the patient has had no admission for HF exacerbation.

Discussion

AV fistula is the preferred choice of dialysis access for hemodialysis patients due to its superior safety profile and higher patency rates. High output heart failure is a well-documented complication of high flow AV fistula [3].

Ideally, an AV fistula should function with enough flow to prevent clotting while maximizing dialysis efficacy. National Kidney Foundation's KDOQI vascular access guidelines recommend a minimum blood flow rate of 500–600 mL/min across the AV fistula for optimal use [4]. There is no consensus on the maximum flow rate across AV fistula. The flow rate over 1500 mL/min has been defined as high flow AV access [5].

There is a sudden decrease in systemic vascular resistance after creating the AV fistula due to the shunting of blood directly from the arterial system to the venous system. This causes a reduction in effective blood volume and pressure, leading to activation of the sympathetic nervous system through baroreceptor activation. This causes peripheral vasoconstriction to increase systemic vascular resistance, most prominent in splenic vasculature, leading to a reduction in renal blood flow. This activates the renin—angiotensin—aldosterone axis and leads to salt and water retention. This, in turn, leads to volume overload and increases venous return, causing an increase in cardiac filling pressure and chamber size. This persistent increase in cardiac fill volume and increased heart rate leads to increased cardiac

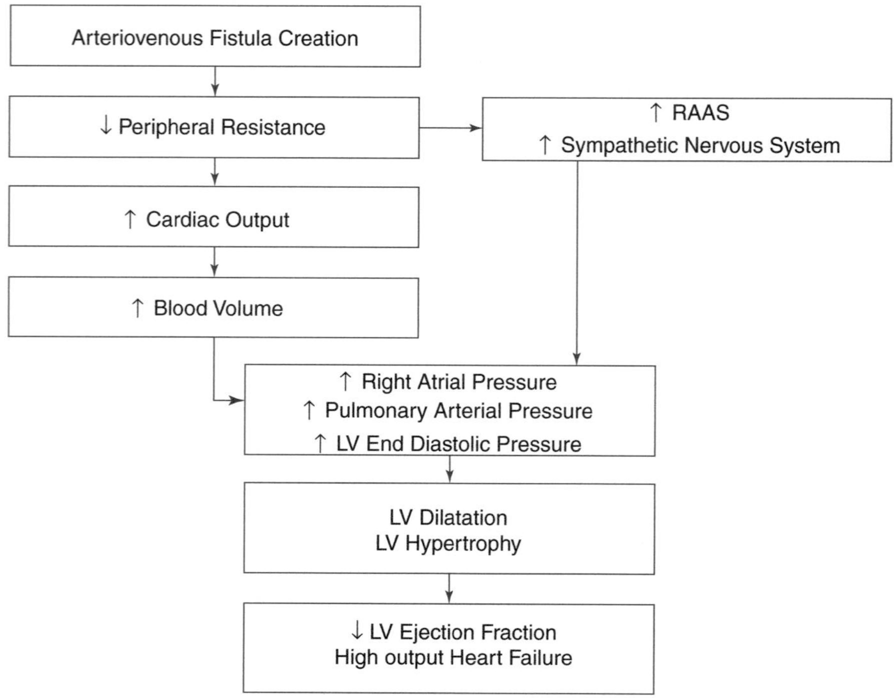

Fig. 55.1 Pathophysiology of high output heart failure

workload and ultimately leads to LV systolic dysfunction [6]. Three months after AVF creation, there is a significant increase in LV mass and left atrial area [7]. (Fig. 55.1).

Symptoms of high output HF are like what is seen in low output HF, specifically dyspnea, tachypnea, peripheral edema, abdominal bloating, nausea, generalized fatigue. Physical exam findings like warm extremities, wide pulse pressure, hyperdynamic precordium can help distinguish high output HF from low output HF.

It is difficult to predict the prevalence of high output HF in this population due to lack of data and relatively low detection rate. In one retrospective study, Schier et al. reported that 25.7% (29 of 113) patients at the medical university of Innsbruck were diagnosed with high output heart failure requiring fistula ligation between years 2005 and 2010 [3].

Multiple data points are required to accurately diagnose high output HF. A high level of suspicion is required on the physician's part as the symptoms are like that of low output cardiac failure. Any patient with newly diagnosed or worsening HF with a functional AV fistula should be evaluated for high output HF.

Due to increased cardiac workload and increased wall stress, there is an increase in BNP levels. A comprehensive echocardiogram is ideally the first step in the evaluation, showing one or more of the following: dilated inferior vena cava, right ventricular enlargement or dysfunction, elevated estimated pulmonary artery pressures, or LV enlargement [8]. LVEF may be normal in the beginning, but over time with ongoing hemodynamic stress, LVEF decreases. Patients should be evaluated for common causes of high output HF, like anemia, obesity, hyperthyroidism apart from AV fistula (Table 55.1). Ultrasound can be helpful to evaluate fistula flow. Fistula flow of more than 2 L/min has been associated with the development of HF, but the flow of fewer than 2 L/min does not exclude hemodynamically significant effects of AV fistula [9]. (Fig. 55.2).

Table 55.1 Etiology of high output heart failure

Physiological conditions
1.   Fever
2.   Exercise/stress
3.   Pregnancy
4.   Anemia
Pathological conditions
1.   Arteriovenous fistula (acquired / congenital)
2.   Obesity
3.   Liver cirrhosis
4.   Myeloproliferative disorders
5.   Hyperthyroidism
6.   Beri-beri
7.   Chronic pulmonary disease

Fig. 55.2 Proposed management algorithm for suspected high output HF due to AVF

Sudden temporary occlusion of the AV fistula would result in bradycardia if it was significantly contributing to increased cardiac output (Nicoladoni–Branham sign) [10]. This serves as a simple, non-invasive test. Right heart catheterization, first with open and then with occluded fistula, should be considered when the suspicion is high. Improvement in cardiac output and reduction in right atrial pressure with fistula occlusion can confirm the diagnosis. Apart from causing high output HF, a high flow AV fistula can lead to the development of distal hypo-perfusion in the extremity by diverting blood away from the distal artery to the fistula, leading to steal syndrome. High fistula flow has also been implicated in central venous stenosis and aneurysm formation [5]. Management of high output HF remains controversial as it should be individualized based on the severity of the patient's HF, cardiac co-morbidities, fistula anatomy, renal graft function, and options for future AV access. (Fig. 55.2). If the patient has excellent graft functions and more options for future vascular access, fistula ligation is reasonable. However, if the graft function is low, dialysis need is anticipated in near future, or there are no further options for vascular access, fistula preserving procedures should be considered. Surgical revision procedures like the MILLER banding technique or revision using distal inflow (RUDI) technique can reduce fistula flow and hence, help preserve AV fistula for future access while improving high output HF [11]. If this fails, fistula ligation would be warranted.

Conclusion

Long-standing high flow AV fistula has been a well-recognized cause of high output HF in the post-transplant population. However, due to the high level of HF rate, high output HF remains an under-recognized entity. A high level of suspicion is warranted to detect high output HF, as the symptoms are like that of low cardiac output HF. Right heart catheterization with and without fistula occlusion is necessary to diagnose high output HF. If confirmed, the fistula may need to be ligated, resulting in loss of dialysis access. However, newer techniques such as MILLER banding and RUDI procedure can help preserve fistula for future access while addressing high output HF.

References

1. Awan AA, Niu J, Pan JS, Erickson KF, Mandayam S, Winkelmayer WC, Navaneethan SD, Ramanathan V. Trends in the causes of death among kidney transplant recipients in the united states (1996–2014). Am J Nephrol. 2018;48(6):472–81. https://doi.org/10.1159/000495081.
2. Ahearn DJ, Maher JF. Heart failure as a complication of hemodialysis arteriovenous fistula. Ann Intern Med. 1972;77(2):201–4. https://doi.org/10.7326/0003-4819-77-2-201. PMID: 4641654
3. Schier T, Göbel G, Bösmüller C, Gruber I, Tiefenthaler M. Incidence of arteriovenous fistula closure due to high-output cardiac failure in kidney-transplanted patients. Clin Transpl. 2013;27(6):858–65. https://doi.org/10.1111/ctr.12248. Epub 2013 Oct 7. 24118251

4. Beathard GA, Lok CE, Glickman MH, Al-Jaishi AA, Bednarski D, Cull DL, Lawson JH, Lee TC, Niyyar VD, Syracuse D, Trerotola SO, Roy-Chaudhury P, Shenoy S, Underwood M, Wasse H, Woo K, Yuo TH, Huber TS. Definitions and end points for interventional studies for arteriovenous dialysis access. Clin J Am Soc Nephrol. 2018;13(3):501–12. https://doi.org/10.2215/CJN.11531116. Epub 2017 Jul 20. PMID: 28729383; PMCID: PMC5967683
5. Sequeira A, Tan TW. Complications of a high-flow access and its management. Semin Dial. 2015;28(5):533–43. https://doi.org/10.1111/sdi.12366. Epub 2015 Mar 23. PMID: 25808428
6. Anand IS. High-output heart failure revisited. J Am Coll Cardiol. 2016;68(5):483–6. https://doi.org/10.1016/j.jacc.2016.05.036. PMID: 27470456
7. Ori Y, Korzets A, Katz M, Erman A, Weinstein T, Malachi T, Gafter U. The contribution of an arteriovenous access for hemodialysis to left ventricular hypertrophy. Am J Kidney Dis. 2002;40(4):745–52. https://doi.org/10.1053/ajkd.2002.35685. PMID: 12324909
8. Reddy YNV, Melenovsky V, Redfield MM, Nishimura RA, Borlaug BA. High-output heart failure: a 15-year experience. J Am Coll Cardiol. 2016;68(5):473–82. https://doi.org/10.1016/j.jacc.2016.05.043. PMID: 27470455
9. Basile C, Lomonte C, Vernaglione L, Casucci F, Antonelli M, Losurdo N. The relationship between the flow of arteriovenous fistula and cardiac output in haemodialysis patients. Nephrol Dial Transplant. 2008;23(1):282–7. https://doi.org/10.1093/ndt/gfm549. Epub 2007 Oct 17. PMID: 17942475
10. BURCHELL HB. Observations on bradycardia produced by occlusion of an artery proximal to an arteriovenous fistula (Nicoladoni-Branham sign). Med Clin North Am. 1958;42(4):1029–35. https://doi.org/10.1016/s0025-7125(16)34255-9. PMID: 13564989
11. Miller GA, Hwang WW. Challenges and management of high-flow arteriovenous fistulae. Semin Nephrol. 2012;32(6):545–50. https://doi.org/10.1016/j.semnephrol.2012.10.005. PMID: 23217334

Chapter 56
Aneurysmal Arteriovenous Fistula in Patients with Kidney Transplant

Ravi V. Patel and Ali Ibrahim Gardezi

Introduction

Arteriovenous (AV) access is the preferred choice of vascular access in patients on hemodialysis (HD) due to its favorable patency rate and association with decreased mortality and morbidity compared to the central venous catheter [1]. Nonetheless, AV fistula is associated with complications such as infection, limb swelling, aneurysm formation, steal syndrome, high output heart failure, and mega fistula formation.

Management of the AV fistula remains a controversial topic amongst transplant nephrologists and vascular access specialists. There is increasing evidence that a patent AV fistula leads to increased cardiac workload and contributes to the development of heart failure [2]. However, there is still insufficient evidence to suggest that pre-emptive closure of a functional AV fistula would reverse the cardiovascular changes and provide cardiovascular mortality benefit in renal transplant recipients [3]. On the other hand, AV fistula would provide readily available access for hemodialysis in case of a failing kidney transplant. The above discussion becomes important, especially when an AVF complication develops in a post-transplant patient. We present a case with a dysfunctional AV fistula in a kidney transplant recipient patient.

R. V. Patel (✉) · A. I. Gardezi
Division of Nephrology, Department of Medicine, University of Wisconsin—Madison School of Medicine and Public Health, Madison, WI, USA
e-mail: rvpatel7@wisc.edu; agardezi@uwhealth.org

© The Author(s), under exclusive license to Springer Nature Switzerland AG 2022

F. Aziz, S. Parajuli (eds.), *Complications in Kidney Transplantation*, https://doi.org/10.1007/978-3-031-13569-9_56

Case

A 55-year-old female with a past medical history of end-stage kidney disease secondary to thin basement membrane disease received a pre-emptive deceased donor kidney transplant with anti-thymocyte globulin induction 7 years before presentation. The patient had a left brachiocephalic AV fistula that was placed before her transplant but never used. Her post-transplant course was complicated by slow graft function (creatinine nadir of 2.06 mg/dL) and recurrent urinary tract infections requiring a reduction in immunosuppression. She subsequently developed antibody-mediated rejection. Transplant kidney biopsy 2 months before presentation showed severe interstitial fibrosis and tubular atrophy with a chronicity score of 9/12. She presented to the clinic with arm swelling, increased size, and pulsation of the right brachiocephalic fistula.

Question 1

What is the next best step in managing this patient?

A. Magnetic Resonance (MR) venogram of the right upper extremity.
B. Computed Tomography (CT) venogram of the right upper extremity.
C. Ultrasound (US) duplex of the AV fistula.
D. Angiogram of the AV fistula.

The correct answer is D.

In this case, the likely cause of the unilateral arm swelling, increasing size, and pulsatility of the fistula is an outflow obstruction. An Angiogram of the fistula cannot only help identify the culprit lesion but also treat it at the same time. Since using iodinated contrast can increase the risk of further deterioration of kidney functions, Carbon Dioxide (CO_2) can be used as the contrast medium to reduce exposure to iodinated contrast.

Aneurysm formation is defined as an abnormal dilatation of the vessel wall (>2 times the diameter of the normal vein). The incidence of aneurysm formation varies between 5 and 28.5% in different studies [4]. An aneurysm can be classified as (1) cannulation site aneurysm, (2) anastomotic aneurysm, or (3) diffuse aneurysmal dilatation of the whole outflow (mega fistula). Different pathological factors are described to influence the development of different types of aneurysms. Repeated trauma from cannulation causes cannulation site aneurysm. The most common cause of an anastomotic aneurysm is infection [5]. Chronic outflow stenosis has been implicated in the mega fistula formation [6].

A mega fistula has multiple aneurysmal segments or generalized dilation of the whole fistula. One proposed definition of an aneurysm is a segment that is >2 times the diameter of the adjacent normal vein size along with high access pressure and blood flow >2000 mL/min. Due to the paucity of published data and no clear definition, it is hard to estimate the incidence.

The interplay between different biological factors and hemodynamic changes influences fistula maturation. The creation of an AV fistula bypasses resistance vessels in the extremity and creates a low-resistance pathway to the heart. This leads to increased blood flow through the newly created AV fistula. This increase in blood flow rate increases walls shear stress (WSS) on both arterial and venous walls. An increase in shear stress leads to increased secretion of vasodilators like nitric oxide and prostacyclin, leading to an increase in vessel size and normalization of the WSS. The increased vessel distention and intraluminal pressure also cause an increase in circumferential wall stress. This is thought to mediate eccentric hypertrophy [7]. In case of uncorrected venous outflow stenosis, the constantly increased intraluminal pressure in the outflow vein would lead to persistent activation of the above mechanism, leading to further outward remodeling of the vessel and, ultimately, aneurysm formation [8].

Case Follow-Up

The patient underwent an angiogram demonstrating 80% stenosis in the cephalic arch and cephalic/subclavian vein junction. (Fig. 56.1) This was reduced to 10% by balloon angioplasty. The patient was later admitted to the hospital with worsening shortness of breath and was diagnosed with disseminated blastomycosis and ganciclovir resistant CMV viremia. Her hospital course was complicated with worsening renal function, and the patient was started on hemodialysis using the existing left brachiocephalic fistula.

The patient returned 4 months after starting hemodialysis with increased pulsatility of the fistula and prolonged bleeding. She underwent another angiogram showing recurrence of stenosis, which was addressed with repeat balloon

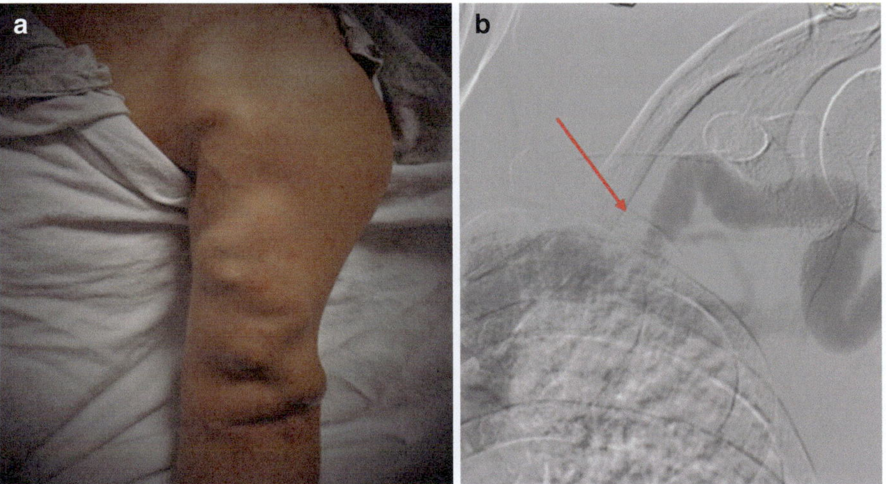

Fig. 56.1 (**a**) Generalized aneurysmal dilatation of the whole fistula resulting in mega fistula formation. (**b**) Angiogram of the fistula showing tight stenosis at the cephalic vein—subclavian vein junction

angioplasty, and the patient was subsequently referred to surgery for fistula revision. However, before the scheduled fistula revision, she presented to the hospital with aneurysm rupture and required emergent fistula ligation. Subsequently, another AVF was placed in the contralateral arm.

Question 2

The decision to preserve or ligate an AVF in a patient with a kidney transplant should depend on what factors?

A. Presence of a fistula associated complication.
B. Available options for future hemodialysis access.
C. Level of graft function.
D. All of the above.

The correct answer is D.

Discussion

Concerning fistula care after kidney transplant, prevention is better than cure. Regular fistula surveillance with early intervention in case of an abnormality can prevent fistula dysfunction and preserve AV access for future use [9]. Once the stenosis and resulting aneurysm develop, it may require multiple interventions to keep the access functional, and even then, failure rates are high. In the above-described case, where the fistula was never used for hemodialysis, trauma from cannulation is not the cause of aneurysm formation.

The patient was found to have outflow stenosis, which is likely the cause of aneurysm formation. Also, the patient did not have any monitoring or intervention in the post-transplant period as the fistula was not being utilized. This allowed for chronic outflow stenosis to go unrecognized for a long time, leading to the development of aneurysm formation.

Figure 56.2 summarizes the management of aneurysmal and mega fistulae in post-transplant patients. Once aneurysms develop, these should be monitored closely for enlargement or rupture, which would then require surgical revision or ligation. In the case of diffusely aneurysmal fistula, it should be evaluated by angiogram to look for any outflow stenosis. In patients with chronic outflow obstruction, further management depends on the risk of needing dialysis shortly and options for future vascular access creation. In patients with well-functioning kidney grafts and the availability of more options for future vascular access, ligation of the fistula would be ideal. In patients at high risk of needing dialysis soon or with no other options for future AV access creation, an attempt to salvage the fistula is reasonable. Balloon angioplasty can be used in urgent situations but is likely to fail. Also, chronic venous stenosis is likely to recur after balloon angioplasty, as in this case. Aneurysm resection and surgical revision of the fistula might yield better results in this scenario [10].

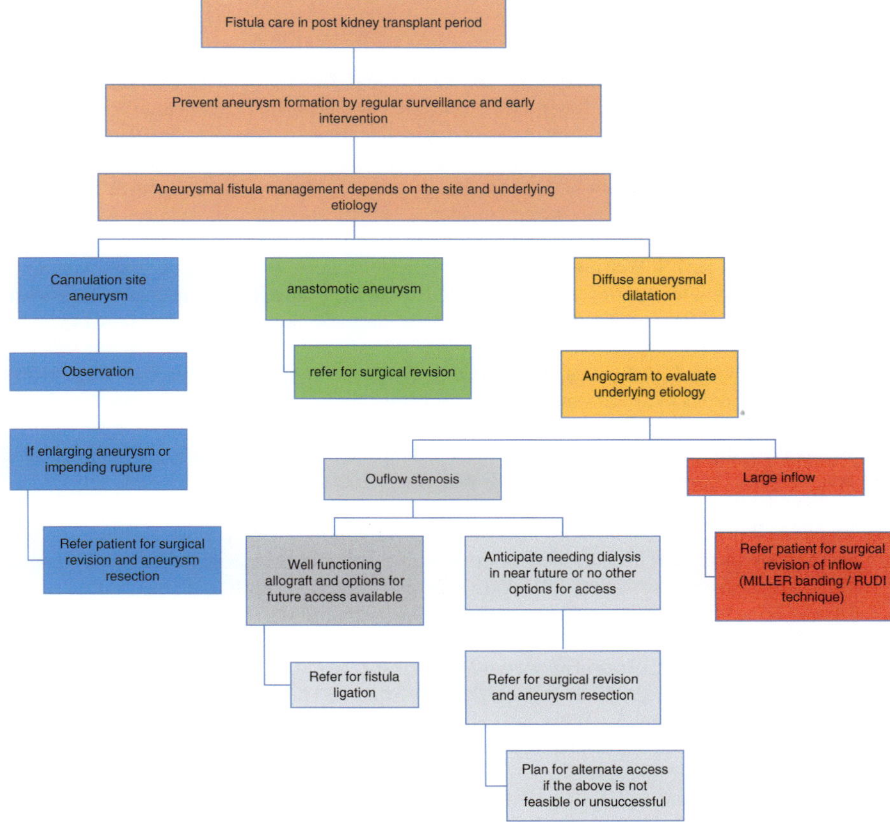

Fig. 56.2 Management of aneurysmal fistula in the post-transplant patient

In case of aneurysmal fistula due to increased blood flow from large anastomosis and without outflow stenosis, surgical revisions like MILLER banding technique or revision using distal inflow (RUDI) technique are required to reduce fistula flow to prevent future complications like high output heart failure [11].

Conclusion

Fistula management in post kidney transplant period remains a controversial topic. Currently, post-transplant AV fistula ligation is reserved for patients with steal syndrome [12]. Pre-emptive monitoring of the fistula and early intervention has shown to help preserve AV access for future use. In the case of a dysfunctional fistula, management decision depends on the severity of the fistula complication, risk of needing hemodialysis shortly, and options for future vascular access.

References

1. Lok CE, Huber TS, Lee T, Shenoy S, Yevzlin AS, Abreo K, Allon M, Asif A, Astor BC, Glickman MH, Graham J, Moist LM, Rajan DK, Roberts C, Vachharajani TJ, Valentini RP, National Kidney Foundation. KDOQI clinical practice guideline for vascular access: 2019 update. Am J Kidney Dis. 2020;75(4 Suppl 2):S1–S164. https://doi.org/10.1053/j.ajkd.2019.12.001.

2. Harnett JD, Foley RN, Kent GM, Barre PE, Murray D, Parfrey PS. Congestive heart failure in dialysis patients: prevalence, incidence, prognosis and risk factors. Kidney Int. 1995;47(3):884–90. https://doi.org/10.1038/ki.1995.132.

3. Unger P, Velez-Roa S, Wissing KM, Hoang AD, van de Borne P. Regression of left ventricular hypertrophy after arteriovenous fistula closure in renal transplant recipients: a long-term follow-up. Am J Transplant. 2004;4(12):2038–44. https://doi.org/10.1046/j.1600-6143.2004.00608.x.

4. Fokou M, Teyang A, Ashuntantang G, Kaze F, Eyenga VC, Chichom Mefire A, Angwafo F 3rd. Complications of arteriovenous fistula for hemodialysis: an 8-year study. Ann Vasc Surg. 2012;26(5):680–4. https://doi.org/10.1016/j.avsg.2011.09.014.

5. Padberg FT Jr, Calligaro KD, Sidawy AN. Complications of arteriovenous hemodialysis access: recognition and management. J Vasc Surg. 2008;48(5 Suppl):55S–80S. https://doi.org/10.1016/j.jvs.2008.08.067.

6. Rajput A, Rajan DK, Simons ME, Sniderman KW, Jaskolka JD, Beecroft JR, Kachura JR, Tan KT. Venous aneurysms in autogenous hemodialysis fistulas: is there an association with venous outflow stenosis. J Vasc Access. 2013;14(2):126–30. https://doi.org/10.5301/jva.5000111.

7. Dixon BS. Why don't fistulas mature? Kidney Int. 2006;70(8):1413–22. https://doi.org/10.1038/sj.ki.5001747.

8. Gardezi AI, Mawih M, Alrawi EB, Karim MS, Aziz F, Chan MR. Mega Fistulae! A case series J Vasc Access. 2021;22(6):1026–9. https://doi.org/10.1177/1129729820968425.

9. Mufty H, Claes K, Heye S, Fourneau I. Proactive surveillance approach to guarantee a functional arteriovenous fistula at first dialysis is worth. J Vasc Access. 2015;16(3):183–8. https://doi.org/10.5301/jva.5000329.

10. Valentine A. Surgical management of aneurysms of arteriovenous fistulae in hemodialysis patients: a case series. Open Access Surgery. 2010;3:9–12. https://doi.org/10.2147/OAS.S9246.

11. Miller GA, Hwang WW. Challenges and management of high-flow arteriovenous fistulae. Semin Nephrol. 2012;32(6):545–50. https://doi.org/10.1016/j.semnephrol.2012.10.005.

12. Hicks CW, Bae S, Pozo ME, DiBrito SR, Abularrage CJ, Segev DL, Garonzik-Wang J, Reifsnyder T. Practice patterns in arteriovenous fistula ligation among kidney transplant recipients in the United States renal data systems. J Vasc Surg. 2019;70(3):842–852.e1. https://doi.org/10.1016/j.jvs.2018.11.048.

Chapter 57
Superior Vena Cava Syndrome Due to Long-Term Central Venous Catheter

Richard Fernandes Almeida and Ali I. Gardezi

Introduction

Central venous occlusion is not uncommon in transplant patients. Many of them have previous dialysis accesses like arteriovenous fistula, graft, or central venous catheter, which increase the risk of central venous occlusion. Additionally, these patients may require central venous catheters in the pre-transplant phase for plasmapheresis as a part of desensitization protocols or post-transplant for long-term intravenous access in case of chronic infections or rejection treatment. Superior Vena Cava (SVC) syndrome represents the most severe presentation of central venous occlusion. This chapter presents a case of SVC syndrome due to a long-term central venous catheter.

Case

A 19-year-old female with a history of ventriculo-pleural shunt due to congenital hydrocephalus, congestive heart failure, and End-Stage Kidney Disease (ESKD) secondary to obstructive uropathy status post second kidney transplantation (15 months before presentation) with estimated GFR of 36 mL/min/1.73 m, complicated by chronic active T-cell mediated, and antibody-mediated rejection was admitted with acute kidney injury in the setting of diarrhea and urinary tract infection. During the hospitalization, she was noted to have worsening facial edema despite discontinuing intravenous fluids and appropriate diuresis with furosemide. Dilated veins were noted over the right chest and neck. Physical exam was otherwise unremarkable for any signs of volume

R. F. Almeida (✉) · A. I. Gardezi
Division of Nephrology, University Of Wisconsin–Madison School of Medicine and Public Health, Madison, WI, USA
e-mail: rfernandesalmeida@uwhealth.org; agardezi@uwhealth.org

© The Author(s), under exclusive license to Springer Nature Switzerland AG 2022

F. Aziz, S. Parajuli (eds.), *Complications in Kidney Transplantation*,
https://doi.org/10.1007/978-3-031-13569-9_57

overload like peripheral edema and crackles or allergic reaction like wheeze or rash. She had a right internal jugular implantable port placed 3 months ago for intravenous infusions and blood draws due to difficult intravenous access. A CT chest performed 1 month after the port placement to evaluate pleural effusion incidentally revealed a chronic partially occlusive calcified thrombus present along the right internal jugular implantable port at the level of right brachiocephalic-SVC junction (Fig. 57.1a, b).

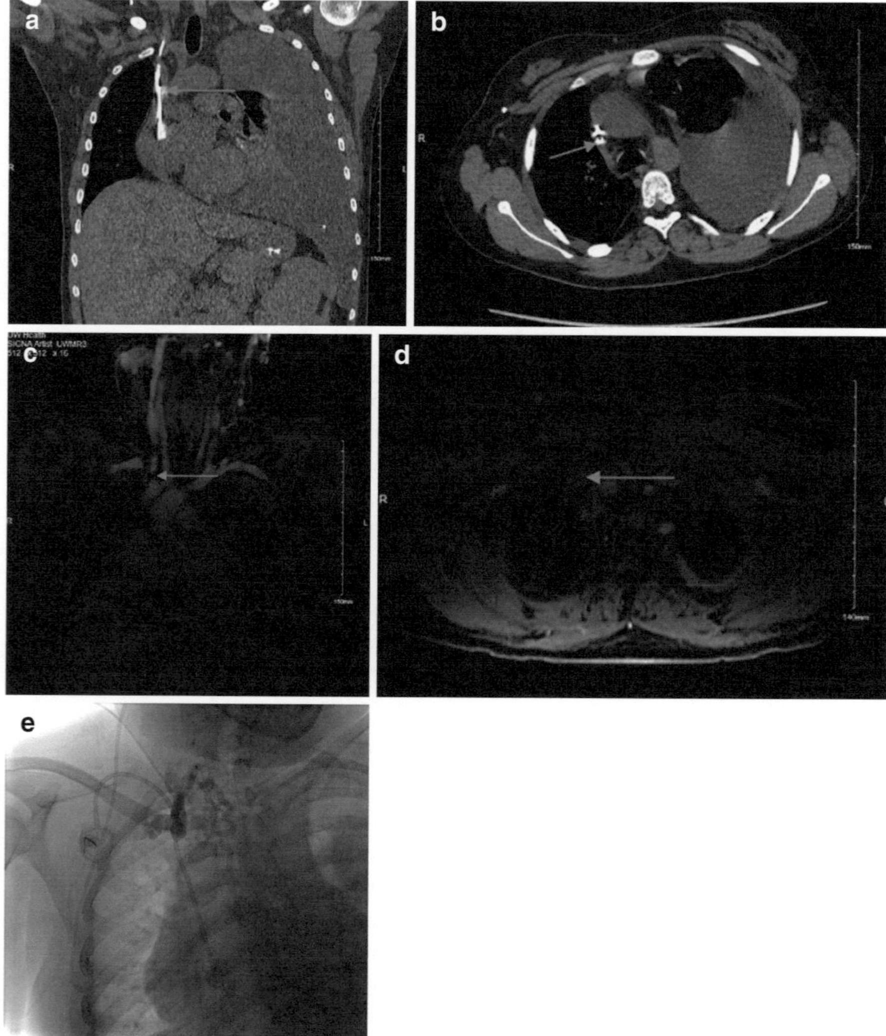

Fig. 57.1 (**a, b**) Coronal and transverse images of CT Chest showing a chronic partially occlusive calcified thrombus present along the right internal jugular implantable port catheter at the right brachiocephalic -SVC junction. (**c, d**) Coronal and transverse images of chest MRA showing a severe focal stenosis in the distal right brachiocephalic vein at its junction with the SVC. The right chest port catheter was found to course through this stenotic area and terminate in the distal SVC. The focal calcification at the area of stenosis on prior CT corresponded to the blooming artifact on MRA. (**e**) Direct Venogram: Reveals complete occlusion at level of right brachiocephalic vein- SVC junction with back flow of contrast into collateral veins

Question 1

What is the most likely diagnosis based on history, physical exam, and previous radiological imaging?

A. Volume overload.
B. Steroid moon facies.
C. Superior Vena Cava (SVC) syndrome.
D. Allergic drug reaction.

The correct answer is C.

This patient's presentation is most compatible with a diagnosis of SVC syndrome given the facial edema, dilated chest wall collateral veins, a precipitating etiology (namely the right internal jugular implantable port), and a prior CT chest showing chronic partially occlusive calcified thrombus at the level of right brachiocephalic-SVC junction. The persistence of facial edema despite adequate diuresis and absence of other signs of volume overload on physical exam makes it an unlikely cause of her presentation. Facial edema is unlikely to represent steroid moon facies as there are no other signs of long-term steroid use. Allergic drug reaction is also an unlikely etiology as there are no other signs of an allergic reaction, including rash or wheezing.

Question 2

What would be the next best step to confirm the diagnosis?

A. No further testing is required. It is a clinical diagnosis.
B. Venous duplex ultrasound.
C. Computed Tomography (CT) or Magnetic Resonance (MR) angiography of the chest.
D. Direct Venography.

The correct answer is C.

Given that this patient's presentation is most consistent with SVC syndrome, there is a risk of progression and considerable resultant morbidity and mortality as described below. In addition, delay in treatment can make the intervention more difficult or even impossible with non-invasive approaches. Thus, no further test is not the appropriate next best step. A non-invasive imaging test with adequate sensitivity should be selected as a screening test which would also give information on the location and severity of the stenosis. This would be either a CT or an MR angiography of the chest depending upon institutional expertise and renal function. Venous duplex ultrasound, although non-invasive, cannot adequately visualize central vasculature and is flawed by reliance on inferred patterns of flow in visualized extra-thoracic veins and is thus not the best next step. Direct venography is an invasive imaging modality and should only be performed when a concomitant intervention is planned.

Case Follow-Up

An MRA of the chest was performed and showed severe focal stenosis in the distal right brachiocephalic vein at its junction with the SVC. The right chest port catheter was found to course through this stenotic area and terminated in the distal SVC. The focal calcification at the area of stenosis on prior CT corresponded to the blooming artifact on MRA (Fig. 57.1c and d).

Discussion

SVC syndrome results from any condition that leads to obstruction of blood flow through the SVC. This can result from extrinsic compression or direct invasion into the vessel, as may be seen with intra-thoracic malignancies/pathologies and intrinsic mechanisms such as stenosis or thrombosis. Indwelling central venous devices like central venous catheters and pacemakers are important risk factors for SVC syndrome.

The incidence of device-related SVC syndrome is rising, mainly due to their increased use [1].

Mechanisms of Obstruction

The development of device-related central venous obstruction may be attributed to three mechanisms:

1. Venous wall thickening: Acutely, venous devices cause local mechanical trauma and result in intimal injury and focal endothelial denudation with or without thrombus formation. Chronic vessel wall irritation by a venous device may result in mural thrombosis that eventually organizes, along with smooth muscle cell proliferation and collagen deposition that encroaches on the vessel lumen [2].
2. Endoluminal obstruction by a thrombus or the endoluminal device itself.
3. Extrinsic arterial and musculoskeletal compression of the venous structures is already compromised due to a vascular access device.

Clinical Presentation

As the flow of blood within the SVC becomes obstructed, venous collaterals form alternative pathways to return venous blood to the right atrium. Depending on the site of the lesion, these collaterals may arise from the azygos, internal mammary, lateral thoracic, paraspinous, and esophageal venous systems to bypass the blockage. The venous collaterals dilate over several weeks. As a result, upper body venous pressure is markedly elevated initially but decreases over time. However, even if well-developed collateral drainage patterns are present, central venous pressures remain elevated, producing the characteristic signs and symptoms of SVC syndrome.

The following signs and symptoms could be seen (in the order of frequency) [1].

1.	Face/neck swelling.
2.	Upper extremity swelling.
3.	Unilateral UE swelling.
4.	Dyspnea at rest.
5.	Cough.
6.	Dilated chest veins.
7.	Chest/shoulder pain.
8.	Flushing/plethora.
9.	Dyspnea only on exertion.
10.	Syncope/presyncope.
11.	Headaches.
12.	Hoarseness.
13.	Hyponatremia.
14.	Weight loss.
15.	Hemoptysis.
16.	Dysphagia.
17.	Dizziness.
18.	Hypoxia.
19.	Confusion.
20.	Night sweats.
21.	No signs or symptoms.
22.	Tinnitus.
23.	Proptosis.
24.	Ischemic stroke.
25.	Epistaxis.

Diagnosis

CT venography is recommended when establishing a diagnosis is critical. In a small study, the sensitivities and specificities of CT venography for the detection of superior vena cava stenosis were 97.5 and 100% [3].

MR angiography is a reasonable alternative to CT. The benefits and risks of gadolinium contrast use in Chronic Kidney Disease (CKD) and ESKD patients, however, need to be weighed before considering an MRA.

Duplex ultrasound is being used extensively to evaluate peripheral venous anatomy. Its main disadvantage is the inability to image the central veins. However, subclavian and internal jugular vein spectral Doppler waveforms can be analyzed for indirect evidence of stenosis or occlusion in the non-visualized central portion of the subclavian vein, brachiocephalic vein, and superior vena cava. This can be inferred by detecting typical patterns of diminished respiratory phasicity and diminished transmitted cardiac pulsatility in the subclavian and jugular veins.

Venography is considered the gold standard for evaluating venous anatomy and is widely used but is an invasive procedure and usually not selected as the initial approach.

Types of SVC Syndrome

Several different classification methods based on the location and degree of obstruction have been proposed [4]. However, Stanford classification is used most commonly [5].

Type 1: Partial occlusion of supra-azygous SVC or bilateral brachiocephalic veins: Venous drainage of upper thorax, upper extremities, and head happens through the usual brachiocephalic to SVC route. There is minimal collateral vein formation and antegrade flow through an azygous vein into SVC. (Fig. 57.2a).

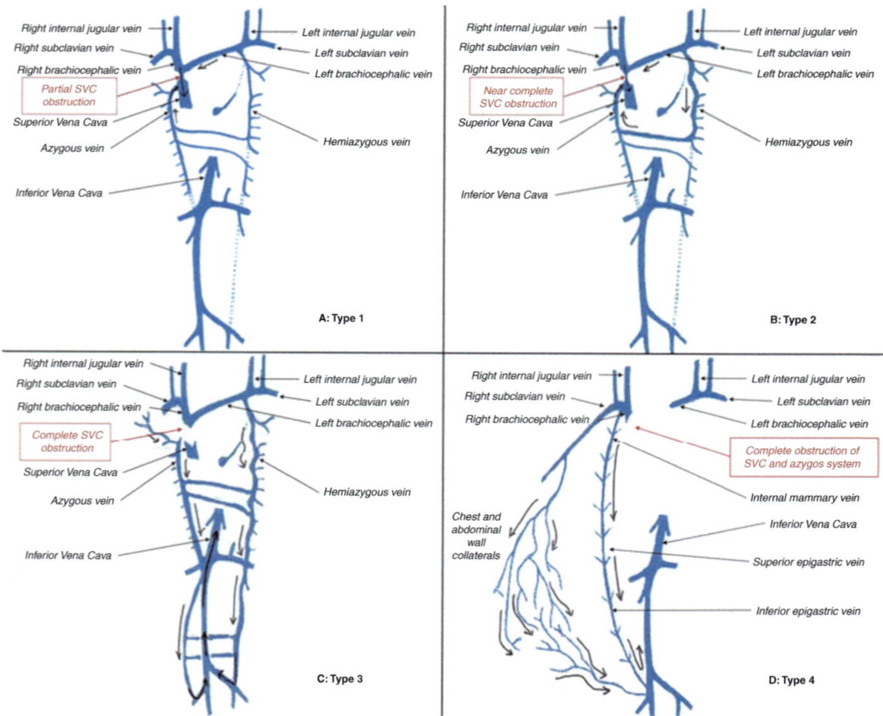

Fig. 57.2 (**a–d**) Stanford Classification of SVC syndrome

Type 2: Near complete occlusion of supra-azygous SVC or bilateral brachiocephalic veins: Venous drainage of upper thorax, upper extremities, and the head is partially shunted via collaterals to hemi-azygous and azygous vein. There is moderate collateral vein formation and antegrade flow through azygous vein into the SVC below the level of obstruction. (Fig. 57.2b).

Type 3: Complete occlusion of SVC at the level of the azygous vein: Azygous system itself is patent. Venous drainage of the upper thorax, upper extremities, and head occurs through azygous and hemiazygos veins. There is extensive collateral vein formation. Because the obstruction is at the level of azygous vein, blood cannot drain into SVC. Consequently, there is a reversal of blood flow in azygous vein where it drains into the inferior vena cava (IVC). (Fig. 57.2c).

Type 4: Complete occlusion of SVC and azygous system: There is moderate to extensive collateral vein formation. The venous drainage of the upper thorax, upper extremities, and head occurs through the chest and abdominal wall collaterals and internal mammary vein into the superior and inferior epigastric vein that ultimately empty into the inferior vena cava. (Fig. 57.2d).

Question 3

What would be the next best step in the management?

A. No further treatment.
B. Venous duplex ultrasound.
C. CTA or MRA chest.
D. Direct venography and angioplasty of the stenosis.

The correct answer is D.

Given the significant morbidity and mortality that can result from SVC syndrome if left untreated, no further treatment is not appropriate. In addition, delay in treatment can make the intervention more difficult or even impossible. Direct venography would be the most appropriate approach as it offers the added benefit of being able to intervene on the lesion (balloon angioplasty with or without stenting).

Case Follow-Up

She underwent an SVC Venogram. (Fig. 57.1e) She was noted to have Type 2 superior vena cava syndrome. Due to the inability to pass the guidewire in the anterograde direction, the right femoral vein was cannulated, and a sheath was advanced to the occlusion. A guidewire was advanced from the femoral vein into the IVC and from there to SVC through the right atrium. It was then successfully passed across the area of stenosis in the retrograde direction. Balloon angioplasty of the lesion was performed. Post balloon angioplasty venogram revealed a 20% residual stenosis at the right brachiocephalic vein-SVC junction and flow of contrast into the right atrium. Angioplasty of the stenosis resulted in the resolution of the signs and symptoms. The right IJ port was subsequently removed after 1 month due to bacteremia.

Management

Indications for treatment include physiologically significant lesions, i.e., venous stenosis with >50% decrease in the luminal diameter and associated clinical or physiological abnormalities [5]. Prophylactic treatment of stenosis that fulfills the anatomic criteria (>50% diameter reduction) but is not associated with a hemodynamic, functional, or clinical abnormality is not warranted and should not be performed [5]. These lesions are better managed by a conservative approach with observation only [6]. If possible, the central venous catheter should be removed to prevent ongoing damage to the vessel.

Treatment approaches include endovascular or surgical.

Endovascular Treatment

Percutaneous Transluminal Angioplasty (PTA) is the initial treatment of choice. Multiple repeated interventions with close surveillance are sometimes required to maintain patency and prevent complete occlusion over the long term. Technical failures may occur in 10–30% of patients treated with PTA.

Stent placement is reserved for acute elastic recoil (>50%) or severe dissection following PTA and recurrent stenosis within 3 months of PTA [4]. It should be noted that in most instances, stenting should be classified as a salvage procedure. Based upon the observational data, stenting does not improve long-term central vein patency; it likely necessitates more reinterventions. Stenting should be avoided as the primary intervention and reserved for the above-mentioned situations only [7, 8].

Surgical Treatment

Direct surgical reconstruction, usually in the form of venous bypass of the occluded central veins, is indicated in patients with symptomatic lesions that are totally occlusive, unresponsive to venoplasty with stenting, or recur rapidly despite angioplasty and stenting.

References

1. Rice TW, Rodriguez RM, Light RW. The superior vena cava syndrome: clinical characteristics and evolving etiology. Medicine (Baltimore). 2006;85(1):37–42. https://doi.org/10.1097/01. md.0000198474.99876.f0.

2. Forauer AR, Theoharis C. Histologic changes in the human vein wall adjacent to indwelling central venous catheters. J Vasc Interv Radiol. 2003;14(9 Pt 1):1163–8. https://doi.org/10.1097/01.rvi.0000086531.86489.4c.
3. Bakhshoude B, Ravari H, Kazemzadeh GH, Rad MP. Diagnostic value of computerized tomography venography in detecting stenosis and occlusion of subclavian vein and superior vena in chronic renal failure patients. Electron Physician. 2016;8(8):2781–6. https://doi.org/10.19082/2781.
4. Azizi AH, Shafi I, Shah N, Rosenfield K, Schainfeld R, Sista A, Bashir R. Superior Vena Cava Syndrome. JACC Cardiovasc Interv. 2020;13(24):2896–910. https://doi.org/10.1016/j.jcin.2020.08.038.
5. Stanford W, Jolles H, Ell S, Chiu LC. Superior vena cava obstruction: a venographic classification. AJR Am J Roentgenol. 1987;148(2):259–62. https://doi.org/10.2214/ajr.148.2.259.
6. Lok CE, Huber TS, Lee T, Shenoy S, Yevzlin AS, Abreo K, Allon M, Asif A, Astor BC, Glickman MH, Graham J, KDOQI Vascular Access Guideline Work Group. KDOQI clinical practice guideline for vascular access: 2019 update. Am J Kidney Dis. 2020;75(4 Suppl. 2):S1–S164.
7. Levit RD, Cohen RM, Kwak A, Shlansky-Goldberg RD, Clark TW, Patel AA, Stavropoulos SW, Mondschein JI, Solomon JA, Tuite CM, Trerotola SO. Asymptomatic central venous stenosis in hemodialysis patients. Radiology. 2006;238(3):1051–6. https://doi.org/10.1148/radiol.2383050119. Epub 2006 Jan 19
8. Ozyer U, Harman A, Yildirim E, Aytekin C, Karakayali F, Boyvat F. Long-term results of angioplasty and stent placement for treatment of central venous obstruction in 126 hemodialysis patients: a 10-year single-center experience. AJR Am J Roentgenol. 2009;193(6):1672–9. https://doi.org/10.2214/AJR.09.2654.

Chapter 58
Venous Access Issues in Kidney Transplant Recipients

Muhammad Sohaib Karim

Introduction

Kidney transplantation has the advantage of improved patient survival [1] and quality of life in end-stage kidney disease (ESKD) [2, 3] patients previously on renal replacement therapy. However, patients previously on hemodialysis for prolonged periods may exhaust their options for vascular access. We describe a typical scenario seen in our interventional nephrology practice.

Patient History

A 76-year-old female with a past medical history of ESKD from diabetic nephropathy on hemodialysis for 12 years before receiving a deceased donor kidney transplant. The patient has a history of multiple failed accesses and was receiving hemodialysis via a tunneled line prior to her successful kidney transplant 3 years back.

The patient is currently admitted for sepsis secondary to osteomyelitis and acute kidney injury thought to be due to acute tubular necrosis requiring intermittent hemodialysis via a tunneled left tunneled jugular catheter.

M. S. Karim (✉)
Division of Nephrology, Department of Medicine, University of Wisconsin, Madison, WI, USA
e-mail: mskarim@medicine.wisc.edu

© The Author(s), under exclusive license to Springer Nature Switzerland AG 2022

F. Aziz, S. Parajuli (eds.), *Complications in Kidney Transplantation*,
https://doi.org/10.1007/978-3-031-13569-9_58

The patient was told that she requires 6 weeks of antibiotics, but it has been challenging to obtain intravenous peripheral access, and currently, she has a 22 G peripheral IV in her left foot.

On exam, you find a frail lady with a left tunneled internal jugular catheter and a pacemaker on her right chest.

Question 1

What possible options are available for short-term intravenous access?

A. Hickman catheter (10 French Single lumen).
B. Tunneled catheter (5 French double lumen).
C. Peripherally Inserted Central Catheter (PICC).

The correct answer is B.

A 5 French tunneled double lumen catheter inserted in a central vein is the correct answer.

Explanation of Answer

The 5 French tunneled double lumen catheter via the right internal jugular vein represents the best option in this case as it is smaller in size as compared to the 10 French Hickman catheter. Also, the catheter is placed in the internal jugular, external jugular, or subclavian vein as compared to the PICC which passes through the basilic, brachial, or cephalic veins in the arm and has the potential to damage these veins (Fig. 58.1).

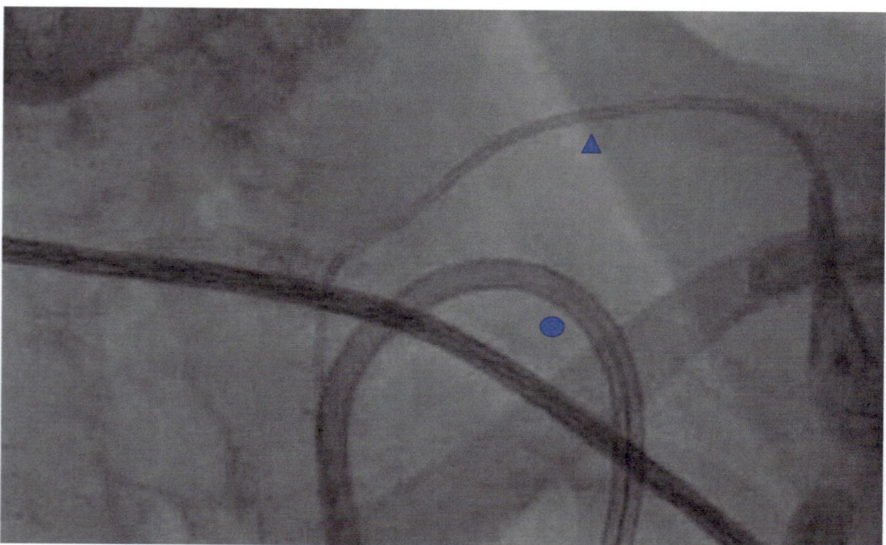

Fig. 58.1 5 French tunneled central catheter inserted in the left jugular vein (▲). Of note, the patient has a tunneled dialysis catheter (●) in the left jugular vein

Question 2
Into which vessel should the catheter be placed?

A. Internal jugular or external jugular vein.
B. Subclavian vein.
C. Brachial vein.

The correct answer is A.
The catheter should be inserted into the internal or external jugular vein.
Explanation of answer
The 5 French tunneled double lumen catheter should be inserted into the external or internal jugular vein, as there is a greater risk of thrombosis with subclavian vein access than internal jugular vein access [4]. The brachial vein is not used for central catheter placement but is possible access for peripherally inserted central catheters (PICC line).

Discussion

Vascular access is important for all patients admitted to the hospital, especially patients with a kidney transplant. Of patients with end-stage kidney disease, only 2.5% are preemptive kidney transplants [5]; therefore, the majority of patients will have received renal replacement therapy via dialysis catheter, arteriovenous access, or peritoneal dialysis catheter. Almost 2/3 of failed kidney transplants will start renal replacement therapy with a dialysis catheter [6].

Past dialysis accesses, both functional and failed, limit the territory available for venous access while in the hospital. Ideally, peripheral vein access in the hands is preferred, but that can lead to complications such as phlebitis, sclerosis, stenosis, or thrombosis [7, 8], and patients cannot leave the hospital with peripheral venous access if they have ongoing access needs.

This leaves a PICC line, tunneled central catheter, or subcutaneous port choices for venous access. A PICC line does have a risk of complication such as stenosis, sclerosis, or thrombosis of vessels in the arm to the superior vena cava [9], which could lead to future nonfunctioning arteriovenous access [10] and compromise the creation of arteriovenous fistula [11] in the future.

A tunneled central line is a 5 F central catheter with a cuff inserted in the external jugular, internal jugular, or subclavian vein with the external portion of the catheter placed in a subcutaneous tunnel. The tunnel length may vary but extends to the anterior chest. Tunneling reduces the risk of infection [12]. As noted above, the risk of thrombosis is higher for subclavian vein access than for internal jugular vein [4]. Therefore, internal jugular vein access is preferred over subclavian vein access.

An implanted device such as a subcutaneous port has a lower risk of infection, fewer complications [8], and should be considered for longer-term access.

References

1. Schnuelle P, Lorenz D, Trede M, Van Der Woude FJ. Impact of renal cadaveric transplantation on survival in end-stage renal failure: evidence for reduced mortality risk compared with hemodialysis during long-term follow-up. J Am Soc Nephrol. 1998;9(11):2135–41. https://doi.org/10.1681/ASN.V9112135.
2. Laupacis A, Keown P, Pus N, Krueger H, Ferguson B, Wong C, Muirhead N. A study of the quality of life and cost-utility of renal transplantation. Kidney Int. 1996;50(1):235–42. https://doi.org/10.1038/ki.1996.307. PMID: 8807593
3. Russell JD, Beecroft ML, Ludwin D, Churchill DN. The quality of life in renal transplantation–a prospective study. Transplantation. 1992;54(4):656–60. https://doi.org/10.1097/00007890-199210000-00018. PMID: 1412757
4. Trerotola SO, Kuhn-Fulton J, Johnson MS, Shah H, Ambrosius WT, Kneebone PH. Tunneled infusion catheters: increased incidence of symptomatic venous thrombosis after subclavian versus internal jugular venous access. Radiology. 2000;217(1):89–93. https://doi.org/10.1148/radiology.217.1.r00oc2789. PMID: 11012428
5. Abecassis M, Bartlett ST, Collins AJ, Davis CL, Delmonico FL, Friedewald JJ, Hays R, Howard A, Jones E, Leichtman AB, Merion RM, Metzger RA, Pradel F, Schweitzer EJ, Velez RL, Gaston RS. Kidney transplantation as primary therapy for end-stage renal disease: a National Kidney Foundation/Kidney Disease Outcomes Quality Initiative (NKF/KDOQITM) conference. Clin J Am Soc Nephrol. 2008;3(2):471–80. https://doi.org/10.2215/CJN.05021107. Epub 2008 Feb 6. PMID: 18256371; PMCID: PMC2390948
6. Chan MR, Oza-Gajera B, Chapla K, Djamali AX, Muth BL, Turk J, Wakeen M, Yevzlin AS, Astor BC. Initial vascular access type in patients with a failed renal transplant. Clin J Am Soc Nephrol. 2014;9(7):1225–31. https://doi.org/10.2215/CJN.12461213. Epub 2014 Jun 5. PMID: 24903392; PMCID: PMC4078970
7. Urbanetto Jde S, Peixoto CG, May TA. Incidence of phlebitis associated with the use of peripheral IV catheter and following catheter removal. Rev Lat Am Enfermagem. 2016;8(24):e2746. https://doi.org/10.1590/1518-8345.0604.2746. PMID: 27508916; PMCID: PMC4990043
8. Cheung E, Baerlocher MO, Asch M, Myers A. Venous access: a practical review for 2009. Can Fam Physician. 2009;55(5):494–6. PMID: 19439704; PMCID: PMC2682308
9. Gonzalez R, Cassaro S. Percutaneous Central Catheter. StatPearls [Internet] Treasure Island (FL): StatPearls Publishing. 2021. Jan 2022. PMID: 29083596.
10. El Ters M, Schears GJ, Taler SJ, Williams AW, Albright RC, Jenson BM, Mahon AL, Stockland AH, Misra S, Nyberg SL, Rule AD, Hogan MC. Association between prior peripherally inserted central catheters and lack of functioning arteriovenous fistulas: a case-control study in hemodialysis patients. Am J Kidney Dis. 2012;60(4):601–8. https://doi.org/10.1053/j.ajkd.2012.05.007. Epub 2012 Jun 15. PMID: 22704142; PMCID: PMC3793252
11. Agarwal AK. Central vein stenosis. Am J Kidney Dis. 2013;61(6):1001–15. https://doi.org/10.1053/j.ajkd.2012.10.024. Epub 2013 Jan 3. PMID: 23291234
12. Timsit JF, Sebille V, Farkas JC, Misset B, Martin JB, Chevret S, Carlet J. Effect of subcutaneous tunneling on internal jugular catheter-related sepsis in critically ill patients: a prospective randomized multicenter study. JAMA. 1996;276(17):1416–20. PMID: 8892717

Chapter 59
Post-Transplant Iliac Venous Thrombosis

Phuoc H. Pham and Eric J. Martinez

Introduction

May-Thurner Syndrome (MTS) is a potential cause of deep vein thrombosis commonly attributed to chronic compression of the left common iliac vein by the right common iliac artery. Despite being a rare phenomenon, it is a cause of venous thrombosis that can detrimentally affect a transplanted renal allograft. Doppler ultrasonography or magnetic resonance venogram (MRV) may assist in diagnosis. Current interventions for the management of MTS include endovascular thrombectomy, stenting, surgical bypass, and anticoagulation therapy. We present the case of a 43-year-old man with ESKD who underwent a living donor kidney allograft retransplantation initially without complication. Early in the post-discharge course, he developed signs of graft failure, left lower extremity edema, and pain. Workup revealed thrombosis in the left common and external iliac vein as well as the allograft renal vein. Thrombectomy was successfully performed; however, the patient continued to have impaired graft function. Endovascular stent placement was performed after MTS diagnosis, allowing successful recovery of the allograft. Excellent graft function was observed at a 2-year follow-up. For graft salvage to remain an option, a high index of suspicion is needed to timely diagnose MTS post-transplant. A review of the diagnosis and management of MTS with consideration of the post-kidney transplant recipient is undertaken.

P. H. Pham
University of Wisconsin School of Medicine and Public Health, Madison, WI, USA

E. J. Martinez (✉)
Annette C. and Harold C. Simmons Transplant Institute, Baylor University Medical Center, Dallas, TX, USA

Baylor Scott & White Transplant Services, Dallas, TX, USA
e-mail: Eric.Martinez1@BSWHealth.org

© The Author(s), under exclusive license to Springer Nature Switzerland AG 2022

F. Aziz, S. Parajuli (eds.), *Complications in Kidney Transplantation*,
https://doi.org/10.1007/978-3-031-13569-9_59

Patient History

A 43-year-old man with a history of ESKD secondary to polycystic kidney disease, hypertension, hypercholesterolemia, pulmonary embolism (PE), and failed kidney allograft transplanted 6 years prior presented for re-transplantation. His pulmonary embolism had occurred 11 years prior after a long flight, and he was treated for 6 months with warfarin. Hypercoagulable workup after anticoagulation completion was negative, and the PE was assumed to be provoked. The patient was also status post bilateral native nephrectomy. Kidney re-transplantation was undertaken with a second living donor renal allograft. At the time of re-transplantation, his panel reactive antibody (PRA) was 56%, and he was negative for preformed donor-specific antibodies. He received anti-thymocyte globulin induction. Maintenance immunosuppression consisted of mycophenolate mofetil, tacrolimus, and prednisone. His serum creatinine (sCr) improved from pretransplant sCr 6.2 to 2.09 mg/dL on postop day 5. He was discharged per institutional protocol on aspirin 81 mg. Five days later, he was readmitted to an outside hospital with acute onset left lower extremity pain and edema, a 2-day history of hematuria, and decreased urine output. Physical exam was remarkable only for extremity tenderness and edema. His initial workup was significant for sodium 130 mmol/L, potassium of 5.8 mmol/L, bicarbonate of 16 mmol/L, and sCr 3.07 mg/dL. Workup at the outside hospital revealed a left-sided deep vein thrombosis extending from the popliteal vein proximally to the femoral vein. Transplant renal doppler on admission is demonstrated in Fig. 59.1.

Question 1

What is the most likely cause of this patient's renal dysfunction?

A. Renal artery thrombosis.
B. Perinephric fluid collection.
C. Acute allograft rejection.
D. Renal vein thrombosis.
E. Renal artery stenosis.

The correct answer is D.

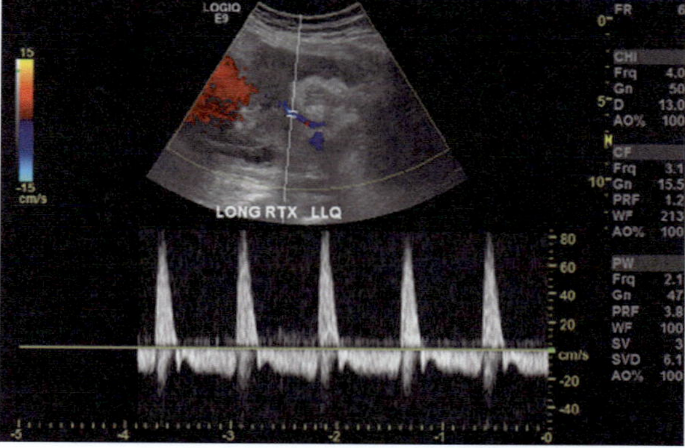

Fig. 59.1 Ultrasound Doppler showed reversal of diastolic flow in the renal artery

Renal vein thrombosis. The most likely cause of the renal dysfunction, in this case, is venous thrombosis as suggested by the elevated sCr, decreased urine output, and renal doppler ultrasound (DUS) showing a patent renal artery with reversal of diastolic flow. DUS also showed no venous outflow in the renal vein, confirming venous thrombosis. Though perinephric fluid collections can cause compression of the renal vein, and a small superior lateral perinephric collection was appreciated on this patient's ultrasound, its size and location were unlikely to result in vascular thrombosis. Fluid collections could also be a sign of retroperitoneal bleeding, which could manifest as elevated sCr though unlikely in this case as the patient initially presented with near-normal hemoglobin and with the improvement since his recent transplant. Renal artery stenosis or thrombosis would manifest with the resistant arterial flow or no arterial flow, respectively, but in this case, the reversal diastolic flow and the absence of venous outflow would not be present. Vascular thrombosis could also occur secondary to acute rejection, however, decreased graft arterial flow would be expected, unlike this.

Hospital Course

The patient underwent surgical exploration with thrombectomy on the same day, which revealed a mottled appearing kidney without signs of ischemia or necrosis. Thrombi were identified in the left common and external iliac veins. The thrombi were extracted at the distal external iliac vein junction with the femoral vein as well as at the anastomosis with the renal vein. A chronic clot was also palpated in the distal inferior vena cava during the procedure. Renal biopsy was taken during the procedure only showed mild to moderate acute kidney injury and was negative for rejection. During the procedure, the patient received 7500 units of intravenous heparin. Postoperatively, the creatinine initially improved to 2.42 mg/dL. He developed anemia and anuric acute kidney injury on the second postoperative day, necessitating blood transfusion and hemodialysis.

Further workup revealed the development of a perinephric hematoma. He underwent surgical re-exploration and evacuation of the hematoma, which revealed intact anastomoses and no identifiable source of bleeding. Due to continuing impaired renal function, renal ultrasound and magnetic resonance venogram (MRV) were ordered to reassess proximal clot burden. His MRV showed a patent renal vein. It, however, demonstrated a severe compression of the left common iliac vein by the right common iliac artery. Additionally, it demonstrated a trace clot from the left saphenous vein proximally to the left femoral vein, as seen in Fig. 59.2.

Question 2
What is the most likely diagnosis that leads to this complication?

A. Compressive hematoma.
B. Aortoiliac aneurysm.
C. Retroperitoneal fibrosis.

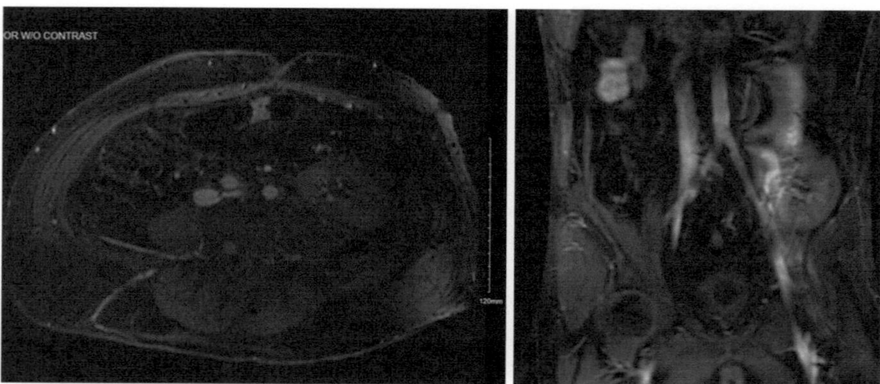

Fig. 59.2 Magnetic resonance venogram shows compression of the left common iliac vein by the right common iliac artery with some trace clot in the venous lumen

D. May-Thurner syndrome.
E. Idiopathic deep vein thrombosis.
F. Osteophyte.

The correct answer is D.

The left common iliac vein compressed by the overlying right common iliac artery is a typical etiology of May-Thurner syndrome (MTS). Perinephric hematoma, though present in this patient and a potential cause of venous compression, is unlikely as the venous findings were present in the operating room even after the evacuation of the hematoma. A perinephric hematoma could, however, potentially exacerbate the obstructed venous flow in the setting of MTS-associated stenosis and thrombosis. Although possible given the previous bilateral nephrectomy, retroperitoneal fibrosis is unlikely in this case as there was no mention of fibrosis during the initial transplant, nor mention of fibrosis seen around the vessels on imaging. Aortoiliac aneurysms and osteophytes are also possible etiologies for extrinsic venous compression; however, these would be more likely detected on imaging. Idiopathic deep vein thrombosis is also a known cause of deep vein thrombosis without precipitating factors. It is unlikely in this case due to the existence of a more likely cause. Furthermore, the patient's previous pulmonary embolism was possibly provoked by a preceding long flight, and subsequent workup for hypercoagulable disorders was negative.

Additional Clinical Course

The patient was diagnosed with MTS and underwent percutaneous venoplasty with the placement of a 12 × 90 mm Wallstent in the left common iliac vein to relieve the compression. Postoperatively, the patient, unfortunately, continued to have kidney injury with a creatinine of 4.70 mg/dL and persistent perinephric hematoma on ultrasound. He had multiple blood transfusions and a second surgical exploration, which again did not reveal an active source of bleeding or blood clots in the renal vein. The renal biopsy sample taken during the operation revealed the mild tubular injury and was negative for rejection. The patient was anticoagulated with a heparin drip bridge to warfarin. His creatinine gradually improved, and he was successfully discharged a week later. One week after discharge, his creatinine improved to 0.73 mg/dL. His renal graft continued to function well at a 2-year follow-up visit.

Discussion

May-Thurner syndrome (MTS) is a rare condition, first identified and described by May and Thurner in 1957, in which the left common iliac vein is compressed by an overriding right common iliac artery [1]. It was hypothesized that the continuous pulsation of the overriding artery and mechanical obstruction leads to intimal hypertrophy, which subsequently obstructs the iliac vein [1]. Later, in retrospective research, the anatomical variant was noted in 25% in a population of 50 patients who had abdominal pain without signs and symptoms of deep vein thrombosis in the lower extremities [2]. In symptomatic lower extremity venous disorder patients, the rates of MTS have varied from 2 to 5%, though some have reported even higher rates [3, 4]. Risk factors for MTS have included female sex, scoliosis, dehydration, hypercoagulable disorders, and radiation exposure [2, 5]. Female patients who are postpartum, multiparous, or using oral contraceptives may have a higher risk of developing symptoms [6]. In the setting of kidney transplantation, Virchow's triad of endothelial injury and immobility (venous stasis) may contribute.

Most of the patients with MTS are asymptomatic. When the venous lesion progresses, a patient can experience acute pain and swelling of the lower extremities. Though the pain and swelling predominantly happen in the left side, right-sided and bilateral symptoms have been reported [4, 7]. Other symptoms included venous claudication and venous insufficiency (edema, discoloration, and skin ulceration)—rare presentations, including ruptured iliac vein and retroperitoneal hematoma, cryptogenic stroke, and pelvic congestion syndrome [8, 9]. The above case had a more typical presentation for MTS with left-sided lower extremity edema and pain. Uniquely, the thrombosis extended into the renal vein of the transplanted kidney, thus causing renal vein thrombosis and acute graft failure. Similar presentations, though rare, have been identified in a small number of case reports [10–13].

Our patient demonstrated the importance of maintaining high suspicion for MTS, especially in patients with lower extremity swelling and graft failure without apparent hypercoagulation risk factors. In some cases, renal dysfunction due to MTS could be masked by a bias toward technical issues if the symptoms occur soon after kidney transplant [11]. The presence of a thrombus in the iliac vein may also make it harder to confirm the diagnosis via imaging [11]. In a case report by Vyas et al., a lymphocele of the transplanted kidney compressed the right iliac vein, thus causing graft dysfunction and lower extremity edema [14]. Though the graft function was restored after drainage of the lymphocele, the patient continued to have left leg swelling, which prompted further investigation, thus revealing MTS. Therefore, maintaining MTS on the differential diagnosis list could help choose appropriate evaluation and management modalities.

In patients with highly suggestive signs and symptoms, duplex ultrasound is the initial noninvasive modality to identify iliac vein stenosis and patency. Signs of stenosis on imaging included post-stenotic turbulence, abnormal Doppler signal at the stenotic area, and sluggish or absence of flow [15]. On the other hand, venography with CT venogram or MR venogram remains the gold standard with >95% sensitivity. While CT venography identifies causes of extrinsic venous compression [15], MR venography can provide better information regarding the pelvic and spinal structures [15]. Alternatively, invasive venous imaging such as catheter-based venography and intravascular ultrasound can be considered to further confirm and assess the chronicity and severity of the lesions [15].

Generally, non-thrombotic MTS with no or mild symptoms such as leg swelling is managed conservatively with compression therapy, leg elevation, and skincare. In the presence of venous thromboembolism, standard treatment with therapeutic anti-coagulation should be initiated. Thrombolytic therapy or thrombectomy may also be needed in the case of severe thrombosis. It is also important to address the root cause, which is the chronic compression of the left iliac vein to prevent long-term sequelae and recurrence of thrombosis. Traditionally, various angioplasty methods, such as vein-patch angioplasty with excision of intraluminal bands, division and relocation of the right common iliac artery, and contralateral saphenous vein graft bypass, can be used to relieve the compression and further prevent long-term sequelae [16]. Stenting with self-expandable or balloon-expandable stents is also an effective treatment. Long-term patency rates are 67%, 89%, and 93% in primary, assisted primary, and secondary cumulative patency at 72 months, respectively. Low in-stent restenosis rates (5% at 72 months), low morbidity, and low mortality are also reported [16, 17].

In renal graft dysfunction with renal vein thrombus, such as our patient, invasive intervention is essential as it can preserve graft function in addition to treating other complications of MTS. Despite being a rare complication, renal vein thrombosis due to MTS in renal transplant has been associated with renal graft injuries and potential failures as described in various case reports [10–13]. The cases included three isolated renal transplants and one simultaneous pancreas and kidney trans-plant. None of the patients had a prothrombic condition. All of them developed renal graft dysfunction from renal vein thrombosis due to underlying MTS ranging from 2 days [11] to 8 weeks [13] post-transplantation. Similar to our case, all patients were managed with thrombectomy followed by self-expanding stent (Wallstent [11, 12] and Smart stent [10]) deployment to the left iliac vein. Therapeutic anticoagulation, primarily warfarin, was started after the stent placement in all four cases. Two of the case reports showed preserved graft function at 1 year follow-up [10, 13] which was consistent with our patient's outcomes. Therefore, despite the limitations of the case-report format, other case studies and our case report have suggested that thrombectomy followed by iliac vein stenting could effectively res-cue graft function.

In summary, maintaining high index of suspicion for MTS in graft failure due to renal vein thrombosis could facilitate prompt diagnosis and intervention, thus successfully salvaging the grafts. There is no literature regarding pretransplant prophylactic stenting in MTS patients nor the frequency of follow-up after stent placement. Postoperatively, Arrazola et al. suggested follow-up intervals of 1 month, 3 months, 6 months, then annually with duplex ultrasound to assess graft function [11]. In our patient's case, we concur with those recommendations as we similarly followed this case.

Disclosures P. Pham has no disclosures. E. Martinez reports employment with the Annette C. and Harold C. Simmons Transplant Institute at Baylor University Medical Center.

Funding None.

References

1. May R, Thurner J. The cause of the predominantly sinistral occurrence of thrombosis of the pelvic veins. Angiology. 1957;8(5):419–27. https://doi.org/10.1177/000331975700800505.
2. Kibbe MR, Ujiki M, Goodwin AL, Eskandari M, Yao J, Matsumura J. Iliac vein compression in an asymptomatic patient population. J Vasc Surg. 2004;39(5):937–43. https://doi.org/10.1016/J.JVS.2003.12.032.
3. Raju S, Neglen P. High prevalence of nonthrombotic iliac vein lesions in chronic venous disease: a permissive role in pathogenicity. J Vasc Surg. 2006;44(1):136–44. https://doi.org/10.1016/j.jvs.2006.02.065.
4. Birn J, Vedantham S. May-Thurner syndrome and other obstructive iliac vein lesions: meaning, myth, and mystery. Vasc Med. 2015;20(1):74–83. https://doi.org/10.1177/1358863X14560429.
5. Marston W, Fish D, Unger J, Keagy B. Incidence of and risk factors for iliocaval venous obstruction in patients with active or healed venous leg ulcers. J Vasc Surg. 2011;53(5):1303–8. https://doi.org/10.1016/j.jvs.2010.10.120.
6. Murphy EH, Davis CM, Journeycake JM, RP DM, Arko FR. Symptomatic ileofemoral DVT after onset of oral contraceptive use in women with previously undiagnosed May-Thurner syndrome. J Vasc Surg. 2009;49(3):697–703. https://doi.org/10.1016/J.JVS.2008.10.002.
7. Moudgill N, Hager E, Gonsalves C, Larson R, Lombardi J, Dimuzio P. May-Thurner syndrome: case report and review of the literature involving modern endovascular therapy. Vascular. 2009;17(6):330–5. https://doi.org/10.2310/6670.2009.00027.
8. Hosn MA, Katragunta N, Kresowik T, Sharp WJ. May-Thurner syndrome presenting as spontaneous left iliac vein rupture. J Vasc Surg Venous Lymphat Disord. 2016;4(4):479–81. https://doi.org/10.1016/j.jvsv.2016.03.007.
9. Kiernan TJ, Yan BP, Cubeddu RJ, et al. May-Thurner syndrome in patients with cryptogenic stroke and patent foramen ovale: an important clinical association. Stroke. 2009;40(4):1502–4. https://doi.org/10.1161/STROKEAHA.108.527366.
10. Vaidya OU, Buersmeyer T, Rojas R, Dolmatch B. Successful salvage of a renal allograft after acute renal vein thrombosis due to May-Thurner syndrome. Case Rep Transplant. 2012;2012:1–3. https://doi.org/10.1155/2012/390980.
11. Arrazola L, Sutherland DER, Sozen H, et al. May-Thurner syndrome in renal transplantation. Transplantation. 2001;71(5):698–702. https://doi.org/10.1097/00007890-200103150-00023.
12. Campsen J, Bang TJ, Kam I, Gupta R. May-thurner syndrome complicating left-sided renal transplant. Transplantation. 2010;89(7):904–6. https://doi.org/10.1097/TP.0B013E3181CD87CE.

13. Gunder M, Lakhter V, Lau K, Karhadkar SS, Di Carlo A, Bashir R. Endovascular intervention for iliac vein thrombosis after simultaneous kidney-pancreas transplant. J Surg Case Reports. 2019;2019(4):1–3. https://doi.org/10.1093/JSCR/RJZ024.
14. Vyas S, Roberti I, McCarthy C. May–Thurner syndrome in a pediatric renal transplant recipient—Case report and literature review. Pediatr Transplant 2008;12(6):708–710. https://doi.org/10.1111/J.1399-3046.2008.00941.X.
15. Brinegar KN, Sheth RA, Khademhosseini A, Bautista J, Oklu R. Iliac vein compression syndrome: clinical, imaging and pathologic findings. World J Radiol. 2015;7(11):375. https://doi.org/10.4329/WJR.V7.I11.375.
16. Ibrahim W, Al SZ, Hasan H, Zeid WA. Endovascular Management of May-Thurner Syndrome. Ann Vasc Dis. 2012;5(2):217. https://doi.org/10.3400/AVD.CR.12.00007.
17. Neglén P, Hollis KC, Olivier J, Raju S. Stenting of the venous outflow in chronic venous disease: long-term stent-related outcome, clinical, and hemodynamic result. J Vasc Surg. 2007;46(5) https://doi.org/10.1016/J.JVS.2007.06.046.

Chapter 60
Pregnancy in Kidney Transplant Recipients

Sam Kant and Sami Alasfar

Introduction

Women with end-stage renal kidney (ESKD) have impaired fertility due to the hypothalamic gonadal axis disruption. Restoration of fertility can occur as soon as 6 months following kidney transplantation. While various transplantation societies recommend avoidance of pregnancy in the first 1–2 years post-transplantation, the allograft, patient, and fetus can be at risk of a myriad of complications. Being cognizant of these risks, expedient diagnosis and management are essential. A concerted multidisciplinary longitudinal follows throughout pregnancy remain the most optimal strategy of surveillance for kidney transplant recipients.

Patient History

A 32-year-old female with a past medical history of end-stage kidney disease (ESKD) secondary to IgA nephropathy who underwent a deceased donor kidney transplantation 4 years ago is seen in the transplant clinic for follow-up. Her immunosuppression regimen consists of tacrolimus 4 mg twice a day, mycophenolate mofetil (MMF) 500 mg BID, and prednisone 5 mg. She has evidence of stable allograft function with a serum creatinine of 1.2 mg/dL with no microscopic hematuria or proteinuria on urinalysis. She wants to discuss aspects relating to pregnancy.

S. Kant (✉) · S. Alasfar
Division of Nephrology, Department of Medicine, The Johns Hopkins University School of Medicine, Baltimore, MD, USA
e-mail: skant1@jhmi.edu; salasfa1@jhu.edu

© The Author(s), under exclusive license to Springer Nature Switzerland AG 2022

F. Aziz, S. Parajuli (eds.), *Complications in Kidney Transplantation*,
https://doi.org/10.1007/978-3-031-13569-9_60

Question 1

What statement is true regarding the appropriate timing of pregnancy post kidney transplantation?

A. It is not advisable to proceed with pregnancy post kidney transplantation.
B. The first-year post-transplantation is the best time to proceed with the pregnancy.
C. Avoidance of contraception is advised to aid in the restoration of the hypothalamic—pituitary—adrenal (HPA) axis after transplantation.
D. Current recommendations advise avoiding conception in the first post-transplant year.

The correct answer is D.

The restoration of the HPA axis is achieved by 6 months post-transplantation, in addition to improvement in fertility and sexual function [1]. The American Society of Transplantation (AST) guidelines recommend avoidance of pregnancy in the first year—thereafter, pregnancy is advised if no rejection within the past year, stable maintenance immunosuppression, no recent acute infections that could impede fetal growth, serum creatinine < 1.5 mg/dL and minimal or no proteinuria [2]. It should be noted, however, that a mean transplant to pregnancy interlude of under 2 years is associated with lower miscarriage rates and higher live birth rates, albeit increased rates of pre-term birth, preeclampsia, gestational diabetes, and allograft loss [3, 4]. It is imperative to communicate these risks clearly to female kidney transplant recipients (KTRs), given low satisfaction with counseling received for this pivotal period [5].

The patient is transitioned from MMF to azathioprine prior to the attempt of conception. She is seen in the clinic 6 months later after being confirmed to be 8 weeks pregnant. She has a blood pressure of 104/65 mmHg, serum creatinine of 1 mg/dL, and unremarkable urinalysis.

Question 2

What is the most frequent medical complication associated with pregnancy in kidney transplant recipients?

A. Preeclampsia.
B. Hypertension.
C. Gestational diabetes.
D. Lower limb edema.

The correct answer is B.

Hypertension is the most common complication associated with pregnancy in KTRs, occurring in over half of pregnant patients [3, 6]. Higher maternal age contributes to the development of hypertension and preeclampsia in this patient group [7]. The onset of hypertension can indicate incipient preeclampsia, with the occurrence of the latter noted in up to 31% of pregnant KTRs [3]. Concerning therapy for hypertension, beta-blockers and calcium channel blockers are more efficacious in comparison to methyldopa for a reduction in risk of severe hypertension [8]. It is important to note that angiotensin-converting enzyme inhibitors and angiotensin receptor blockers are contraindicated given the higher risk of fetal kidney injury [9].

Additional Clinical Course

The patient was diagnosed with hypertension at 21 weeks of pregnancy, which was subsequently well controlled on nifedipine 30 mg daily. Kidney function was consistently at baseline with serum creatinine ranging between 1.1 and 1.3 mg/dL and no proteinuria on urinalysis. At 33 weeks, however, she developed worsening hypertension with the evolution of proteinuria quantified at 1.7 g on a spot urine protein to creatine ratio. A week later, serum creatinine worsened to 2.3 mg/dL. After discussing with the obstetrics team, the decision was made to proceed with induction and delivery. Within 2 days of C-section, blood pressure progressively improved, and her serum creatinine decreased to 1.6 mg/dL.

Discussion

Successful childbirth in KTRs dates back to 1958 when Edith Holmes became the first woman to give birth after transplantation [10]. In addition to numerous associated advantages, transplantation provides improved fertility and higher chances of live birth in comparison to dialysis [11, 12]. The recommendations for optimal time for attempting conception post-transplantation differ as per the US (avoiding conception in the first year) and European society guidelines (avoidance during first 2 years) [2, 13]. In the first post-transplant year, pregnancy is independently associated with an increased risk of graft loss [4].

It is recommended that alterations in the immunosuppression regime be made before conception. Most immunosuppressive medications are category C (animal studies have shown an adverse effect on the fetus or are lacking, and there are no adequate and well-controlled studies in humans) or D (evidence of human fetal risk) in Food and Drug Administration pregnancy safety classification. Calcineurin inhibitors and corticosteroids are listed as category C and can be safely used with close monitoring of levels. Anti-metabolites (mycophenolate mofetil and azathioprine) are listed as category D; however, azathioprine can be safely used during pregnancy with a recommendation that it be substituted for mycophenolate mofetil prior to conception.

The complications in pregnant KTRs span the spectrum of maternal and fetal complications. Hypertension and preeclampsia are the most frequent maternal complications, with the distinction between the two often difficult to achieve. The risk

Table 60.1 Complications associated with pregnancy in kidney transplant recipients

Maternal complications	Fetal complications
Hypertension	Low birth weight
Preeclampsia	Stillbirths
Gestational diabetes	Pre-term delivery
Miscarriage	Neonatal death
Allograft rejection	Birth defects

of preeclampsia in KTRs is over six times higher than in the general population [3]. Chronic hypertension, previous preeclampsia, and elevated serum creatinine (> 1.5 mg/dL) at the beginning of pregnancy are factors predictive for the development of preeclampsia [14]. Low-dose aspirin should be initiated between 12 and 18 weeks of pregnancy, given its protective effect in preventing and delaying the onset of preeclampsia [15]. It is recommended that anti-hypertensives be commenced if blood pressure is consistently elevated above 140/90 mmHg (medical treatment discussed above). Close discussion with high-risk obstetrics should be maintained if preeclampsia is associated with end-organ dysfunction for consideration of delivery based on gestational age.

It can also be challenging to distinguish preeclampsia from allograft rejection; however, the former is associated with increased proteinuria, while the latter is associated with higher creatinine levels [16]. It should be noted that pregnancy creates a milieu of immunological tolerance, and most registry data has not shown a higher risk of rejection, except in sensitized patients [17]. However, high serum creatinine, rejection before pregnancy, and sub-optimal immunosuppressive drug levels are associated with a higher risk of rejection during pregnancy [18]. An ultrasound-guided allograft biopsy can be safely performed during pregnancy, with expedient utilization in the event of worsening creatinine and/or proteinuria [19]. High-dose steroids can be used safely in treatment rejection, with sparse data on the use of anti-thymocyte globulin and rituximab [20].

With regard to fetal outcomes, the rate of pre-term delivery is higher in KTRs in comparison to the general population and has been mostly attributed to fetal or maternal compromise [21]. Higher serum creatinine levels (> 1.7 mg/dL) and maternal hypertension are associated with pre-term delivery [22]. In addition, a higher risk for small for gestation and low birth weight offspring has also been reported in KTRs [23]. Table 60.1 lists maternal and fetal complications in pregnant KTRs.

In conclusion, the optimal management of prospective pregnancy in KTRs begins prior to conception. A concerted effort involving transplant nephrology and high-risk antenatal obstetrics is required to preempt and closely monitor for a myriad of complications that could afflict the allograft, patient, and fetus.

Disclosures S. Kant reports employment with the Johns Hopkins University.

Sami Alasfar reports employment with the Johns Hopkins University; receiving research funding from CareDx and the World Health Organization (WHO).

Funding None.

References

1. Saha M, Saha HHT, Niskanen LK, Salmela KT, Pasternack AI. Time course of serum prolactin and sex hormones following successful renal transplantation. Nephron. 2002;92(3):735–7. Available from https://www.karger.com/Article/Abstract/64079
2. McKay DB, Josephson MA. Reproduction and transplantation: report on the AST consensus conference on reproductive issues and transplantation. Am J Transplant. 2005;5(7):1592–9. Available from http://www.ingentaconnect.com/content/mksg/ajt/2005/00000005/00000007/art00004
3. Deshpande NA, James NT, Kucirka LM, Boyarsky BJ, Garonzik-Wang JM, Montgomery RA, Segev DL. Pregnancy outcomes in kidney transplant recipients: a systematic review and meta-analysis. Am J Transplant. 2011;11(11):2388–404. https://doi.org/10.1111/j.1600-6143.2011.03656.x.
4. Rose C, Gill J, Zalunardo N, Johnston O, Mehrotra A, Gill JS. Timing of pregnancy after kidney transplantation and risk of allograft failure. Am J Transplant. 2016;16(8):2360–7. https://doi.org/10.1111/ajt.13773.
5. Yoshikawa Y, Uchida J, Akazawa C, Suganuma N. Outcomes of and perspectives on pregnancy counseling among kidney transplant recipients. Transplantation. 2019;4(1):100019. Available from https://explore.openaire.eu/search/publication?articleId=doajarticles::cb04bb74b6c6dd53b5d49cb187e19d73
6. Shah S, Venkatesan RL, Gupta A, Sanghavi MK, Welge J, Johansen R, Kean EB, Kaur T, Gupta A, Grant TJ, Verma P. Pregnancy outcomes in women with kidney transplant: meta-analysis and systematic review. BMC nephrol. 2019;20(1):24. Available from: https://www.ncbi.nlm.nih.gov/pubmed/30674290
7. McDonald SP. Australia and New Zealand dialysis and transplant registry. Kidney Int Suppl. 2015;5(1):39–44. Available from: https://www-sciencedirect-com.proxy1.library.jhu.edu/science/article/pii/S2157171615321067
8. Abalos E, Duley L, Steyn DW. Anti-hypertensive drug therapy for mild to moderate hypertension during pregnancy. Cochrane Database Syst Rev. 2014;(2):CD002252. Available from https://www.ncbi.nlm.nih.gov/pubmed/24504933
9. Bullo M, Tschumi S, Bucher B, Bianchetti M, Simonetti G. Pregnancy outcome following exposure to angiotensin-converting enzyme inhibitors or angiotensin receptor antagonists: a systematic review. Hypertension. 2012;60(2):444–50. Available from http://ovidsp.ovid.com/ovidweb.cgi?T=JS&NEWS=n&CSC=Y&PAGE=fulltext&D=ovft&AN=00004268-201208000-00031
10. Ong SC, Kumar V. Pregnancy in a kidney transplant patient. Clin J Am Soc Nephrol. 2020;15(1):120–2. Available from https://www.ncbi.nlm.nih.gov/pubmed/31451514
11. Gill JS, Zalunardo N, Rose C, Tonelli M. The pregnancy rate and live birth rate in kidney transplant recipients. Am J Transplant. 2009;9(7):1541–9. Available from: http://www.ingentaconnect.com/content/mksg/ajt/2009/00000009/00000007/art00014
12. Piccoli GB, Cabiddu G, Daidone G, Guzzo G, Maxia S, Ciniglio I, Postorino V, Loi V, Ghiotto S, Nichelatti M, Attini R, Coscia A, Postorino M, Pani A. The children of dialysis: live-born babies from on-dialysis mothers in Italy—an epidemiological perspective comparing dialysis, kidney transplantation and the overall population. Nephrol Dial Transplant. 2014;29(8):1578–86. Available from https://www.ncbi.nlm.nih.gov/pubmed/24759612
13. EBPG Expert Group on Renal Transplantation. European best practice guidelines for renal transplantation. Section IV: long-term management of the transplant recipient. IV.10. Pregnancy in renal transplant recipients. Nephrol Dial Transplant. 2002;17(Suppl 4):50–5. Available from https://www.ncbi.nlm.nih.gov/pubmed/12091650
14. Majak GB, Reisæter AV, Zucknick M, Lorentzen B, Vangen S, Henriksen T, Michelsen TM. Preeclampsia in kidney transplanted women; outcomes and a simple prognostic risk score system. PloS one. 2017;12(3):e0173420. Available from https://www.ncbi.nlm.nih.gov/pubmed/28319175

15. ACOG committee opinion no. 743: Low-dose aspirin use during pregnancy. Obstet Gynecol. 2018;132(1):e44–52. Available from: http://ovidsp.ovid.com/ovidweb.cgi?T=JS&NEWS=n&CSC=Y&PAGE=fulltext&D=ovft&AN=00006250-201807000-00057
16. Yin O, Kallapur A, Coscia L, Constantinescu S, Moritz M, Afshar Y. Differentiating acute rejection from preeclampsia after kidney transplantation. Obstet Gynecol. 2021;137(6):1023–31. Available from https://www.ncbi.nlm.nih.gov/pubmed/33957644
17. Richman K, Gohh R. Pregnancy after renal transplantation: a review of registry and single-center practices and outcomes. Nephrol Dial Transplant. 2012;27(9):3428–34. Available from https://www.ncbi.nlm.nih.gov/pubmed/22815546
18. Armenti VT, McGrory CH, Cater JR, Radomski JS, Moritz MJ. Pregnancy outcomes in female renal transplant recipients. Transplantation. 1998;30(5):1732–4. https://doi.org/10.1016/S0041-1345(98)00408-4.
19. Davidson JM, Lindheimer MD. Maternal-fetal medicine: principles and practice. Philadelphia, PA, USA: Saunders; 2004.
20. Shah S, Verma P. Overview of pregnancy in renal transplant patients. Int J nephrol. 2016;2016:4539342–7. Available from https://www.airitilibrary.com/Publication/alDetailedMesh?DocID=P20151210006-201612-201704180003-201704180003-93-99
21. Coscia LA, Constantinescu S, Moritz MJ, Frank AM, Ramirez CB, Maley WR, Doria C, McGrory CH, Armenti VT. Report from the national transplantation pregnancy registry (NTPR): outcomes of pregnancy after transplantation. Clin transpl. 2010:65–85. Available from: https://www.ncbi.nlm.nih.gov/pubmed/21698831
22. Sibanda N, Briggs JD, Davison JM, Johnson RJ, Rudge CJ. Pregnancy after organ transplantation: a report from the UK transplant pregnancy registry. Transpl Int. 2007;83(10):1301–7. Available from: https://www.ncbi.nlm.nih.gov/pubmed/17519778
23. Bramham K, Nelson-Piercy C, Gao H, Pierce M, Bush N, Spark P, Brocklehurst P, Kurinczuk JJ, Knight M. Pregnancy in renal transplant recipients: a UK national cohort study. CJSAN. 2013;8(2):290–8. Available from http://cjasn.asnjournals.org/content/8/2/290.abstract

Chapter 61
Post-Transplant Diabetes Mellitus

Manoj Bhattarai and Suverta Bhayana

Introduction

Post-transplant diabetes mellitus (PTDM) is one of the important metabolic complications occurring in about 10–20% of the patients following kidney transplantation [1]. In addition, about 30% of patients develop prediabetes after kidney transplantation [2]. It is crucial for physicians taking care of transplant patients to be familiar with this common clinical condition with prognostic significance, as the prevalence of PTDM is expected to increase due to an increase in the lifespan of transplant recipients [1]. Here we describe a case of PTDM and discuss risk factors, diagnosis, and management of PTDM.

Case

A 60-year-old male with a past medical history of end-stage kidney disease secondary to IgA nephropathy underwent a deceased donor kidney transplant. The patient was on dialysis for 5 years before the transplant. Past medical history was also

M. Bhattarai (✉)
Division of Nephrology/Department of Medicine, University of Texas Health San Antonio,
San Antonio, TX, USA
e-mail: bhattaraim@uthscsa.edu

S. Bhayana
Kidney and Pancreas Transplant Program, Department of Medicine, Transplant Center,
University of Texas Health San Antonio, San Antonio, TX, USA

Kidney and Pancreas Transplant Program, Department of Surgery, Transplant Center,
University of Texas Health San Antonio, San Antonio, TX, USA
e-mail: bhayana@uthscsa.edu

© The Author(s), under exclusive license to Springer Nature
Switzerland AG 2022

F. Aziz, S. Parajuli (eds.), *Complications in Kidney Transplantation*,
https://doi.org/10.1007/978-3-031-13569-9_61

391

significant for hypertension, hyperlipidemia, and morbid obesity with a BMI of 36 at the time of transplant. He received basiliximab for induction (20 mg on day 0 intraoperative and 4). He also received steroids per-protocol (Solu-Medrol 500 mg intraoperatively on days 1 and 2, Solu-Medrol 250 mg on day 3, prednisone 40 mg on day 4 followed by prednisone 5 mg indefinitely). Maintenance immunosuppression regimen consisted of tacrolimus, mycophenolate mofetil, and prednisone. He had immediate graft function and was discharged on postoperative day # 5 with a serum creatinine of 1.3 mg/dL. The early postoperative course was uncomplicated, but the patient was found to have worsening kidney function with a serum creatinine of 2.1 mg/dL on postoperative day 21. A kidney biopsy was performed after the usual causes of kidney dysfunction were ruled out. The biopsy showed interstitial inflammation involving 20% of the core and grade 2 tubulitis. Banff 1A T-cell mediated rejection was diagnosed, and the patient was treated with pulse steroids (Methylprednisolone 500 mg intravenous daily for 3 days) followed by oral steroid taper for 4 weeks. (After completion of pulse dose, prednisone 40 mg daily, decrease dose by 10 mg every week until a patient at 10 mg P.O. daily). There was no evidence of antibody-mediated rejection on the biopsy, and donor-specific antibodies were negative. The patient had an excellent response to therapy, and the kidney function improved with serum creatinine at 1.3 on day # 7 after the first dose of IV solumedrol. During follow-up, he was found to have fasting blood glucose (FBG) of 178 mg/dL. Repeat laboratory test results 4 days later showed FBG of 169 mg/dL. A diagnosis of steroid-induced hyperglycemia was made.

Question 1

Along with lifestyle modification and dietary education, what is the next best step in managing this patient?

A. Check HbA1C to confirm the diagnosis of PTDM.
B. Do an oral glucose tolerance test (OGTT) to confirm the diagnosis of PTDM.
C. Initiate insulin therapy.
D. Initiate sodium-glucose co-transporter 2 (SGLT2) inhibitor.

The correct answer is C.

This patient's post-transplant hyperglycemia is related to steroid use during the early post-transplant period. Until the kidney function stabilizes, treatment with insulin (basal with sliding scale) is recommended. Since insulin requirements typically go down with the tapering dose of steroids, a sliding scale insulin regimen is recommended. The dose of long-acting insulin can be easily adjusted based on the blood glucose readings. Insulin also helps to preserve beta-cell mass [3]. SGLT2 inhibitors are an excellent option for managing diabetes mellitus, especially due to cardiovascular and renal protective effects, as shown by multiple large randomized controlled trials [4, 5]. But these drugs are not optimal for our patients due to the uncertain degree and duration of hyperglycemia in the current situation. Also, this patient is within the first 6 weeks of transplant and has an elevated risk of urinary tract infection that can be further compounded by these agents. These drugs also cause a benign drop in GFR by decreasing glomerular filtration pressure. Since clinicians rely on serum creatinine, among other parameters, to gauge the response to rejection treatment, fluctuation of creatinine due to these agents may create difficulty in management. HbA1C is an unreliable diagnostic test for the diagnosis of PTDM during an early post-transplant period. Though OGTT is considered the best test for use in post-transplant patients, our patient already had two readings of high FBG, leading to diagnosis.

Course   He was started on insulin glargine injection and sliding scale, dose adjusted as per his glucose level, and his glycemic control improved over time. The patient consistently achieved FBG less than 100 mg/dL with an insulin regimen. The patient continued to do well during his subsequent follow-up visits. His graft function remained stable, with serum creatinine ranging from 1.1 to 1.3. Insulin requirement decreased gradually as steroids were tapered to a prednisone dose of 5 mg daily (that he would take indefinitely). He was able to come off insulin glargine injection on day 20 post rejection treatment and was maintained on a sliding scale alone over the next one and half months when he was taken off the sliding scale. By month 3 (8 weeks post-treatment with pulse steroids), he consistently maintained FBG < 110 mg/dL without antidiabetic agents. Lifestyle modifications were recommended, including exercise and dietary advice. His allograft function was excellent during the 6-month follow-up visit, with a serum creatinine of 1.2 without any proteinuria. He did not have any infectious complications during the first 6 months after the transplant. However, it was noted that he had gained about 25 lbs. during this time frame and was found to have an FBG of 135 mg/dL. On reviewing his monthly labs, his FBG was gradually trending up with 112, 117, and 122 mg/dL values in the preceding 3 months, respectively.

Question 2

What is the next best step in managing this patient?

A. Continue to monitor glucose for the next few months.
B. Change immunosuppression regimen.
C. Initiate insulin therapy.
D. Initiate oral antidiabetic agents.

The correct answer is D.

Initiate oral antidiabetic agents. Since he is on a stable and low dose of steroids and other immunosuppressive medications, it is reasonable to start him on oral antidiabetic agents at this point. One clear advantage of newer oral agents like SGLT2 inhibitor and GLP-1 agonist over insulin is weight loss and long-term cardiovascular and renal benefits [1]. Metformin is also a reasonable option and is weight neutral. Since he has had high FBG for the last 3 months, it is inappropriate to wait further before starting treatment. Although calcineurin inhibitors are associated with post-transplant diabetes, these agents are instrumental in preventing rejections and typically continue throughout the life of the graft [6]. Also, no clear-cut evidence exists that changing immunosuppression medications will decrease the risk of PTDM [7]. Moreover, the international consensus meeting on post-transplantation diabetes mellitus recommended choosing an immunosuppressive medication regimen to maximize patient and allograft survival regardless of risk for development of PTDM [8].

Discussion

PTDM was previously known as new-onset diabetes after transplant (NODAT). In 2014, the international consensus meeting on post-transplantation diabetes mellitus recommended changing the terminology to PTDM [8]. PTDM has an adverse outcome on the long-term survival of post-transplant patients due to infection-related complications, cardiovascular events, and death-censored graft failure [9]. In addition, impaired glucose tolerance (IGT) is also associated with the risk of premature death [1]. Both IGT and PTDM are reversible, so timely diagnosis and intervention are extremely important, which may help to reduce the complications and poor outcome [10].

Risk Factors

In addition to traditional risk factors for type 2 diabetes mellitus, PTDM is associated with some transplant-specific risk factors. The risk factors in our patient included hispanic ethnicity, age, obesity with additional weight gain, steroid use (during induction and treatment of rejection), and tacrolimus use. The risk factors for PTDM are listed in Table 61.1 below.

As listed above in Table 61.1, several immunosuppressive medications, including steroids, have been associated with risk for the development of PTDM. Steroids can increase the risk of PTDM by multiple mechanisms, including the stimulation of gluconeogenesis in the liver and insulin resistance in peripheral tissues. In

Table 61.1 Risk factors for post-transplant diabetes [1, 10, 11]

Pre-transplant risk factors	Post-transplant specific risk factors
Age > 40 years	Glucocorticoids
Race: African American and Hispanic	Calcineurin inhibitors (tacrolimus, cyclosporin, rapamycin, and everolimus)
Obesity	Infections (HCV, CMV)
Family history of diabetes	Specific HLA alleles (A30, B27, and B42)
Genetic factors	Cause of ESKD (PCKD)
Dyslipidemia	Hypomagnesemia
IGT	

IGT Impaired glucose tolerance; *HCV* Hepatitis C Virus; *CMV* Cytomegalovirus; *ESKD* End-stage kidney disease; *PCKD* Polycystic kidney disease.

addition, they impair hepatic glycogen synthesis and directly affect beta cells, leading to inhibition of glucose-induced insulin release. On the other hand, calcineurin inhibitors (CNIs) contribute to PTDM mainly by inhibiting insulin release [12, 13]. CNIs, through inhibition of calcineurin phosphatase, leading to prevention of calcineurin—nuclear factor of activated T cells (NFAT) activated transcription of the insulin gene and other genes that help beta cells proliferation [1]. Tacrolimus, which is more frequently used than cyclosporine in transplant patients, has a higher incidence of PTDM [14]. mTOR inhibitors may have an effect similar to CNIs in beta-cell proliferation and insulin release. In addition, they can exacerbate lipotoxicity to beta cells [1]. Hepatitis C virus has been implicated as a risk factor for PTDM, mainly from enhancing insulin resistance, whereas CMV infection may cause insulin secretion impairment from beta cells [12].

Diagnosis

PTDM is diagnosed by the same diagnostic criteria recommended by the American Diabetes Association (ADA) for diagnosis of diabetes mellitus in the general population, which includes (1) FPG $\geq$ 126 mg/dL or (2) 2-hour plasma glucose $\geq$ 200 mg/dL during an oral glucose tolerance test (OGTT) or (3) HbA1c $\geq$ 6.5% or (4) random plasma glucose $\geq$ 200 mg/dL in the presence of classic symptoms of hyperglycemia or hyperglycemic crisis [15]. However, a few issues warrant discussion when it comes to the diagnosis of PTDM. First, transient hyperglycemia is very common during the immediate post-transplant period and can be present in 80–90% of the patients [16]. This is attributed to multiple factors, including high dose steroids, CNI, perioperative stress, and restoration of kidney function. Due to this reason, it is recommended not to diagnose PTDM during the first 45 days post-transplant. After 45 days, if kidney function and immunosuppression medications doses are stable and in the absence of infection, PTDM can be diagnosed using an oral glucose tolerance test (OGTT), fasting, and random glucose criteria. HbA1C should not be used alone to screen for diagnosis of PTDM within the first year after transplant because it underestimates the diagnosis of DM [17]. ADA recommends OGTT as the preferred test to diagnose PTDM [15].

Management

There have been significant advancements in diabetes management with newer therapies, but data in kidney transplant patients is lacking. Although insulin remains the mainstay therapy for managing PTDM, the use of newer antidiabetic agents is increasing. We use insulin as the initial therapy for managing hyperglycemia in the immediate post-transplant period and slowly add non-insulin therapies if the hyperglycemia persists. We also wait for the kidney and liver function to stabilize before adding oral agents. The insulin dose is gradually lowered as the oral agents are added to achieve euglycemia with minimal insulin need. We commonly use metformin, thiazolidinediones, an SGLT2 inhibitor, and GLP1RA in addition to insulin. DPP-4 inhibitors and sulfonylurea are used less commonly in our practice. Patients are encouraged to make lifestyle changes and consult with a diabetes educator and registered dietician.

The American Society of Endocrinology has recommended metformin as the preferred initial glucose-lowering medication and lifestyle changes. Although gastrointestinal (G.I.) side effects like nausea, vomiting, and diarrhea area concern, these drugs are safe and well tolerated by kidney transplant recipients. G.I. side effects can be minimized with the use of extended-release formulation. Metformin use is avoided in patients with eGFR <30 mL/min due to the risk of lactic acidosis [18].

Thiazolidinediones (TZDs) decrease insulin resistance by acting on adipose tissue, muscle, and to a lesser extent, the liver to increase glucose utilization and decrease glucose production. Although TZDs markedly reduce insulin requirements, these drugs are associated with various side effects, most notably heart failure exacerbation. These drugs are well tolerated in kidney transplants [18], and we routinely use them as add-on therapy on appropriate candidates.

Sodium-glucose co-transporter 2 (SGLT2) inhibitors have gained popularity in recent years. These drugs act by inhibiting SGLT2, which is present in the proximal tubule of the nephron. SGLT2 mediates the reabsorption of filtered glucose; thus, by inhibiting SGLT2, these drugs promote the renal excretion of glucose, resulting in reduced serum glucose levels and osmotic diuresis. In addition to lowering blood glucose, these drugs help reduce systolic blood pressure, weight loss and offer cardiac and renal benefits to patients with type 2 diabetes mellitus. EMPA-REG OUTCOME was a multicenter, placebo-controlled trial involving 7020 participants which showed that empagliflozin was associated with a reduction in major adverse cardiac events.

Credence trial showed that when compared with placebo, canagliflozin resulted in a 30% reduction in the composite endpoint of end-stage kidney disease, doubling of serum creatinine from baseline, and death from renal or cardiovascular disease [4, 5]. These drugs are associated with a higher incidence of genital yeast infections, but the risk of urinary tract infections is comparable to the placebo group. Genital yeast infections can be minimized with proper personal hygiene, and treatment consists of topical or oral antifungal medications. Euglycemic diabetic ketoacidosis is another significant side effect of these drugs, and the risk can be mitigated by concomitant use of low-dose insulin. Although transplant patients were excluded in these major trials, some small studies of SGLT2 inhibitors have been in the transplant population. Empagliflozin use showed a weak antihyperglycemic effect with a drop in eGFR during the initial period followed by stabilization. Its use was associated with weight reduction and no increased risk of UTI [7]. Due to the limited sample size and duration of follow-up, renal and cardiovascular benefits could not be corroborated. Although further studies are needed to explore the long-term safety and efficacy of SGLT2 inhibitors in diabetic kidney transplant patients, current data in the general population is compelling. We routinely use these drugs in our practice in appropriate patients.

Glucagon-like peptide-1 receptor agonists (GLP1RA) are another class of drugs that are shown to be effective in reducing the risk of complications associated with T2DM in non-transplant recipients. Endogenous GLP1 potentiates glucose-dependent insulin secretion and inhibits glucagon secretion in pancreatic islet cells, minimizing the risk of hypoglycemia. GLP1RA bind and activate GLP-1 receptors, mimicking the action of the naturally secreted GLP-1. These drugs delay gastric emptying and reduce postprandial hyperglycemia. The benefits of GLP1RA have translated to improved cardiovascular and renal outcomes in clinical trials. LEADER trial showed lower rates of cardiovascular events and death from any cause than placebo [19]. These drugs are also associated with significant weight loss. A small study showed that these drugs might be a relatively safe and effective treatment for kidney transplant recipients with type 2 diabetes that reduces insulin requirements [20].

At our transplant center, we use the following guideline to treat PTDM patients based on the guidelines for non-transplant patients and the data available in the transplant patients. Common medications, their side effects, and dosing are provided in Table 61.2 below from the adult kidney transplant protocol from our center.

1. We start with insulin monotherapy initially until the patient's kidney function is stable.
2. Metformin and SGLT2 inhibitors are the first-line therapy for patients who are suitable candidates for the initiation of oral agents.
3. We add GLP1RA followed by TZDs if adequate blood glucose control is not achieved with the first-line therapy.
4. We try to minimize the insulin dose but maintain low-dose insulin with SGLT2 inhibitors to prevent diabetic ketoacidosis.

Prevention

Identifying risk factors before transplant and correcting modifiable risk factors like obesity, prediabetes, and metabolic syndrome may help prevent PTDM. However, so far, data with exercise and other interventions before transplant is not available. The evolution of late-onset PTDM in most post-transplant patients is from prediabetes, so targeting patients with IGT early in the course and treatment with metformin is a good strategy to prevent PTDM [10]. Since steroid and CNIs are risk factors for the development of PTDM, it may appear reasonable to use steroid and CNI sparing regimens; however, we must weigh the risk of rejection versus development of PTDM while using these regimens. Multiple studies involving early steroid withdrawal, rapid steroid tapering, and steroid-free regimen have shown decreased incidence of PTDM [9]. A small retrospective analysis has shown that switching from tacrolimus to cyclosporin decreased HbA1C and FBG [22]. However, the

Table 61.2 Treatment of post-transplant diabetes [21]

Medications	Potential side effects	Dosing
Metformin (Glucophage) Metformin ER (Glucophage XR, Fortamet, Glumetza)	Nausea and diarrhea Potential for vitamin B12 deficiency in patients with gastric bypass surgery Lactic acidosis	Initial dose 500 mg daily Titrate every 1–2 weeks to maximum dose based on eGFR: eGFR ≥ 45 mL/min—2000 mg/day eGFR 30–45 mL/min—max dose 1000 mg daily eGFR < 30 mL/min—contraindicated Discontinue 24 h prior to intravenous iodinated contrast administration And during hospital admission
Thiazolidenediones • Pioglitazone (Actos)	Fluid retention and peripheral edema Heart failure exacerbation Increased risk for fractures Macular edema	Initial dose 15 mg daily Titrate to 30 mg daily after 3 months May increase to 45 mg daily
SGLT2 inhibitors • Dapagliflozin (Farxiga) • Empagliflozin (Jardiance) • Canagliflozin (Invokana)	Genitourinary fungal infection Volume depletion Hypotension/orthostatic symptoms Euglycemic diabetic ketoacidosis	*Dapagliflozin* Initial dose 5 mg once daily May increase to 10 mg daily Discontinue if eGFR < 45 mL/min/1.72 m² *Empagliflozin* Initial dose 10 mg once daily May increase to 25 mg once daily eGFR> 30: No dose adjustment eGFR < 30 use not recommended *Canagliflozin* Initial dose 100 mg once daily (prior to the first meal of the day) May increase to 300 mg once daily eGFR 30 to <60: 100 mg once daily eGFR < 30: Not recommended

(continued)

Table 61.2 (continued)

Medications	Potential side effects	Dosing
GLP-1 receptor agonists • Liraglutide (Victoza) • Exenatide (Byetta) • Semaglutide (Ozempic) • Semaglutide (Rybelsus) • Exenatide ER (Bydureon) • Dulaglutide (Trulicity)	Nausea, vomiting, diarrhea Local reaction at the injection site Contraindicated in patients with medullary carcinoma of the thyroid, multiple endocrine neoplasia, or pancreatic disease	*Liraglutide*: Starting dose 0.6 mg daily Titrate every 2–4 weeks to 1.2 then 1.8 mg as tolerated. *Semaglutide* (oral formulation) Starting dose 3 mg/day May increase to 7 mg/day after 30 days Can increase to 14 mg/day after an additional 30 days if needed Administer 30 min before a meal *Semaglutide* (subcutaneous formulation) Initial 0.25 mg once weekly for 4 weeks, then increase to 0.5 mg once weekly May increase to 1 mg once weekly after an additional 4 weeks No renal adjustments are necessary *Exenatide I.R.:* 5 µg twice daily within 60 min prior to morning and evening meal Increase to 10 µg twice daily after 30 days based on response/side effects Use with caution for eGFR between 30 and 50 *Exenatide E.R.:* 2 mg once weekly (without regard to meals) eGFR > 45: No dose adjustment eGFR < 45: Use not recommended *Dulaglutide* Initial 0.75 mg once weekly Increase to 1.5 mg once weekly after 4–8 weeks May increase to 3 mg once weekly after at least 4 weeks on 1.5 mg once weekly (max: 4.5 mg) No renal adjustments

international consensus meeting on post-transplantation diabetes mellitus in 2014 made recommendations to use the best immunosuppression regimen based on patient and graft survival irrespective of risk for development of PTDM [8]. Calcineurin inhibitor minimization and steroid avoidance should be considered when possible. Calcineurin inhibitor sparing protocols that utilize belatacept (CD80/86—CD28 co-stimulation blocker) are now being used. BENEFIT study showed that belatacept use had been associated with a superior glomerular filtration rate as compared to cyclosporin but a higher risk of acute rejection. Additionally, belatacept avoids the metabolic side effects like diabetes, hypertension, and dyslipidemia caused by a CNI-based-regimen [23]. CNI and steroid-sparing regimens are associated with an increased risk of rejection and should not be used in high immunological risk patients.

Acknowledgments The authors would like to thank Helen Sweiss, PharmD, for providing information on the medications listed above in Table 61.2.

References

1. Jenssen T, Hartmann A. Post-transplant diabetes mellitus in patients with solid organ transplants. Nat Rev Endocrinol. 2019;15(3):172–88.
2. Porrini EL, et al. Clinical evolution of post-transplant diabetes mellitus. Nephrol Dial Transplant. 2016;31(3):495–505.
3. Gerstein HC, et al. Basal insulin and cardiovascular and other outcomes in dysglycemia. N Engl J Med. 2012;367(4):319–28.
4. Perkovic V, et al. Canagliflozin and renal outcomes in type 2 diabetes and nephropathy. N Engl J Med. 2019;380(24):2295–306.
5. Zinman B, et al. Empagliflozin, cardiovascular outcomes, and mortality in type 2 diabetes. N Engl J Med. 2015;373(22):2117–28.
6. Ekberg H, et al. Reduced exposure to calcineurin inhibitors in renal transplantation. N Engl J Med. 2007;357(25):2562–75.
7. Hecking M, et al. Management of post-transplant diabetes: immunosuppression, early prevention, and novel antidiabetics. Transpl Int. 2021;34(1):27–48.
8. Sharif A, et al. Proceedings from an international consensus meeting on post-transplantation diabetes mellitus: recommendations and future directions. Am J Transplant. 2014;14(9):1992–2000.
9. Aziz F. New onset diabetes mellitus after transplant: the challenge continues. Am Soc Nephrol. 2021:1212–4.
10. Rodríguez-Rodríguez AE, et al. Post-transplant diabetes mellitus and prediabetes in renal transplant recipients: an update. Nephron. 2021;145(4):317–29.
11. Räkel A, Karelis AD. New-onset diabetes after transplantation: risk factors and clinical impact. Diabetes Metab. 2011;37(1):1–14.
12. Langsford D, Dwyer K. Dysglycemia after renal transplantation: definition, pathogenesis, outcomes and implications for management. World J Diabetes. 2015;6(10):1132–51.
13. Delaunay F, et al. Pancreatic beta cells are important targets for the diabetogenic effects of glucocorticoids. J Clin Invest. 1997;100(8):2094–8.
14. Vincenti F, et al. Results of an international, randomized trial comparing glucose metabolism disorders and outcome with cyclosporine versus tacrolimus. Am J Transplant. 2007;7(6):1506–14.
15. Classification and diagnosis of diabetes: standards of medical Care in Diabetes-2018. Diabetes Care. 2018;41(Suppl 1):S13–s27.
16. Chakkera HA, et al. Hyperglycemia during the immediate period after kidney transplantation. Clin J Am Soc Nephrol. 2009;4(4):853–9.
17. Shivaswamy V, Boerner B, Larsen J. Post-transplant diabetes mellitus: causes, treatment, and impact on outcomes. Endocr Rev. 2016;37(1):37–61.
18. Kurian B, Joshi R, Helmuth A. Effectiveness and long-term safety of thiazolidinediones and metformin in renal transplant recipients. Endocr Pract. 2008;14(8):979–84.

19. Marso SP, et al. Liraglutide and cardiovascular outcomes in type 2 diabetes. N Engl J Med. 2016;375(4):311–22.
20. Kukla A, et al. The use of GLP1R agonists for the treatment of type 2 diabetes in kidney transplant recipients. Transplant Direct. 2020;6(2):e524.
21. University transplant center. Adult Kidney Transplant Protocol. San Antonio, Texas.
22. Ghisdal L, et al. Conversion from tacrolimus to cyclosporine a for new-onset diabetes after transplantation: a single-Centre experience in renal transplanted patients and review of the literature. Transpl Int. 2008;21(2):146–51.
23. Vincenti F, et al. A phase III study of belatacept-based immunosuppression regimens versus cyclosporine in renal transplant recipients (BENEFIT study). Am J Transplant. 2010;10(3):535–46.

Chapter 62
Tertiary Hyperparathyroidism Post-Renal Transplant

Margaret Bloom and Sandesh Parajuli

Introduction

Secondary hyperparathyroidism occurs almost ubiquitously in the ESRD population. Renal transplant usually corrects secondary hyperparathyroidism; however, a small percentage of patients may develop tertiary hyperparathyroidism as early as 1-year post-transplant. There is currently a lack of evidence and guidelines for treating tertiary hyperparathyroidism, specifically regarding the use of calcimimetics versus parathyroidectomy. Conflicting evidence also exists regarding optimal timing for parathyroidectomy.

Patient History

A 63-year-old female with a past medical history of end-stage renal disease (ESRD) due to membranoproliferative glomerulonephritis type 1 underwent a deceased donor kidney transplant. Prior to the transplant, she was on hemodialysis for 4 years. Her other pertinent past medical history includes secondary hyperparathyroidism requiring cinacalcet and seizure disorder with non-convulsive status epilepticus diagnosed the year before transplant controlled with levetiracetam. Within the first week post-transplant, she developed hypercalcemia with a serum calcium of 11.6 mg/dL. Her PTH was 1309 pg/dL at this time.

M. Bloom (✉) · S. Parajuli
Department of Medicine, University of Wisconsin, Madison, WI, USA
e-mail: mbloom@uwhealth.org; sparajuli@medicine.wisc.edu

© The Author(s), under exclusive license to Springer Nature Switzerland AG 2022
F. Aziz, S. Parajuli (eds.), *Complications in Kidney Transplantation*,
https://doi.org/10.1007/978-3-031-13569-9_62

403

Question 1

What should the initial management be for this patient's hypercalcemia immediately post-transplant?

A. Calcitonin.
B. Continue cinacalcet and obtain weekly serum calcium levels at discharge.
C. Aggressive intravenous fluid resuscitation.
D. Nothing, her serum calcium, and PTH will improve as GFR increases over the next 12 months.

The correct answer is B.

Given this patient's PTH level with concomitant hypercalcemia, it is reasonable to continue cinacalcet post-transplant. Moreover, some evidence suggests that discontinuing calcimimetics at the time of transplant could lead to rebound hyperparathyroidism and a higher PTX rate [1]. Though answers A and C may be used as immediate interventions for hypercalcemia, they do not address the underlying issue of this patient's known secondary hyperparathyroidism. The extent to which her PTH and calcium are elevated warrants treatment, making answer D incorrect.

Hospital Course

Cinacalcet 60 mg daily was resumed before hospital discharge. She reached a nadir creatinine of 1.4 mg/dL within 6 weeks post-transplant.

Approximately 2 months post-transplant, this patient was re-admitted with altered mental status after a family member found her obtunded at home. Initial laboratory workup was notable for elevated renal indices, hypercalcemia, and elevated inflammatory markers (Table 62.1).

Her chest X-ray was notable for patchy ground-glass opacities, and EEG was consistent with the ictal-interictal continuum pattern. Initial treatment included

Table 62.1 Lab work of the patient

Chemistry	
Sodium	140 mmol/L
Potassium	3.8 mmol/L
BUN	43 mg/dL
Creatinine	2.3 mg/dL
Calcium	16.0 mg/dL
Complete blood count	
WBC	14 K/µL
Hgb	9.5 g/dL
Hct	29%
Inflammatory markers	
CRP	437 mg/dL
Lactic acid	3.1 mg/dL

WBC white blood cell count, *Hgb* hemoglobin, *Hct* hematocrit, *CRP* C reactive protein

empiric antibiotics for presumed aspiration pneumonia, antiepileptic drugs, isotonic intravenous fluids for a pre-renal acute kidney injury (AKI), and calcitonin for the hypercalcemic crisis. She was admitted to the neurointensive care unit for further studies and management.

An extensive workup was performed, including CT abdomen/pelvis, neuroimaging, lumbar puncture, nuclear medicine bone scan, serum protein electrophoresis (SPEP), and free light chains, all negative.

Question 2

What is the most likely cause for this patient's presentation?

A. Post-transplant lymphoproliferative disease (PTLD).
B. Hypercalcemia related to immobility.
C. Tertiary hyperparathyroidism.
D. Bacterial meningitis.

The correct answer is C.

When reviewing this patient's initial postoperative course, she should be considered high risk for tertiary hyperparathyroidism, given her postoperative hypercalcemia and significantly elevated PTH level (>1000 pg/dL). Though PTLD should be considered, her unremarkable imaging and negative serum studies (SPEP, free light chains) ruled out this differential. Her neuroimaging and lumbar puncture were also unrevealing, making bacterial meningitis unlikely.

Additional Hospital Course

With a diagnosis of tertiary hyperparathyroidism as the primary etiology for this patient's hypercalcemic crisis and altered mental status, endocrine surgery was consulted, and she underwent a subtotal parathyroidectomy. She developed the hungry bone syndrome post-operatively, which required close monitoring and repletion of her calcium, magnesium, and phosphorus. Her serum creatinine increased approximately 0.5 mg/dL post-operatively but returned to her nadir of 1.4 mg/dL by post-operative day 4. She was started on calcitriol 0.25 µg at discharge with bi-weekly monitoring of calcium, phosphorus, and PTH levels. She maintained normal transplant allograft function 1-year post-parathyroidectomy with a GFR of 50 mL/min and serum creatinine of 1.1 mg/dL. Her PTH and calcium levels remained normal at 53 pg/mL and 9.0 mg/dL, respectively.

Discussion

Secondary hyperparathyroidism (sHPT) frequently occurs in individuals with ESRD and carries significant morbidity and mortality due to increased coronary artery disease and renal osteodystrophy. Though kidney transplant usually corrects sHPT, as many as 25% of patients will have tertiary hyperparathyroidism (tHPT)

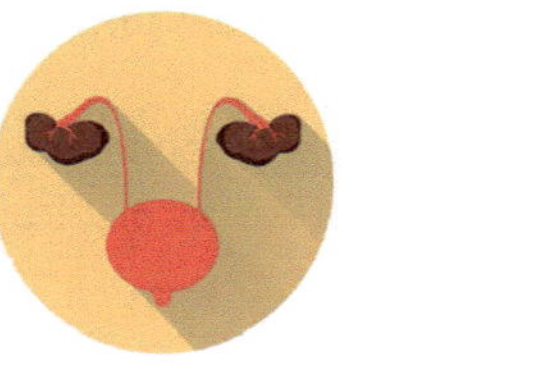
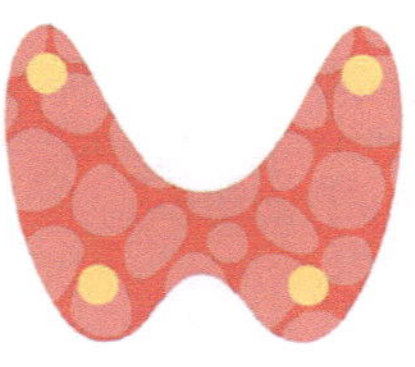
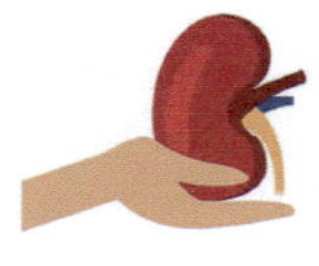

Fig. 62.1 Secondary Hyperparathyroidism vs. Tertiary Hyperparathyroidism

1 year after transplant [2, 3] (Fig. 62.1). Risk factors for tHPT post-transplant include prolonged time on dialysis, enlarged parathyroid glands, immediate post-transplant hypercalcemia, and female gender with high serum levels of PTH, calcium, phosphate, and alkaline phosphatase [2, 3].

Treatment for tHPT after transplant remains controversial due to lack of evidence, specifically regarding the use of calcimimetics versus PTX. Though calcimimetics are often a first-line therapeutic for tHPT in this context, as many as 50% of these patients might ultimately be referred for PTX for various reasons, including medication cost, tolerance, and overall poor calcium control [4]. Moreover, evidence suggests that surgical treatment with PTX is superior to calcimimetic therapy alone to correct metabolic disorders seen in tHPT [5]. Thus, providers may want to consider referral for PTX earlier in the post-transplant course of patients with evidence of tHPT.

Currently, no guidelines exist regarding the timing of parathyroidectomy, and studies show conflicting evidence on this topic. For example, Littbarski and colleagues' single-center retrospective analysis concluded that PTX within 1 year of kidney transplant is an independent risk factor for impaired graft function—possibly due to direct hemodynamic effects of PTH and tubulointerstitial damage caused by prolonged hypercalcemia [3, 6, 7]. Okada et al. demonstrated similar findings, concluding that pre-transplant PTX should be considered in severe sHPT to prevent hypocalcemia and renal graft dysfunction that may be more likely in post-transplant PTX [6]. Conversely, Meng and colleagues demonstrated that acute renal allograft dysfunction post-PTX is temporary and usually returns to pre-surgery levels within 1 year, as seen in this case study [7].

Several studies suggest proactively avoiding tHPT by referring patients with severe sHPT for PTX before transplants, such as individuals with PTH > 1000 pg/

mL and no calcimimetic use or 500 pg/mL with calcimimetic use [8, 9]. Overall, taking a multidisciplinary approach with the involvement of nephrology, transplant surgery, and endocrine surgery could prove highly beneficial in developing clear treatment guidelines regarding the prevention and management of tHPT in kidney transplant patients.

Disclosures M. Bloom reports employment with the University of Wisconsin Medical Foundation.

References

1. Evenepoel P, et al. Mineral metabolism in renal transplant recipients discontinuing cinacalcet at the time of transplantation: a prospective observational study. Clin Transpl. 2018;26(3):393–402. https://doi.org/10.1111/j.1399-0012.2011.01524.x.
2. Finnerty BM, et al. Parathyroidectomy versus cinacalcet in the management of tertiary hyperparathyroidism: surgery improves renal transplant allograft survival. J Surgery. 2019;165:129–34. https://doi.org/10.1016/j.surg.2018.04.090.
3. Littbarski SA, Kaltenborn A, Gwiasda J, et al. Timing of parathyroidectomy in kidney transplant candidates with early secondary hyperparathyroidism: effect of pretransplant versus early or late post-transplant parathyroidectomy. J Surgery. 2018;163:373–80. https://doi.org/10.1016/j.surg.2017.10.016.
4. Dream S, Chen H, Lindeman B. Tertiary hyperparathyroidism why the delay? Ann Surg Open. 2020;273(3):120–2. https://doi.org/10.1097/SLA.0000000000004069.
5. Giollo Rivelli G, Lopes de Lima M, Mazzali M. Therapy for persistent hypercalcemic hyperparathyroidism post-renal transplant: cinacalcet versus parathyroidectomy. J Bras Nefrol. 2020;42(3):315–22. https://doi.org/10.1590/2175-8239-JBN-2019-0207.
6. Okada M, Hiramitsu T, Ichimori T, et al. Comparison of pre- and post-transplant parathyroidectomy in renal transplant recipients and the impact of parathyroidectomy timing on calcium metabolism and renal allograft function: a retrospective single-center analysis. World J Surg. 2020;44:498–507. https://doi.org/10.1007/s00267-019-05124-6.
7. Meng C, Martins P, Frazao J, Pestana M. Parathyroidectomy in persistent post-transplantation hyperparathyroidism—single-center experience. Transplant Proc. 2017;49:795–8. https://doi.org/10.1016/j.transproceed.2017.01.067.
8. Delos Santos R, Rossi A, Coyne D, Maw TT. Management of post-transplant hyperparathyroidism and bone disease. Drugs. 2019;79:501–13. https://doi.org/10.1007/s40265-019-01074-4.
9. Patel R, Delos Santos R. The conundrum of parathyroidectomy vs cinacalcet for treatment of post-transplant hyperparathyroidism. J Bras Nefrol. 2020;42(3):264–5. https://doi.org/10.1590/2175-8239-JBN-2020-0107.

Chapter 63
Joint Replacement Surgery Comparing Patients with End-Stage Renal Disease and Post Kidney Transplant

Ban Dodin and Sandesh Parajuli

Introduction

Patients with ESKD often suffer from osteoarthritis, renal osteodystrophy, and osteonecrosis of the femoral neck secondary to chronic immunosuppressive medication use that necessitates consequent joint replacement. Despite these comorbidities, the timing of joint replacement in transplant recipients has been largely debated. We present a case of a patient with ESKD needing joint replacement surgery with a review of the recent literature.

Patient History

A 65-year-old female with end-stage kidney disease (ESKD) due to diabetes on dialysis is experiencing severe hip pain secondary to osteoarthritis that has hindered her quality of life. She is being considered for a right hip replacement surgery. She has been managing her pain with oxycodone a few times a day, as acetaminophen is not able to control her pain, and she is hesitant to take non-steroidal anti-inflammatory medications. She is also being considered for a potential living donor kidney transplant from her husband, who is not yet approved for the living kidney donor but undergoing evaluation. Her pain has persisted; however, orthopedic surgeons are hesitant to perform a hip replacement surgery on her due to her being on dialysis and recommended that she wait until after her kidney transplant.

S. Parajuli · B. Dodin (✉)
University of Wisconsin School of Medicine and Public Health, Department of Medicine, Madison, WI, USA
e-mail: bdodin@wisc.edu

© The Author(s), under exclusive license to Springer Nature Switzerland AG 2022

F. Aziz, S. Parajuli (eds.), *Complications in Kidney Transplantation*,
https://doi.org/10.1007/978-3-031-13569-9_63

Question 1

The aforementioned patient has not been scheduled for a kidney transplant yet, as her husband is still not cleared for a donation; the expected timeframe to transplant is 10–12 months. However, she is considering the option of having a hip replacement before her kidney transplant. What is the best option for this patient going forward?

A. Joint replacement surgeries are contraindicated in kidney transplant patients, and so this patient can only undergo hip replacement surgery before she undergoes a kidney transplant.
B. She should have her kidney transplant done before having her hip replacement to avoid deleterious kidney transplant outcomes.
C. Patients on dialysis tend to have better orthopedic outcomes compared to their kidney transplant counterparts, so she should consider having her joint replacement done before her kidney transplant.
D. Kidney transplant recipients tend to have better orthopedic outcomes compared to their dialysis counterparts, so she should consider having her joint replacement done after her kidney transplant.

The correct answer is D.

Current literature has focused more on the viability of orthopedic implants in kidney transplant recipients relative to their dialysis counterparts. Most studies have concluded that joint replacements have better long-term outcomes in kidney transplant recipients relative to patients on dialysis, noting lower infection rates, lower rates of revision, and fewer postoperative complications [1–4].

Patient Course

Subsequently, the patient underwent successful kidney transplantation and was doing well with a serum creatinine of 0.9 mg/dL 18 months post-transplant. Following her transplant, she was maintained on a triple immunosuppressant regimen, which consisted of prednisone, tacrolimus, and mycophenolate. The patient remained stable from a kidney transplant perspective, but her hip pain continued to be a nuisance for her.

Question 2

Her hip pain continued to worsen, limiting her activities of daily living. Her orthopedic surgeon recommended getting hip replacement surgery. However, she is worried about the postoperative risks and the risk of losing her kidney graft, as she adamantly opposes returning to dialysis after hip replacement surgery. This prompts questioning what risks hip replacement surgery pose on kidney transplant viability and whether joint replacement surgery outcomes will result in detrimental transplant-specific outcomes. What risks are associated with joint replacement surgery in kidney transplant recipients?

A. The patient is at a significantly increased risk of suffering from death censored graft failure but not acute graft rejection if she undergoes joint replacement at this time.
B. The patient is not at a significantly increased risk of suffering from acute graft rejection, death censored graft failure, or death if she undergoes joint replacement at this time.
C. The patient is at increased risk of acute graft rejection but not death censored graft failure if she undergoes joint replacement surgery.
D. The patient is at an increased risk of death but not acute graft rejection if she undergoes joint replacement surgery.

The correct answer is B.

A recent single-center study by Dodin et al. found that kidney transplant recipients who require subsequent joint replacement surgery do not appear to be at increased risk of acute graft rejection, death censored graft failure (DCGF), or death following joint replacement surgery [5]. Although more studies in the field are required, these data suggest that joint replacement surgery can be safely recommended for selected kidney transplant recipients (KTRs).

Clinical Course

The patient recovered well from surgery after her hip replacement and did not suffer any complications post-operatively. She is ambulatory and has had excellent pain relief following joint replacement. She has an excellent range of motion and has been handling her physical therapy regimen well.

Discussion

Patients with ESKD often suffer from osteoarthritis, renal osteodystrophy, and osteonecrosis of the femoral neck secondary to chronic immunosuppressive medication use that necessitates consequent joint replacement [1]. The overarching mechanism responsible for avascular necrosis of the femoral head involves apoptosis of bone marrow and bone-forming cells; this results in femoral head collapse and subsequent damage of the overlying cartilage. With this loss of cartilage, the rounded femoral head flattens, resulting in osteoarthritis [6]. Despite these comorbidities, the timing of joint replacement in transplant recipients has been largely debated. Our patient serves as a prime example of countless KTRs who require subsequent joint replacement, yet the risks and incidences of kidney graft failure, acute rejection, and patient survival remain unclear. The majority of literature in the field has assessed orthopedic outcomes among patients on dialysis compared with KTRs; some studies have assessed orthopedic outcomes among non-transplant

Table 63.1 Selected studies of joint replacement surgery

Reference	Year of publication	Sample size	Findings
Dodin et. al	Dec 2021	382	Joint replacement was not associated with acute graft rejection, death censored graft failure, or patient death in KTRs
Douglas et. al	July 2021	2864	Lower risk of mortality and revision rates in KTRs compared to dialysis patients
Popat et. al	March 2021	797	Higher deep infection rates were observed in patients on hemodialysis relative to KTRs. Higher revision rates were seen in cemented implants in the hemodialysis group vs. KTRs; KTRs had a higher revision rate in uncemented implants.
Li et. al	Dec 2020	N/A	Lower risk of mortality detected in KTRs relative to dialysis; KTRs had less risk for periprosthetic infection
Inoue et.al	April 2020	107	Significantly higher rates of post-op infection in dialysis patients vs. kidney transplant patients.
Labaran et. al	Jan 2020	1020	Kidney transplant patients experience higher morbidity and mortality compared to non-transplant patients when undergoing revision joint arthroplasty
Tornero et. al	March 2015	114	Long-term hemodialysis patients and KTRs experienced higher rates of early post-op complications relative to non-transplant patients; hemodialysis patients experienced higher periprosthetic fracture; KTRs experienced higher prosthetic joint infection.
Debarge et. al	May 2007	37	Kidney transplant recipients achieved good results following joint arthroplasty and morbidity similar to the general population; dialysis patients experienced greater perioperative morbidity.
Lieberman et. al	Apr 1995	46	The higher deep infection rate in patients undergoing joint replacement on chronic dialysis

patients and KTRs as well and are summarized in Table 63.1. The consensus delineates better joint replacement outcomes, lower infection rates, fewer postoperative complications, and lower risk of mortality in KTRs relative to patients on dialysis [1, 2, 4]. Moreover, patients on dialysis may experience higher rates and the earlier timing of joint replacement surgery revisions, more hospital readmissions by 90 days, and more mechanical complications following surgery [7–9]. One study compared orthopedic outcomes in KTRs relative to non-kidney transplant matched controls and found that patients with kidney transplants who undergo revision joint arthroplasty experienced increased morbidity and mortality compared to non-transplant recipients [3] who underwent revision arthroplasty.

The aforementioned patient was part of a single-center study conducted at the University of Wisconsin Hospitals, where all of our patients underwent kidney transplantation, some of whom underwent subsequent joint replacement surgery post-transplant. Incidence of acute graft rejection, DCGF, and patient mortality was compared among both groups of patients. Our results suggest no increased risk of acute graft rejection, DCGF, or patient mortality in patients who undergo joint replacement post kidney transplantation relative to matched controls who did not undergo joint replacement. These data suggest that joint replacement can be safely recommended for a select patient population who have undergone kidney transplantation.

In selected kidney transplant recipients who require subsequent joint replacement, joint replacement surgery can be safely recommended for patients suffering from hip and/or knee pain without risking adverse kidney transplant outcomes.

References

1. Li J, Li M, Peng BQ, Luo R, Chen Q, Huang X. Comparison of total joint arthroplasty outcomes between renal transplant patients and dialysis patients-a meta-analysis and systematic review. J Orthop Surg Res. 2020;15(1):590.
2. Inoue D, Yazdi H, Goswami K, Tan TL, Parvizi J. Comparison of postoperative complications and survivorship of Total hip and knee arthroplasty in dialysis and renal transplantation patients. J Arthroplast. 2020;35(4):971–5.
3. Labaran LA, Amin R, Bolarinwa SA, Puvanesarajah V, Rao SS, Browne JA, et al. Revision joint arthroplasty and renal transplant: a matched control cohort study. J Arthroplast. 2020;35(1):224–8.
4. Debarge R, Pibarot V, Guyen O, Vaz G, Carret JP, Bejui-Hugues J. Total hip arthroplasty in patients with chronic renal failure transplant or dialysis. Rev Chir Orthop Reparatrice Appar Mot. 2007;93(3):222–7.
5. Dodin B, Breyer I, Osman F, Alstott J, Aziz F, Garg N, et al. Kidney transplant outcomes among recipients with post-transplant hip or knee joint replacement surgery. Clin Transpl. 2021:e14564.
6. Guerado E, Caso E. The physiopathology of avascular necrosis of the femoral head: an update. Injury. 2016;47(Suppl 6):S16–26.
7. Popat R, Ali AM, Holloway IP, Sarraf KM, Hanna SA. Outcomes of total hip arthroplasty in haemodialysis and renal transplant patients: systematic review. Hip Int. 2021;31(2):207–14.
8. Douglas SJ, Pervaiz SS, Sax OC, Mohamed NS, Delanois RE, Johnson AJ. Comparing primary total hip arthroplasty in renal transplant recipients to patients on dialysis for end-stage renal disease: a nationally matched analysis. J Bone Joint Surg Am. 2021;
9. McCleery MA, Leach WJ, Norwood T. Rates of infection and revision in patients with renal disease undergoing total knee replacement in Scotland. J Bone Joint Surg Br. 2010;92(11):1535–9.

Chapter 64
Obstructive Sleep Apnea in Kidney Transplant Recipient

Rachna Tiwari and Camilla K. B. Matthews

Introduction

Obstructive sleep apnea (OSA) is a common condition characterized by recurrent episodes of partial or complete obstruction of respiratory passages during sleep. Repeated episodes during sleep may cause sleep fragmentation and nonrestorative sleep. Untreated OSA can cause symptoms such as daytime sleepiness or morning headaches, but many people may be asymptomatic [1].

We are presenting a case of a pediatric kidney transplant recipient who was noted to have severe OSA post-transplant.

Case

A 3-year and 5 months-old boy with a medical history significant for preterm birth at 35 weeks, Eagle Barrett triad (formally known as Prune belly syndrome with associated medical issues including pulmonary hypoplasia, global developmental delay, and bilateral congenital hydronephrosis due to obstructive uropathy) is now status post-living-related kidney transplant from his mother at the age of 20 months.

R. Tiwari (✉)
Department of Medicine, University of Wisconsin—Madison School of Medicine and Public Health, Madison, WI, USA
e-mail: rtiwari3@wisc.edu

C. K. B. Matthews
Department of Pediatrics, University of Wisconsin—Madison School of Medicine and Public Health, Madison, WI, USA
e-mail: ckmatthews@pediatrics.wisc.edu

© The Author(s), under exclusive license to Springer Nature Switzerland AG 2022

F. Aziz, S. Parajuli (eds.), *Complications in Kidney Transplantation*,
https://doi.org/10.1007/978-3-031-13569-9_64

He is currently on mycophenolate mofetil and tacrolimus as a part of post-transplant care. He was referred to a sleep clinic due to snoring, witnessed apneas, daytime and nighttime mouth breathing, and restless sleep. In early infancy, he required oxygen therapy which was discontinued at 6 months of age. The clinical examination on presentation to the sleep clinic showed 3+ enlarged tonsils bilaterally. Abdominal exam revealed dry G tube site and Mitrofanoff covered with band-aid. Due to concern for obstructive sleep apnea, a sleep study was ordered, which showed severe obstructive sleep apnea (OSA) with apnea–hypopnea index (AHI) of 47.4 events per hour (pediatric normative AHI is 1.5 events per hour or under), as well as findings of severe intermittent hypoxemia with the lowest oxygen saturation at 61% (time spent below 90% was 84.1 min) along with hypercarbia. Sleep study further revealed frequent snoring, mouth breathing, gasping, frequent repositioning, sitting up out of sleep, body movements, and increased respiratory effort contributing to sleep fragmentation. Urgent management for severe OSA was recommended. ENT was consulted for drug-induced sleep endoscopy (DISE), which is a sedated examination of the upper and lower airway. DISE showed 4+ tonsils with a significant posterior extension of the tonsils, causing posterior epiglottis displacement resulting in total airway obstruction, 80% adenoid enlargement, and a large tongue base. Adenotonsillectomy was performed with post-operative inpatient admission. A follow-up sleep study to check for residual OSA was recommended.

Question 1

What are the kidney-specific outcomes for patients who have post-transplant OSA versus those who do not have OSA?

A. There is a significant increase in death-censored graft failure (DCGF) and acute rejection (AR).
B. There are not enough studies to assess the clinically significant effects of OSA among kidney transplant recipients both in the adult and pediatric world.
C. Underdiagnoses of OSA is common in our general population, and the risk it poses is often underestimated.
D. Both B and C are correct.

The Correct Answer Is D

Overall, there are few studies regarding kidney transplants and OSA, and even fewer among pediatric kidney transplants. A pilot study of 27 patients aged 6–17 years showed that sleep-disordered breathing (SDB) among children with CKD was 10-times higher than the general pediatric population [2].Adult patients with chronic kidney disease (CKD) are highly likely to have OSA. It is thought that the relationship is bi-directional. OSA leads to episodic desaturations and activation of the sympathetic nervous system; the renin—angiotensin—aldosterone system alters cardiovascular hemodynamics leading to free radical generation. This leads to endothelial dysfunction, atherosclerosis, fibrosis leading to adverse cardiovascular events, and likely renal damage. OSA is also associated with hypertension and maybe an independent predictor of proteinuria. On the other hand, ESKD fluid overload plays an essential role in the pathogenesis of OSA. OSA is associated with accelerated loss of kidney function. Continuous positive airway pressure (CPAP) helps in eliminating patients' symptoms and improving their quality of life and may have beneficial effects on kidney function [3] [4, 5].

One cross-sectional study among 200 adult kidney transplant recipients showed that the prevalence of OSA and restless leg syndrome (RLS) was higher in kidney transplant recipients when compared to the general population [6]. The apnea—hypopnea index (AHI), which measures the severity of OSA, was noted to worsen over time and was directly related to an increase in BMI in renal transplant patients [7]. In an observational cohort study done in 823 adult patients, high risk of OSA was an independent predictor of graft loss among females after adjusting for age, comorbidities, HTN, BMI, and kidney function (HR:3.05; CI: 1.24–7.51; $p = 0.015$) while the high risk for OSA did not predict graft survival among males [8]. On the other hand, another study analyzed records of 415 adult kidney transplant recipients with pretransplant OSA, which was not associated with risk of death and no significant increase in death-censored graft failure (DCGF) and acute rejection (AR). Similar results were noted on de novo OSA. However, the risk might have been underestimated due to the underdiagnosis of OSA [9]. Another study has found no association between the presence of OSA and all-cause mortality in kidney transplant recipients or the rate of progression of CKD [10].

Question 2
Do kidney transplants help with OSA, especially in ESKD and OSA patients?

A. Unknown.
B. Yes.
C. No.

The correct answer is A
Although there are theories that claim that renal transplantation may help improve OSA in patients with ESKD, information about sleep apnea in patients post-transplant is not consistent [11].

Further course: Due to the severity of initial findings of OSA on this patient's diagnostic polysomnogram, he is at high risk for residual OSA. If a repeat sleep study shows residual OSA, further surgical treatment options can include referral to ENT for possible lingual tonsillectomy [12]and tongue base reduction [13] or nasal inferior turbinate reduction in a patient with inferior turbinate hypertrophy [14]. For possible medication treatment options, a trial of montelukast for mild OSA, due to its anti-inflammatory property [15], could be considered. In addition, CPAP is deemed to be first-line treatment in patients who have residual moderate to severe OSA without a surgically correctible cause [16]. Other treatment options can include a trial of orofacial myofunctional therapy (OMT) which not only helps with residual OSA but also improves adherence in CPAP treated OSA patients [17].

Discussion

OSA prevalence in the adult population ranges from 9% to 12%, 13% to 33% in men, 6% to 19% in women. The prevalence of OSA increases with advancing age and is higher with obese individuals when compared to overweight individuals [1]. Symptoms and clinical findings of OSA can include loud or irregular snoring, daytime sleepiness, nonrestorative sleep, morning headache, nocturia, and increased neck circumference. These reported symptoms should trigger suspicion of obstructive sleep apnea. OSA is an independent risk factor for cardiovascular disease and motor vehicle accidents. First-line therapy for symptomatic or moderate to severe OSA in adults is a continuous positive airway pressure (CPAP) machine, whereas alternative therapies can be used in patients who decline or are unable to use CPAP [18].

The prevalence of obstructive sleep apnea in children is 2–4%, with the overall prevalence increasing associated with the increase in childhood obesity. Obstructive sleep apnea syndrome (OSAS) is associated with cardiovascular morbidity, poor quality of life, and neurobehavioral effects in children. The American Academy of Pediatrics (AAP) recommends screening for OSAS during routine visits. Typical symptoms can include snoring, restless sleep, daytime hyperactivity, bedwetting, dry mouth, and headaches. For patients who have increased risk factors like craniofacial disorders, neurological disorders, or genetic disorders, screening should be done annually as part of routine preventative care. Although the pathophysiology is multifactorial, the most common cause is an overgrowth of adenoids and tonsils, leading to upper airway obstruction during sleep [19]. The primary treatment is adenotonsillectomy which can result in improvements in attention, daytime behaviors, and likely cognitive abilities [20]. The anatomical abnormalities contributing to OSA differ with different age groups [21]. The success rate of surgical treatment (T &A) alone varies depending on the population type. Findings of residual OSA after adenotonsillectomy can be as high as 40–75% in children. For children with persistent OSA, alternative forms of treatment like CPAP, medication treatment options, or further surgical options are used [22].

There is a significant difference in OSA symptoms between children and adults [23]. The STOP-Bang questionnaire is a useful screening tool for OSA in the adult population (Fig. 64.1) [24]. The higher the score on the STOP-BANG questionnaire, the higher likelihood of moderate to severe OSA [25].

The pediatric sleep questionnaire (PSQ) has been a valuable and reliable tool to screen for OSA in the pediatric population for ages 2–18 [26] Other methods can also be used to screen for pediatric OSA screening, one of which is as follows: (Fig. 64.2).

Although clinically significant effects of obstructive sleep apnea among kidney transplant patients are not known, sleep disorders may have deleterious effects on the kidney allograft, and hence screening and management are important [27]. Routine screening for obstructive sleep apnea in both pediatric and adult kidney transplant patients is an area for improved clinical care of renal transplant patients with a need for ongoing longitudinal research in this area.

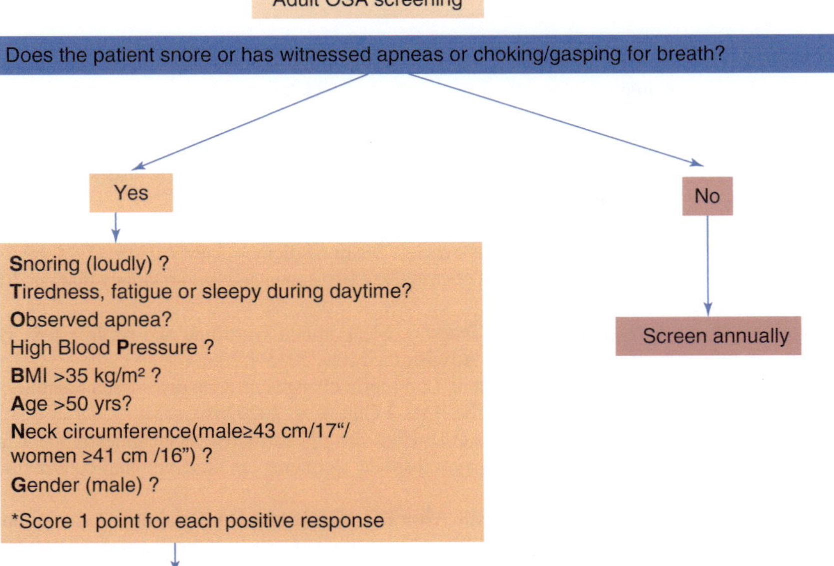

Fig. 64.1 Adult OSA screening

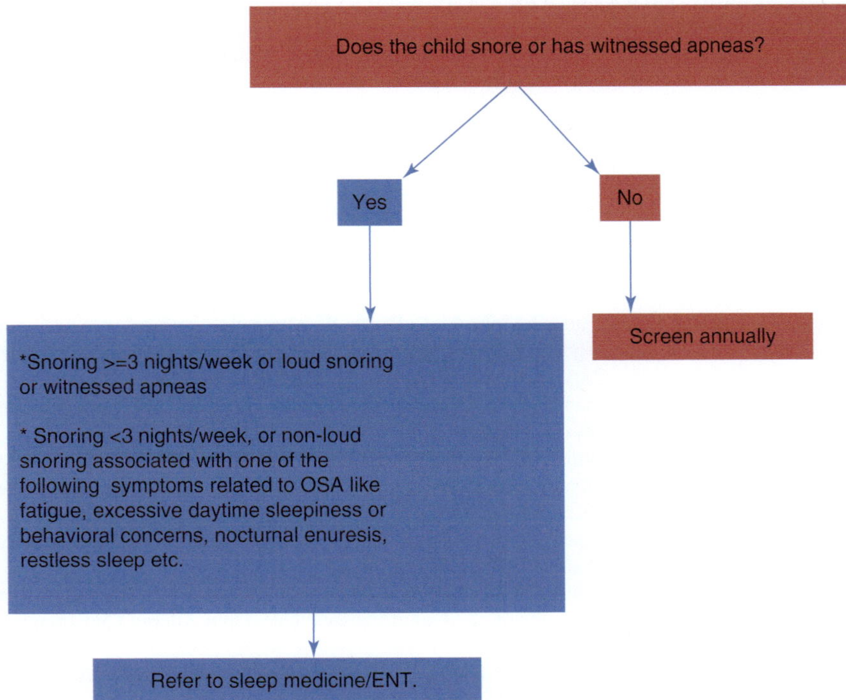

Fig. 64.2 Pediatric OSA screening

References

1. Senaratna CV, Perret JL, Lodge CJ, et al. Prevalence of obstructive sleep apnea in the general population: a systematic review. Sleep Med Rev. 2017;34:70–81.
2. Lelii M, Senatore L, Morello W, et al. Sleep-disordered breathing in children with chronic kidney disease: a pilot study. Eur Respir J. 2020;56(suppl 64):1229.
3. Lin C-H, Perger E, Lyons OD. Obstructive sleep apnea and chronic kidney disease. Curr Opin Pulm Med. 2018;24(6):549–54.
4. Voulgaris A, Marrone O, Bonsignore MR, Steiropoulos P. Chronic kidney disease in patients with obstructive sleep apnea. A narrative review Sleep medicine reviews. 2019;47:74–89.
5. Adeseun GA, Rosas SE. The impact of obstructive sleep apnea on chronic kidney disease. Curr Hypertens Rep. 2010;12(5):378–83.
6. Naini AE, Amra B, Mahmoodnia L, Taheri S. Sleep apnea syndrome and restless legs syndrome in kidney transplant recipients. Adv Biomed Res. 2015;4:206.
7. Mallamaci F, Tripepi R, D'Arrigo G, et al. Long-term changes in sleep disordered breathing in renal transplant patients: relevance of the BMI. J Clin Med. 2020;9(6):1739.
8. Szentkiralyi A, Czira ME, Molnar MZ, et al. High risk of obstructive sleep apnea is a risk factor of death censored graft loss in kidney transplant recipients: an observational cohort study. Sleep Med. 2011;12(3):267–73.
9. Tiwari R, Lyu B, Alagusundaramoorthy S, Astor BC, Mandelbrot DA, Parajuli S. Association of diagnosed obstructive sleep apnea with kidney transplant outcomes. Clin Transpl. 2019;33(12)
10. Fornadi K, Ronai KZ, Turanyi CZ, et al. Sleep apnea is not associated with worse outcomes in kidney transplant recipients. Sci Rep. 2014;4:6987.
11. Daabis R, El-Gohary E. Sleep apnea in kidney transplant patients: clinical correlates and comparison with pretransplant patients. Egypt J Chest Dis Tuberc. 2012;61(4):453–8.
12. Kang KT, Koltai PJ, Lee CH, Lin MT, Hsu WC. Lingual tonsillectomy for treatment of pediatric obstructive sleep apnea: a meta-analysis. JAMA otolaryngology–head & neck surgery. 2017;143(6):561–8.
13. Ulualp S. Outcomes of tongue base reduction and lingual tonsillectomy for residual pediatric obstructive sleep apnea after Adenotonsillectomy. Int Arch Otorhinolaryngol. 2019;23(4):e415–21.
14. Cheng PW, Fang KM, Su HW, Huang TW. Improved objective outcomes and quality of life after adenotonsillectomy with inferior turbinate reduction in pediatric obstructive sleep apnea with inferior turbinate hypertrophy. Laryngoscope. 2012;122(12):2850–4.
15. CADTH Rapid Response Reports. Montelukast for sleep apnea: a review of the clinical effectiveness, cost effectiveness, and guidelines. Ottawa, ON: Canadian Agency for Drugs and Technologies in HealthCopyright © 2014 Canadian Agency for Drugs and Technologies in Health; 2014.
16. Rana M, August J, Levi J, Parsi G, Motro M, DeBassio W. Alternative approaches to adenotonsillectomy and continuous positive airway pressure (CPAP) for the management of pediatric obstructive sleep apnea (OSA): a review. Sleep disord. 2020;2020:7987208.
17. Koka V, De Vito A, Roisman G, et al. Orofacial Myofunctional therapy in obstructive sleep apnea syndrome: a pathophysiological perspective. Medicina. 2021;57(4):323.
18. Veasey SC, Rosen IM. Obstructive sleep apnea in adults. N Engl J Med. 2019;380(15):1442–9.
19. Bitners AC, Arens R. Evaluation and management of children with obstructive sleep apnea syndrome. Lung. 2020;198(2):257–70.
20. Marcus CL, Brooks LJ, Draper KA, et al. Diagnosis and management of childhood obstructive sleep apnea syndrome. Pediatrics. 2012;130(3):e714–55.
21. Vos WG, De Backer WA, Verhulst SL. Correlation between the severity of sleep apnea and upper airway morphology in pediatric and adult patients. Curr Opin Allergy Clin Immunol. 2010;10(1):26–33.
22. Thomas S, Patel S, Gummalla P, Tablizo MA, Kier C. You cannot hit snooze on OSA: sequelae of pediatric obstructive sleep apnea. Children. 2022;9(2)

23. Alsubie HS, BaHammam AS. Obstructive sleep apnoea: children are not little adults. Paediatr Respir Rev. 2017;21:72–9.
24. Hardy Tabet C, Lopez-Bushnell K. Sleep, snoring, and surgery: OSA screening matters. J Perianesth Nurs. 2018;33(6):790–800.
25. Nagappa M, Liao P, Wong J, et al. Validation of the STOP-Bang questionnaire as a screening tool for obstructive sleep apnea among different populations: a systematic review and meta-analysis. PLoS One. 2015;10(12):e0143697.
26. Chervin RD, Hedger K, Dillon JE, Pituch KJ. Pediatric sleep questionnaire (PSQ): validity and reliability of scales for sleep-disordered breathing, snoring, sleepiness, and behavioral problems. Sleep Med. 2000;1(1):21–32.
27. Parajuli S, Tiwari R, Clark DF, Mandelbrot DA, Djamali A, Casey K. Sleep disorders: serious threats among kidney transplant recipients. Transplant Rev (Orlando). 2019;33(1):9–16.

Chapter 65
Transplanted Kidney Failure After Prolonged Kidney Graft Survival

Abish Kharel and Sandesh Parajuli

Introduction

After transplantation, prolonging kidney graft survival becomes the goal of care. Increasing long-term graft survival would reduce the number of retransplantations, reduce patients returning to dialysis, and therefore increase available kidneys to those awaiting first transplantation. Our patient case and discussion will review determinants of prolonged survival over the pre-transplantation and post-transplantation periods.

Patient History

A 65-year-old man with a history of end-stage kidney disease due to congenital nephropathy underwent a deceased-donor kidney transplant in 1988. Post-transplantation complications included: early acute rejection 35 days post-transplant, which was treated with prednisone, and CMV viral infection in 1990 treated with ganciclovir. When followed in 2020 for a regular post-transplant follow-up, his maintenance immunosuppression consisted of prednisone and cyclosporine. Other

A. Kharel (✉)
University of Wisconsin-Madison School of Medicine and Public Health,
Madison, WI, USA
e-mail: kharel2@wisc.edu

S. Parajuli
Department of Medicine, Division of Nephrology, University of Wisconsin-Madison School
of Medicine and Public Health, Madison, WI, USA
e-mail: sparajuli@medicine.wisc.edu

© The Author(s), under exclusive license to Springer Nature
Switzerland AG 2022
F. Aziz, S. Parajuli (eds.), *Complications in Kidney Transplantation*,
https://doi.org/10.1007/978-3-031-13569-9_65

medications included amlodipine, atenolol, and simvastatin for other comorbidities and hypertension and hyperlipidemia.

Question 1

What will be the most likely cause of graft failure in this man?

A. Rejection.
B. Death with a functioning graft.
C. Cyclosporine toxicity.
D. BK nephropathy.

The correct answer is B.

Death is the leading cause of graft failure. Specifically, cardiovascular disease is the most common cause of death with a functioning graft. Individual risk factors such as obesity, hyperlipidemia, hypertension, and diabetes are highly prevalent in kidney transplant recipients resulting in cumulative burden over time [1]. Therefore, pharmacologic and nonpharmacologic interventions such as exercise, weight loss, and dietary restrictions are recommended. In addition, all adults and adolescents are recommended to be screened for dyslipidemia regularly and after adjusting immunosuppressive medications. Graft failure due to rejection is also a major contributor to graft failure, and hence the search for newer modalities of screening and treatment is ongoing. Many immunosuppressive agents have well-described side effects, including cyclosporine; however, it is not a major contributor to graft failure. BK nephropathy is a complication due to BK virus infection in transplant patients managed with viremia screening and immunosuppression reductions. However, most BK nephropathy happens usually within the first 1–2 years of transplant.

Patient Course

The patient returns to your office, in 2021 (33 years post-transplantation), for routine post-transplant follow-up. The creatinine was elevated at 2.2 mg/dL (baseline 1.2–1.4 mg/dL). An allograft biopsy was performed the next week, which showed chronic active antibody-mediated rejection (ABMR), with severe chronic changes. The patient was started treatment with intravenous immunoglobulin (IVIG) and steroid taper. Two weeks later, the patient still had persistently elevated creatinine at 2.8 mg/dL, with eGFR of 19.

Question 2

Given the concern for allograft failure, what is the best treatment option for this patient going forward?

A. Retransplantation.
B. Dialysis.
C. Increase immunosuppression.
D. No changes to the treatment plan.

The correct answer is A.

Retransplanting, especially preemptively after graft failure, has a similar survival rate compared to first transplantation and less adverse outcomes such as acute rejection, delayed graft functioning, and death with functioning graft when compared to patients who undergo retransplantation after a period of dialysis. Reinitiation of dialysis is an option for patients in immediate need or those not a candidate for retransplantation. However, restarting dialysis after graft failure has shown to have a higher mortality risk compared to retransplantation [2]. Immunosuppression management is challenging after allograft failure. For patients planning on retransplantation, maintenance of low dose immunosuppression is recommended for the risk of de novo allosensitization. However, in patients with significant comorbid conditions and ineligibility for retransplantation, immunosuppression withdrawal should be considered [2].

Discussion

Kidney transplantation remains the treatment of choice for patients with End-Stage Kidney Disease (ESKD). Compared to dialysis, successful transplantation yields an improved quality of life and a lower mortality risk [3, 4]. However, after many years, most kidney grafts fail. Despite excellent 1-year kidney graft survival, the long-term graft survival rate remains low, improving over time. The 10-year overall graft survival rate of deceased-donor kidney transplants from 1996 to 1999 was 42.3% and increased to 53.6% from 2008 to 2011 [5] (Fig. 65.1).

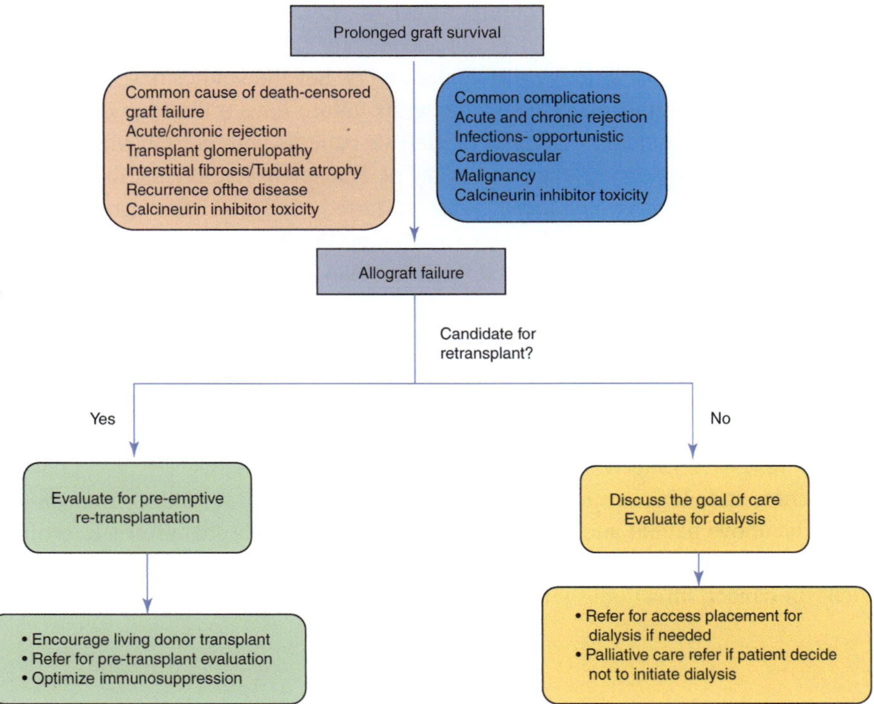

Fig. 65.1 Approach to the graft failure after prolonged kidney graft survival

There are multiple determinants of long-term graft survival over the pre-transplantation and post-transplantation periods. In the pre-transplantation period, the risk of graft rejection and patient mortality are reduced by cross-matching techniques and prudent use of engrafting. New data from 2019 shows that for DDKT, 5-year graft survival was 64.6% with Kidney Donor Profile Index (KDPI) > 85%, 82.1% with KDPI 21–35%, and 83.9% with KDPI $\leq$ 20 [6]. Thus, the challenge is to balance these variables while addressing the increasing need for transplantation. Increased degree of Human Leukocyte Antigen (HLA) mismatching has been associated with a 13% higher risk of graft failure with one HLA mismatch and 64% higher risk with six HLA mismatch [7]. New obstacles during the post-transplant period include delayed graft function, episodes of acute rejection, viral infections, and metabolic comorbidities, including hypertension, hyperlipidemia, cancer, and cardiovascular disease. The leading causes of death after the first year post-transplantation are malignancies (29%), cardiovascular disease (23%), and infections (12%) [5]. Malignancies in KTRs are three to five times higher than in the general population [8]. Skin cancers, especially squamous cell and basal cell carcinomas, are the most common. Overall cardiovascular mortality is approximately two times higher in KTRs compared to the general population [9]. Hypertension and hyperlipidemia are established risk factors for atherosclerosis and subsequently impact long-term graft survival. Infection risks are much higher in KTRs than in the general population [5, 8]. Cytomegalovirus infection is the most common opportunistic infection after transplantation and a risk factor for acute rejection and graft failure [5]. However, effective antiviral treatment is available, and therefore prevention, early recognition, and treatment are essential.

Most KTRs, after allograft failure, either return to dialysis or are re-listed for transplantation. Currently, failed grafts account for 5% of the dialysis population and 15% waitlisted for kidney transplantation [2]. Several studies have highlighted that patients who return to dialysis after graft failure have a higher mortality rate than patients with functioning grafts or dialysis patients with no transplantation. In one study analyzing the Scientific Registry of Transplant Recipients, the mortality risk was 78% higher in those who restarted dialysis after graft failure. Retransplantation offers significantly lower mortality rates compared to dialysis. Furthermore, preemptive transplantation rather than transplantation after a period of dialysis has shown better overall graft and patient survival. In a recent analysis of US Renal Data System report of 17,584-second KTRs, those who had preemptive retransplanting had less acute rejection (12% versus 16%; $p < 0.0001$), delayed graft function (DGF) (8% versus 23%; $p < 0.0001$), and lower death with functioning graft [10].

The long-term survival of kidney transplantation remains a major goal for researchers and clinicians to address the increasing demand for kidney transplantation. The above patient and review of the literature highlight that efforts to prolong graft survival should focus on better organ quality and early prevention and treatment for cancer, infections, and cardiovascular diseases.

References

1. US Renal Data System. In: Bethesda MD, editor. USRDS 2008 annual data report: atlas of chronic kidney disease and end-stage renal disease in the United States. National Institutes of Health, National Institute of Diabetes and Digestive and Kidney Diseases; 2008.
2. Fiorentino M, Gallo P, Giliberti M, Colucci V, Schena A, Stallone G, Gesualdo L, Castellano G. Management of patients with a failed kidney transplant: what should we do? Clin Kidney J. 2021;14(1):98–106. https://doi.org/10.1093/ckj/sfaa094.
3. Fiebiger W, Mitterbauer C, Oberbauer R. Health-related quality of life outcomes after kidney transplantation. Health Qual Life Outcomes. 2004;2:2.
4. Parajuli S, Clark DF, Djamali A. Is kidney transplantation a better state of CKD? Impact on diagnosis and management. Adv Chronic Kidney Dis. 2016;23:287–94.
5. Hariharan S, et al. Long-term survival after kidney transplantation. NEJM. 2021;385(8):729–43. https://doi.org/10.1056/NEJMra2014530.
6. Hart A, Lentine KL, Smith JM, Miller JM, Skeans MA, Prentice M, Robinson A, Foutz J, Booker SE, Israni AK, Hirose R, Snyder JJ. OPTN/SRTR 2019 annual data report: kidney. Am J Transplant. 2021;21:21–137. https://doi.org/10.1111/ajt.16502.
7. Williams RC, et al. The risk of transplant failure with HLA mismatch in first adult kidney allografts from deceased donors. Transplantation. 2016;100(5):1094–102. https://doi.org/10.1097/TP.0000000000001115.
8. Parajuli S, et al. Characteristics and outcomes of kidney transplant recipients with a functioning graft for more than 25 years. Kidney diseases. 2018;4(4):255–61. https://doi.org/10.1159/000491575.
9. Sarnak MJ, Levey AS. Cardiovascular disease and chronic renal disease: a new paradigm. Am J Kidney Dis. 2000;35(4 suppl 1):S117–31.
10. United S renal data system. In: Bethesda MD, editor. USRDS 2011 annual data report. National Institutes of Health, National Institute of Diabetes and Digestive and Kidney Diseases; 2015.

Chapter 66
Failed Allograft Due to Persistent BKV

Sriram Sriperumbuduri and Bushra Syed

Introduction

BK virus nephropathy (BKVN) is an opportunistic infection in the post-kidney transplantation period with a prevalence of up to 3–5% [1]. It can lead to allograft dysfunction, ureteral strictures, de novo DSA due to the reduction of immunosuppression, graft rejection, and rarely urological malignancies. The net state of immunosuppression is the most important risk factor for BKVN, and there is a higher risk with the use of anti-thymocyte globulin (ATG) and mycophenolate mofetil (MMF) or tacrolimus [2]. Prior allograft loss attributed to BKVN is not a contraindication for re-transplantation [3, 4]. We will explore some of the considerations in retransplantation amongst this patient population.

Case

A 58-year-old male with ESKD secondary to diabetic nephropathy had a deceased donor kidney transplant. He had a cPRA of 0 and a negative HLA cross match. A cumulative dose of 4.5 mg/kg of thymoglobulin was used for induction. Maintenance immunosuppression included tacrolimus with a target trough of 6–8 ng/mL, CellCept (MMF) 1 g twice daily, and prednisone 5 mg daily. His serum creatinine (Cr) nadir was 1.2 mg/dL.

S. Sriperumbuduri · B. Syed (✉)
University of Mississippi Medical Center, Jackson, MS, USA
e-mail: ssriperumbuduri@umc.edu; bsyed@umc.edu

© The Author(s), under exclusive license to Springer Nature Switzerland AG 2022

F. Aziz, S. Parajuli (eds.), *Complications in Kidney Transplantation*,
https://doi.org/10.1007/978-3-031-13569-9_66

Three months post-transplant, Cr increased to 1.6 mg/dL. Evaluation showed elevated serum BKV PCR titer at 109,000 copies/mL. Despite the discontinuation of MMF and lowering of tacrolimus dose, serum BKV titer worsened to 244,000 copies/mL and Cr to 2 mg/dL. Tacrolimus was switched to everolimus, and IV immunoglobulin was started every 2 weeks for four doses. Subsequently, serum BKV titer decreased to 15,700 copies/mL, and Cr improved to 1.6 mg/dL.

After 8 months of stable renal function, Cr again worsened to 2.3 mg/dL, and serum BKV titer had risen to 106,000 copies/mL. Kidney graft biopsy showed class 3 BK virus nephropathy with 60% interstitial fibrosis. Four doses of intravenous cidofovir were given with a decline in serum BKV titer to 50,000 copies/mL. The Cr continued to worsen despite this, and he was initiated on hemodialysis 18 months post-transplant. Subsequently, all the immunosuppression was discontinued.

He returned to the transplant clinic 6 months after reinitiating dialysis to be re-evaluated for a second kidney transplant.

Question 1

Which of the following factors in the inter-transplant period will reduce the risk of recurrence of BKVN in the second transplant?

A. Undetectable BKV PCR at time of retransplantation.
B. Allograft nephrectomy.
C. Discontinuation of all immunosuppression while he is on dialysis.
D. A & C.

The correct answer is D.

Achieving clearance of BK viremia is the ideal target prior to retransplant to decrease the risk of viral recurrence. The reactivation of BK virus of recipient origin is a dominant mechanism of recurrent disease after retransplant [5, 6]. Continuing immunosuppression after the graft failure was shown to be associated with a higher risk of viral reactivation [7]. Although some studies have highlighted the donor origin of the virus, no conclusive data exist to suggest routine graft nephrectomy. Nephrectomy may facilitate the temporary cessation of immunosuppression, allowing specific T-cell immune responses to clear the virus, with decreased risk of reactivation after the retransplant.

Question 2

What immunosuppression options are available for retransplantation following graft loss from BKVN?

A. Use of non-depleting agents for induction in the setting of low allosensitization.
B. Transitioning from CNI to mTOR for maintenance immunosuppression.
C. Do not use cell depleting agents regardless of the degree of allosensitization.
D. A &B.

The correct answer is D.

The choice of induction agent in the setting of re-transplant is influenced by the BK viral load, previous rejection episodes, and the presence of donor-specific antibodies (DSAs). Persistent BK viral titers should prompt the use of non-depleting induction therapy [8, 9]. A recent prospective study looking at the conversion from standard dose calcineurin inhibitors (CNI) and MMF to everolimus and reduced exposure CNI following biopsy-proven BKVN has shown benefit with the combined endpoint graft loss and 57% eGFR reduction ($p = 0.02$) [10].

Discussion

Graft loss due to BKVN is not a contraindication for retransplantation. Available data is convincing for good graft outcomes with decreased risk of BK virus recurrence following the retransplant, as shown in Table 66.1. Recurrence risk can be mitigated by assuring clearance of viremia before retransplantation [5, 6], minimization of immunosuppression in the inter-transplant period [7], and selecting an induction and maintenance immunosuppression regimen that best balances the risk of recurrence with the risk of rejection [8–10].

There are no set guidelines for the optimal immunosuppression regimen in this setting, and an individualized approach must be adopted. Some considered factors include recipient BK serostatus, recipient age, prior sensitization and number of rejection episodes, and degree of HLA mismatch at the time of retransplantation. Even though existing data supports retransplantation, more research is required to clarify the optimal peri-transplant immunosuppression options to maximize allograft survival.

Table 66.1 Table showing the various studies that looked at graft survival and BKVN following retransplant with initial allograft failure due to BKVN

Study	No. of subjects	The median duration of follow up	Graft survival after retransplantation	No. of cases of recurrent BK virus reactivation, including viruria, viremia, and BKVN- n (%)	Graft failures due to BKVN- n (%)
Leeaphorn et al. [8]	341	4.7 years	90.6% at 5 years	Data not available	7 (15.2%)
Dharnidharka et al. [9]	126	Follow between 2004 and 2009	93.6% at 3 years	22 (17.6%)	1 (0.79%)
Duvuru et al. [5]	31	30 months	Data not available	11 (35.4%)- Viruria-5, Viremia-6. 2 developed BKVN	Nil
Dong et al. [7]	13	5.9 years	92.3% at the end of study period	1 (7.7%)	Nil

References

1. Myint TM, Chong CHY, Wyld M, Nankivell B, Kable K, Wong G. Polyoma BK virus in kidney transplant recipients: screening, monitoring, and management. Transplantation. 2022;106(1):e76–89.
2. Dharnidharka VR, Cherikh WS, Abbott KC. An OPTN analysis of national registry data on treatment of BK virus allograft nephropathy in the United States. Transplantation. 2009;87(7):1019–26.
3. Hirsch HH, Randhawa PS, AST Infectious diseases Community of Practice. BK polyomavirus in solid organ transplantation-guidelines from the American society of transplantation infectious diseases community of practice. Clin Transpl. 2019;33(9):e13528.
4. Nguyen K, Diamond A, Carlo AD, Karhadkar S. Characterization of kidney Retransplantation following graft failure due to BK virus nephropathy. J Surg Res. 2021;269:110–8.
5. Geetha D, Sozio SM, Ghanta M, et al. Results of repeat renal transplantation after graft loss from BK virus nephropathy. Transplantation. 2011;92(7):781–6.
6. Hirsch HH, Knowles W, Dickenmann M, et al. Prospective study of polyomavirus type BK replication and nephropathy in renal-transplant recipients. N Engl J Med. 2002;347(7):488–96.
7. Dong R, Shetty A, Tambur AR, Ison MG. Outcomes of repeat kidney transplantation following prior graft failure secondary to BK nephropathy: a single-center retrospective study. Transpl Infect Dis. 2021;23(4):e13672.
8. Leeaphorn N, Thongprayoon C, Chon WJ, Cummings LS, Mao MA, Cheungpasitporn W. Outcomes of kidney retransplantation after graft loss as a result of BK virus nephropathy in the era of newer immunosuppressant agents. Am J Transplant. 2020;20(5):1334–40.
9. Dharnidharka VR, Cherikh WS, Neff R, Cheng Y, Abbott KC. Retransplantation after BK virus nephropathy in prior kidney transplant: an OPTN database analysis. Am J Transplant. 2010;10(5):1312–5.
10. Bussalino E, Marsano L, Parodi A, et al. Everolimus for BKV nephropathy in kidney transplant recipients: a prospective, controlled study. J Nephrol. 2021;34(2):531–8.

Chapter 67
Retransplantation After Kidney Graft Failure Due to BK Polyomavirus Nephropathy

Isabel Breyer and Sandesh Parajuli

Introduction

The topic of repeat transplantation after graft loss due to BK nephropathy (BKN) is important, as clinicians are managing the care of an increasing number of patients with BKN in this era of potent immunosuppressive use. A recent study estimates that 750–1500 kidney transplants in the US develop BKN each year, with 50–80% of these patients progressing to graft failure [1]. The efficacy, safety, and optimization of retransplantation in this patient population are an important area of ongoing research.

Patient History

A 52-year-old man with a history of stage IV CKD due to autosomal dominant polycystic kidney disease underwent bilateral native nephrectomies and living-related donor kidney transplantation. He was not on dialysis and was making normal amounts of urine. He did not have preformed donor-specific antibodies, and his calculated panel reactive antibody (cPRA) was 0% at the time of transplant. The patient received alemtuzumab for induction and underwent early steroid withdrawal. He was discharged on an immunosuppressive maintenance regimen of tacrolimus 6 mg BID and mycophenolic acid 720 mg BID. His postoperative course was complicated by delayed graft function.

I. Breyer (✉) · S. Parajuli
Division of Nephrology, Department of Medicine, University of Wisconsin School of Medicine and Public Health, Madison, WI, USA
e-mail: ibreyer@wisc.edu; sparajuli@medicine.wisc.edu

© The Author(s), under exclusive license to Springer Nature Switzerland AG 2022
F. Aziz, S. Parajuli (eds.), *Complications in Kidney Transplantation*,
https://doi.org/10.1007/978-3-031-13569-9_67

433

This patient's post-transplant course was further complicated by numerous hospital admissions for acute kidney injury, antibody-mediated rejection (ABMR), and COVID-19 pneumonia. Shortly after these events, routine lab monitoring revealed BK polyomavirus infection approximately 13 months post-transplant. BK viremia was diagnosed with a BK plasma viral load of 5.5 $\log_{10}$ copies/mL (306,000 copies/mL). Serum creatinine and eGFR were 2.64 mg/dL and 25 mL/min/1.73 m², respectively.

In response to the diagnosis of BK viremia, the patient's mycophenolic acid was decreased to 360 mg BID. Additionally, a kidney biopsy was performed, which showed evidence of both ABMR and BKN.

Question 1

In the setting of concurrent BKN and rejection, which of the following treatments take priority?

A. Reduce immunosuppressive regimen.
B. Intravenous immunoglobulin (IVIG) and corticosteroids.
C. No change in immunosuppression.

The correct answer is B.

In the setting of both acute rejection and BKN, the rejection episode must take priority and be treated following rejection protocols [2]. Once there is evidence that the rejection episode has responded to treatment, the immunosuppressive regimen may be reduced to allow BK-specific immune reconstitution and viral clearance.

Additional Clinical Course

After the biopsy findings, the rejection episode was treated with dexamethasone and IVIG, and the immunosuppressive regimen was kept the same.

Approximately 5 weeks after the treatment of rejection, the patient's BK plasma viral load peaked at 5.9 $\log_{10}$ copies/mL (849,000 copies/mL). Serum creatinine and eGFR were 3.75 mg/dL and 17 mL/min/1.73 m², respectively. Despite treatment for his most recent episode of rejection, the patient's kidney function did not recover, and his graft began to fail due to both rejection and BKN. His BK viremia persisted, as the immunosuppressive regimen was challenging to adjust given the concurrent graft rejection. He was referred for another transplant, pending BK viral clearance.

At the time of the last follow-up, the patient has achieved BK viral clearance, has resumed dialysis, and a living donor workup is being completed for retransplantation.

Question 2

After retransplantation, what is the risk that this patient's new graft will again fail due to BKN?

A. Less than 5%.
B. 5–10%

C. 15–20%
D. 25–30%.

The correct answer is A.

Results from two large studies discussed below suggest that retransplantation after graft loss due to BKN is safe and effective, as only 2% of patients experienced the loss of the second graft due to BKN [3, 4].

In a large study by Leeaphorn et al., patients who underwent retransplantation after graft loss due to BKN experienced good outcomes [3]. Overall, 13.5% of patients had their second graft fail during the follow-up period (4.70 year median follow-up time), and 15.2% of these grafts failed due to BKN once again. In total, 2.1% (7 of 341) of patients experienced repeated graft failure due to BKN. This is in comparison to patients whose first graft failed for reasons other than BKN, of which 18.5% had their second graft fail during follow-up, and only 2.2% of the second failures were due to BKN. Although there was a greater risk of repeat graft failure due to BKN in patients whose first failure was due to BKN, this group experienced less graft failure overall than the other group, and there were no significant differences in acute rejection or patient survival between the two groups.

In another large study by Nguyen et al., information from 495 patients who underwent retransplantation after graft failure due to BKN over the past 30 years was collected from the OPTN/UNOS database and analyzed [4]. Graft failure was noted in 63 (12.7%) patients, of which 10 patients experienced repeat graft failure due to BKN. In total, 2.0% (10 of 495) of patients again experienced graft failure due to BKN upon retransplantation. Additionally, the repeat transplant provided patients with a longer graft lifespan on average (10.44 years) than the original transplant, which failed due to BKN did (3.70 years), and rates of rejection were lower in the repeat transplants compared to the originals. The findings of this study support retransplantation after graft failure due to BKN. Table 67.1 summarizes the findings of these two large studies and two additional smaller studies.

While there is a risk of repeat graft failure due to BKN after retransplantation, there may be ways to optimize patients prior to retransplantation to lower this risk. For example, Geetha et al. found that patients who achieved BK viral clearance prior to retransplantation were less likely to experience BK viral replication post-transplant [5]. BK viral clearance is achieved via the reduction in immunosuppression ± allograft nephrectomy. In cases where allograft nephrectomy is performed, there is the added benefit of being able to completely hold immunosuppression to

Table 67.1 Studies of retransplantation after graft loss due to BKN

Reference	Publication year	Sample size retransplanted	Repeat graft failure due to BKN (%)
Nguyen et al. [4]	2021	495	2.0
Leeaphorn et al. [3]	2020	341	2.1
Dharnidharka et al. [7]	2010	126	0.008
Ramos et al. [8]	2004	10	0

allow the patient to develop BK-specific immunity prior to their retransplantation [6]. Thus, retransplantation after graft loss due to BKN is preferably done post-BK viral clearance.

Multiple studies are in agreement that retransplantation after graft loss due to BKN is safe and effective for the majority of patients. Recent guidelines from the American Society of Transplantation Infectious Diseases Community of Practice support retransplantation after graft loss due to BKN in the setting of BK viral clearance and independent of allograft nephrectomy [2]. In cases where viral clearance cannot be achieved, and BK viremia is persistent, the guidelines recommend a decline in the viral load of at least 2 $\log_{10}$ copies/mL prior to retransplantation.

In conclusion, the risk of a second graft failure due to BKN following retransplantation for graft loss due to BKN is small, approximately 2.0% in the large studies that have been conducted. Therefore, patients such as the one presented in this chapter should be recommended for retransplantation as they are likely to experience favorable outcomes. BK viral clearance should be achieved prior to retransplantation in order to optimize outcomes, but whether or not allograft nephrectomy is necessary remains unclear.

References

1. Kotla SK, Kadambi PV, Hendricks AR, Rojas R. BK polyomavirus-pathogen, paradigm, and puzzle. Nephrol Dial Transplant. 2021;36(4):587–93. https://doi.org/10.1093/ndt/gfz273.
2. Hirsch HH, Randhawa PS, Practice AIDCo. BK polyomavirus in solid organ transplantation-Guidelines from the American Society of Transplantation Infectious Diseases Community of Practice. Clin Transplant. 2019;33(9):e13528. https://doi.org/10.1111/ctr.13528.
3. Leeaphorn N, Thongprayoon C, Chon WJ, Cummings LS, Mao MA, Cheungpasitporn W. Outcomes of kidney retransplantation after graft loss as a result of BK virus nephropathy in the era of newer immunosuppressant agents. Am J Transplant. 2020;20(5):1334–40. https://doi.org/10.1111/ajt.15723.
4. Nguyen K, Diamond A, Carlo AD, Karhadkar S. Characterization of kidney Retransplantation following graft failure due to BK virus nephropathy. J Surg Res. 2021;269:110–8. https://doi.org/10.1016/j.jss.2021.07.047.
5. Geetha D, Sozio SM, Ghanta M, et al. Results of repeat renal transplantation after graft loss from BK virus nephropathy. Transplantation. 2011;92(7):781–6. https://doi.org/10.1097/TP.0b013e31822d08c1.
6. Dong R, Shetty A, Tambur AR, Ison MG. Outcomes of repeat kidney transplantation following prior graft failure secondary to BK nephropathy: a single-center retrospective study. Transpl Infect Dis. 2021;23(4):e13672. https://doi.org/10.1111/tid.13672.
7. Dharnidharka VR, Cherikh WS, Neff R, Cheng Y, Abbott KC. Retransplantation after BK virus nephropathy in prior kidney transplant: an OPTN database analysis. Am J Transplant. 2010;10(5):1312–5. https://doi.org/10.1111/j.1600-6143.2010.03083.x.
8. Ramos E, Vincenti F, Lu WX, et al. Retransplantation in patients with graft loss caused by polyoma virus nephropathy. Transplantation. 2004;77(1):131–3. https://doi.org/10.1097/01.TP.0000095898.40458.68.

Chapter 68
Sensitization After Failed Kidney Transhplant

Douglas J. Norman

Introduction

It is estimated that failed kidney grafts account for 5% of the dialysis population and 15% of the patients waitlisted for kidney transplantation. If a living donor is not available, these patients have to wait for many years before receiving another transplant. All of these recipients would have been on immunosuppressive medication at the time of graft failure. However, the continuation or discontinuation of immunosuppression following a failed kidney transplant is controversial. Retained, failed kidney allografts in the absence of immunosuppression can lead to sensitization and graft intolerance syndrome. Graft intolerance syndrome can cause a systemic inflammatory state that usually requires an allograft nephrectomy. Even after a kidney allograft has been removed, it is not clear whether and for how prolonged immunosuppression should be continued. Allograft tissue cannot be removed completely, and there is usually a small donor vessel retained. We will discuss various approaches after failed kidney allograft based on this case.

Patient History

The patient is a 22-year-old woman who developed steroid-sensitive nephrotic syndrome at two. At age 17, her kidney disease had become resistant to steroids, tacrolimus, and mycophenolate, and a kidney biopsy showed FSGS. She began peritoneal dialysis that year and received 1 unit of packed red blood cells. Later that year, she received a deceased donor kidney transplant. The donor was standard criteria,

D. J. Norman (✉)
Oregon Health and Science University, Portland, OR, USA
e-mail: normand@ohsu.edu

© The Author(s), under exclusive license to Springer Nature Switzerland AG 2022

F. Aziz, S. Parajuli (eds.), *Complications in Kidney Transplantation*,
https://doi.org/10.1007/978-3-031-13569-9_68

437

Public Health Service (PHS) low risk, and the Kidney Donor Profile Index (KDPI) was 14%. The cold ischemia time was 14.5 h. The HLA mismatch was 4 (1 A, 2 B, and 1 DR). Donor and recipient were both CMV and EBV seropositive.

At the time of transplant, the patient's HLA Class I and II panel reactive antibodies (PRAs) were both 0%, and the calculated PRA (cPRA) based on a Luminex single antigen bead assay was also 0%. A thrombophilia workup before the transplant was negative.

Immunosuppression included basiliximab for induction and tacrolimus, mycophenolate, and prednisone for maintenance. The new kidney made urine for a few hours following the transplant, but the patient became anuric. A Doppler ultrasound showed no arterial blood flow. Surgical exploration found an allograft renal artery thrombosis. The pathologic diagnosis was renal arterial thrombosis and no other abnormalities. Specifically, there was no evidence of recurrent FSGS. A discussion ensued regarding managing immunosuppression in this patient.

Question 1

What is the most appropriate way to manage immunosuppression following a failed kidney transplant?

A. Stop all immunosuppression immediately because the kidney has failed.
B. Continue immunosuppression indefinitely because a failed kidney transplant left in place can lead to anti-HLA sensitization in the recipient.
C. Remove the kidney and stop immunosuppression immediately since there is no longer donor tissue that can stimulate anti-HLA antibody production.
D. Remove the kidney and maintain immunosuppression because there is always some donor tissue that remains.
E. Weigh the risks and benefits of maintaining or discontinuing immunosuppression based on whether the patient is a candidate for another transplant and how long it is likely that the patient will wait for another transplant.

The correct answer is E.

Weigh the risks and benefits of maintaining immunosuppression. The continuation of immunosuppression following a failed kidney transplant is controversial [1]. Retained, rejected kidney transplants in the absence of immunosuppression can lead to sensitization and graft intolerance syndrome [2]. Graft intolerance syndrome can cause a systemic inflammatory state that usually requires an allograft nephrectomy [3]. After a kidney allograft has been removed, it is not clear whether and for how prolonged immunosuppression should be continued. Allograft tissue cannot be removed completely, and there is usually a small donor vessel retained [4].

Further Course

The kidney was removed at surgical exploration because the arterial thrombosis was extensive, and blood flow could not be restored. The patient required a total of 5 units of packed red blood cells, given on postoperative days, 2, 5, 10, 14, and 23, due to hemoglobin that repeatedly dropped to between 6.0 and 6.5 mg/dL.

Prednisone was stopped on postoperative day 40 to promote wound healing, and tacrolimus (1 mg twice daily) and mycophenolate (750 mg twice daily) were maintained. The plan was to maintain immunosuppression until at least 4 weeks after the final red blood cell transfusion. On a postoperative day 53 (30 days after the last transfusion), the mycophenolate was reduced to 250 mg twice daily, and the tacrolimus dose was kept at 1 mg twice daily. A serum sample obtained on postoperative day 57 demonstrated that her HLA Class I and II PRAs were 0%. The single antigen bead assay was negative for any anti-HLA antibodies.

On postoperative day 60, she was given another 2 units of packed red blood cells for hemoglobin that had again dropped to 6.0 mg/dL. The mycophenolate was resumed at 750 mg twice daily. The tacrolimus level on postoperative day 65 was 4.6 ng/mL.

An immunosuppression taper began on a postoperative day 90 (4 weeks after the last blood transfusion). The mycophenolate was reduced to zero over 6 weeks, and the tacrolimus was reduced to zero after an additional 4 weeks. Immunosuppression withdrawal spanned 10 weeks.

Six months after her first transplant, she was referred for a second transplant. During that evaluation, which was 30 days after completing immunosuppression withdrawal, the HLA Class I PRA was 71%, and Class II was 96%. The calculated cPRA based on the single antigen bead assay was 100%.

Question 2

What is the likely cause of this patient's anti-HLA antibody sensitization?

A. Multiple blood transfusions following kidney transplantation and removing all immunosuppression.
B. Removing prednisone on postoperative day 40 to help wound healing.
C. Removing the kidney at graft loss because a retained kidney will act as a sponge and sop up any antibodies that might be produced.
D. Patient likely became pregnant in the intervening months, and pregnancy is known to cause anti-HLA antibody production.
E. The antibodies are likely to be autoantibodies and should not be considered important.

The correct answer is A.

Multiple blood transfusions following a kidney transplant and removal of immunosuppression. The usual causes of anti-HLA antibody production are previous transplants, blood transfusions, and prior pregnancies [5]. The patient had never been pregnant but required many blood transfusions. In retrospect, immunosuppression should have been extended for longer and probably maintained indefinitely even though the kidney was removed at transplant. Another consideration for maintaining immunosuppression is the fact that the patient is young and likely to be re-transplanted relatively quickly. Maintaining immunosuppression while on dialysis would not have put her at significant risk for infection.

Further Course

She was activated on the deceased donor waiting list. Two months later, she was transplanted with a second deceased donor kidney. This was a standard criteria, KDPI 11% imported donor kidney with a zero antigen HLA mismatch (0 HLA A, 0 HLA B, 0 HLA DR). The cold ischemia time was 23 h. The T, B, and antiglobulin cytotoxic cross matches were negative, and the Flow T and B cell cross matches were negative.

Question 3

Why was she transplanted so quickly after listing for a second transplant even though she was highly sensitized?

A. Patients who lose a kidney allograft within 90 days after transplant can maintain their status on the waiting list and the waiting time points they had accrued.
B. The Organ Procurement and Transplantation Network (OPTN) rules prioritize patients with a zero antigen mismatch with a potential donor from anywhere in the U.S.
C. Transplant centers are required to list in the OPTN computer (UNet) the antigens against which patients have developed antibodies, so donors with those antigens are never offered to those patients.
D. The OPTN prioritizes patients with a cPRA of 100% by giving them a large number of points for kidney allocation when a donor that lacks all of the unacceptable antigens put into UNet is identified.
E. All of the above.

The answer is E.

Since patients often wait for several years for a transplant, the OPTN allows waiting time points to be maintained if a kidney fails within 90 days after transplant. This is considered to be out of the control of the patient. Patients with a zero antigen mismatch (A, B, DR) with a potential donor receive a national priority. Kidneys that are a zero mismatch with a patient must be shipped to that patient regardless of where in the U.S. the donor resides. The Kidney Allocation System (KAS) implemented by the OPTN in December 2014 made several changes that benefit sensitized patients. First, unacceptable antigens, based on anti-HLA antibody analysis, must be entered into UNet to calculate the PRA. As a result, donors with HLA antigens considered unacceptable are never offered to patients. A patient with a cPRA of 100% has a multitude of antigens that are deemed unacceptable; therefore, it is extremely unlikely a donor could be found in a small local donor pool. The new KAS prioritizes patients with a cPRA of 100%, thus significantly expanding a pool of potential donors. When a donor is identified who has none of the unacceptable antigens listed in UNet for a patient with a CPRA of 100%, that donor kidney must be sent to the patient's transplant center if no other patients are considered higher priority based on other determinants of allocation. As a result of all of these OPTN rules (6), our patient was given the highest priority for an excellent and well-matched imported kidney.

Further Course

Immunosuppression was thymoglobulin for induction, and tacrolimus, mycophenolate, and prednisone were given for maintenance. Sera were tested for donor-specific antibodies weekly × 4 and at 3 and 12 months posttransplant using single antigen beads, and none was found. Surveillance biopsies at 3 and 12 months after transplant showed no rejection, no evidence of recurrent FSGS, and minimal nonspecific changes. The serum creatinine was 0.88 mg/dL at 3 months and 0.82 mg/dL at 3 years posttransplant. While this patient suffered the complications of graft thrombosis and sensitization after her first transplant, she benefitted from an organ allocation system that prioritizes highly sensitized patients who are well-matched with a potential deceased donor; therefore, she was able to receive a well-matched second transplant.

Discussion

This patient developed anti-HLA antibodies despite removing her failed graft and continuing full dose immunosuppression for 4 weeks after her last transfusion, and then tapering off immunosuppression slowly over 10 weeks. While on immunosuppression, no anti-HLA antibodies developed despite having a failed kidney and receiving several transfusions. After tapering immunosuppression, she became highly sensitized. Immunosuppression should have been kept on longer or not stopped.

At our center, we prefer to continue immunosuppression after a kidney fails because we believe that a retained rejected kidney transplant is likely to cause sensitization, graft intolerance syndrome, or both. Our policy has also been to give about 4 weeks of immunosuppression to patients who receive blood transfusions before transplant to minimize the risk of sensitization. Continuing immunosuppression after a kidney fails remains a controversial issue because of the risks of immunosuppression for a dialysis patient. The decision about maintaining immunosuppression should be based on the likelihood that a patient will be a candidate for another transplant and the amount of time a patient will wait for another transplant. If a patient has a living donor at our center, we will continue triple immunosuppression to ensure no anti-HLA antibodies will develop. If a patient is placed on a waiting list, we will taper one of the agents (usually the calcineurin inhibitor) and maintain the patient on dual therapy. When the kidney is explanted, we generally have removed immunosuppression. This case suggests that, even after removing a failed graft, immunosuppression should be tapered slowly and perhaps not if blood transfusions have also been given.

References

1. Langone AJ, Chuang P. The management of the failed renal allograft: an enigma with potential consequences. Semin Dial. 2005;18(3):185–7. https://doi.org/10.1111/j.1525-139X.2005.18305.x. PMID: 15934959
2. Woodside KJ, Schirm ZW, Noon KA, Huml AM, Padiyar A, Sanchez EQ, Sarabu N, Hricik DE, Schulak JA, Augustine JJ. Fever, infection, and rejection after kidney transplant failure. Transplantation. 2014;97(6):648–53. https://doi.org/10.1097/01.TP.0000437558.75574.9c.
3. López-Gómez JM, Pérez-Flores I, Jofré R, Carretero D, Rodríguez-Benitez P, Villaverde M, Pérez-García R, Nassar GM, Niembro E, Ayus JC. Presence of a failed kidney transplant in patients who are on hemodialysis is associated with chronic inflammatory state and erythropoietin resistance. J Am Soc Nephrol. 2004;15(9):2494–501. https://doi.org/10.1097/01.ASN.0000137879.97445.6E.
4. Akoh JA. Transplant nephrectomy. World J Transplant. 2011;1(1):4–12. https://doi.org/10.5500/wjt.v1.i1.4.
5. Weinstock C, Schnaidt M. Human leucocyte antigen sensitisation and its impact on transfusion practice. Transfus Med Hemother. 2019;46:356–69. https://doi.org/10.1159/000502158. https://optn.transplant.hrsa.gov/media/eavh5bf3/optn-policies-effective-as-of-dec-6-2021-e-signature.pdf

Chapter 69
Transplant Nephrectomy for Malignancy in the Setting of a Failing Allograft

David C. Cron and Joel T. Adler

Introduction

This is a case of a 55-year woman with a failing kidney transplant diagnosed with extramedullary plasmacytoma involving her kidney allograft. She underwent a transplant nephrectomy as part of her treatment. We discuss the indications for transplant nephrectomy and the surgical approach. We discuss the role of preoperative renal artery angioembolization as a strategy to minimize blood loss during transplant nephrectomy.

Case

The patient is a 55-year-old woman with a history of hypertension, type 2 diabetes, and focal segmental glomerulosclerosis status post living unrelated kidney transplant 10 years ago, now with failing graft. Her post-transplant course was complicated with papillary thyroid cancer metastatic to lymph nodes (5 years ago, s/p thyroidectomy and modified radical neck dissection). She was also diagnosed with an extramedullary plasmacytoma involving her kidney allograft 2½ years ago. This IgG kappa plasmacytoma was treated with chemotherapy (cyclophosphamide/

D. C. Cron
Department of Surgery, Massachusetts General Hospital, Boston, MA, USA
e-mail: dcron@partners.org

J. T. Adler (✉)
Division of Transplant Surgery, Department of Surgery and Perioperative Care, Dell Medical School at the University of Texas at Austin, Austin, TX, USA
e-mail: joel.adler@austin.utexas.edu

© The Author(s), under exclusive license to Springer Nature Switzerland AG 2022
F. Aziz, S. Parajuli (eds.), *Complications in Kidney Transplantation*,
https://doi.org/10.1007/978-3-031-13569-9_69

bortezomib/dexamethasone completed 2 years ago) with an initial clinical response until she was found to have recurrence restricted to her allograft in the last 6 months. A transplant nephrectomy was considered. Given the plasmacytic infiltration of her allograft and her need for eventual re-transplant based on her declining graft function, it was recommended that she undergoe a transplant nephrectomy to minimize immunosuppression needs and ensures adequate treatment response of her plasmacytoma prior to re-transplant. At this time, she was on low-dose prednisone, tacrolimus, and mycophenolate mofetil.

A staged approach to nephrectomy was planned. To aid with vascular control and minimize the potential for blood loss during the nephrectomy, she first underwent embolization of her transplant renal artery with interventional radiology the day before surgery. Her pre- and post-embolization images are shown in Fig. 69.1a, b. The kidney transplant artery was Gelfoam and coil embolized with good response, with only sluggish flow remaining in a small proximal arterial branch to the lower pole, which was not technically amenable to intervention.

The next day, she underwent a transplant nephrectomy. Her prior incision was opened, and the dissection was performed in the extra-capsular plane. The ureter was divided. Approximately 2 h were spent lysing adhesions to mobilize the kidney. The hilar vessels were identified and isolated, and the transplant renal artery and vein were individually ligated. Estimated blood loss was 100 cc. The patient tolerated the procedure well without intraoperative complications. She resumed hemodialysis during her uncomplicated postoperative stay, and she was discharged home on postoperative day 6. She is now undergoing surveillance from a plasmacytoma standpoint with no evidence of recurrence, and she is waitlisted for re-transplant.

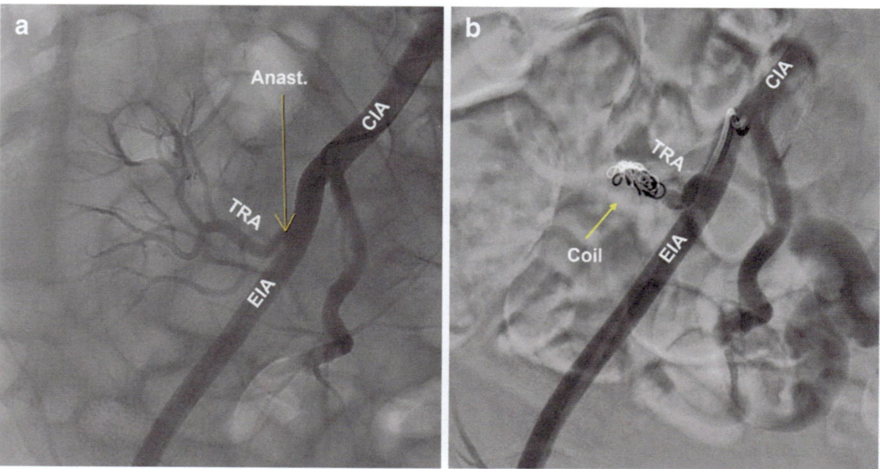

Fig. 69.1 (**a**) Initial angiogram of transplant kidney. (**b**) Angiogram of transplant kidney after Gelfoam and coil embolization of the transplant renal artery. *Anast* = transplant renal artery anastomosis. *CIA* common iliac artery. *EIA* external iliac artery. *TRA* transplant renal artery

Question 1

Which of the following is NOT an indication for transplant nephrectomy?

A. Early allograft failure (within weeks to months of transplant).
B. Ruptured allograft with hemorrhage.
C. Allograft failure beyond 1-year post-transplant, asymptomatic.
D. Allograft failure beyond 1-year post-transplant, with persistent symptoms (pain, hematuria).

The correct answer is C.

Failed allografts are not routinely removed unless associated with persistent symptoms refractory to medical management. However, early allograft failure is a common indication for nephrectomy, though practices vary by the center. Kidney allograft rupture is a rare complication usually seen in the early postoperative setting in the presence of acute rejection, renal vein thrombosis, or acute tubular necrosis; nephrectomy is generally required for this life-threatening complication.

Indications for Transplant Nephrectomy

Indications for transplant nephrectomy are summarized in Table 69.1. Early graft failure (within 1 year of transplant) is an indication for transplant nephrectomy, but this practice varies between transplant centers. This allows cessation of immunosuppression and prevents symptomatic rejection in the failed allograft. Between 1995 and 2003, 56% of early graft failures (within 1 year of transplant) and 27% of later graft failures (beyond 1 year) underwent transplant nephrectomy in the United States [1]. Symptomatic rejection, also termed graft intolerance syndrome, is the most common indication for transplant nephrectomy of a failed graft. Pain is the most common symptom associated with a failed allograft, but additional symptoms

Table 69.1 Indications for transplant nephrectomy

Early graft failure (within 1 year)
Specific graft complications
Primary non-function
Transplant rupture
Pseudoaneurysm rupture
Recurrent infections
Symptomatic rejection
Pain over graft
Hematuria
Chronic inflammation (e.g., fever, anemia)
Malignancy in allograft

include hematuria, chronic inflammatory signs/symptoms (e.g., fever, anemia), and infections. Refractory symptoms necessitating nephrectomy are more common with early graft failure than later graft failure (e.g., beyond 1 year). Initial treatment options for graft intolerance syndrome include pulse dose steroids and transient increases in immunosuppression regimens. The decision to perform a nephrectomy must be carefully weighed, as the procedure can be morbid and the vascular dissection challenging, particularly in later graft failure.

Malignancy in the transplanted kidney is another indication for transplant nephrectomy in the delayed setting. Transplant recipients are at increased risk of malignancy due to their immunosuppressed state. The incidence of solid tumors in transplant kidneys is estimated at 0.2% [2]. Renal cell carcinoma is the most common tumor (91% of all solid tumors), with clear cell renal cell carcinoma being the most common specific histology (51% of renal cell carcinomas) [2]. Management of these tumors is similar to the non-transplant population, with options including percutaneous ablation, partial transplant nephrectomy, and radical transplant nephrectomy. The post-transplant lymphoproliferative disorder can also directly involve the kidney allograft, and this is typically treated with a reduction in immunosuppression and often chemotherapy, but nephrectomy is sometimes needed for localized involvement of the allograft [3].

Preoperative Workup and Considerations

Preoperative imaging is critical to define the vascular anatomy prior to transplant nephrectomy. A kidney transplant ultrasound is used to assess flow through the transplant vasculature, informing the decision to pursue preoperative transplant renal artery embolization (discussed below). Computed tomography scans are also helpful to evaluate the anatomy of the kidney transplant vessels relative to the iliac vessels. Plans must be formulated for postoperative dialysis. At the time of surgery, packed red blood cells should be available as there is potential for significant blood loss.

Question 2

Dense scar tissue is usually encountered during transplant nephrectomy, especially when the patient is further out from transplant. Which of the following are options to minimize blood loss during transplant nephrectomy?

A. Angioembolization of transplant renal artery, preoperatively.
B. Angioembolization of transplant renal artery, intraoperatively.
C. Transection along the hilum leaving a small amount of kidney parenchyma, rather than individually isolating and ligating the transplant vessels.
D. All of the above.

The correct answer is D.

Angioembolization of the transplant renal artery is associated with less intraoperative blood loss and lower transfusion requirement. This procedure can be done in a staged approach prior to nephrectomy, and at some centers, it is done concurrently with the nephrectomy operation. In the setting of dense adhesions, dissection around the kidney transplant allograft can be perilous, and it may not be possible to individually isolate the transplant renal artery and vein. In this case, it is acceptable to leave a small amount of hilar tissue behind by clamping across the hilum and ligating the vascular pedicle as a whole.

Surgical Approach

The prior kidney transplant incision is opened, and the dissection is performed extra-peritoneally, if possible, down to the kidney allograft. Dense adhesions can be expected for patients farther out from their transplant. In these cases, dissection is carried out in the subcapsular plane when possible, as this plane, though prone to bleeding, should be unviolated and free of adhesions. The transplant ureter is identified and ligated. Before dissecting out the hilum containing the transplant renal artery and vein, the iliac artery and vein must be identified, with proximal and distal control secured if possible. Management of the hilum is dictated by the degree of adhesions, as this can be a perilous dissection. For later nephrectomies, it is often not possible to individually isolate and ligate the transplant renal artery and vein. Often it is safest to leave a small amount of kidney hilum on the transplant renovascular pedicle. In this case, the entire pedicle is clamped to minimize the chance of vascular compromise during dissection. Care is taken to avoid injury to the iliac vessels. The kidney is sharply excised along a line close to the hilum (as depicted in Fig. 69.2). This may leave a small amount of parenchyma, but this is not felt to pose a significant immunologic risk. The hilar remnant and pedicle are oversewn, and hemostasis is assured.

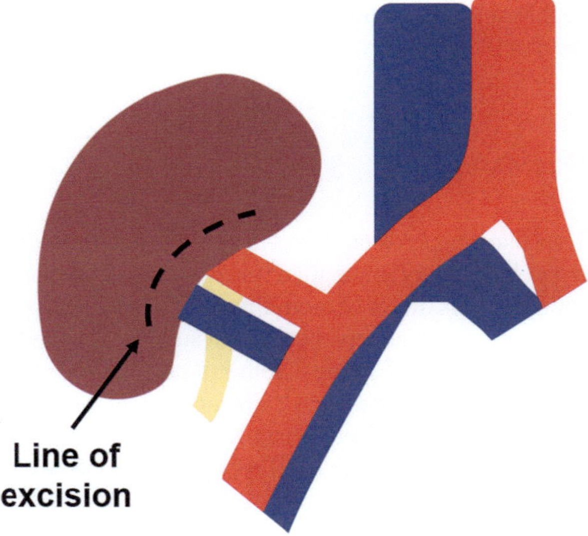

Fig. 69.2 Depiction of a transplanted kidney in situ. It is often necessary and safest to leave a small amount of hilar tissue by excising along a line close to the hilum (dashed line)

Preoperative Angioembolization for Vascular Control

As demonstrated in the patient case above, preoperative angioembolization of the transplant renal artery is an option to decrease the potential for blood loss during the transplant nephrectomy. This can be done via a staged approach or concurrent with the nephrectomy procedure. This technique is associated with lower intraoperative estimated blood loss [4–6] and lower transfusion requirements [4, 6]. This technique is even used by some as a stand-alone treatment for graft intolerance syndrome and can be effective in avoiding the need for transplant nephrectomy in this setting [7].

Renal artery embolization is used in other non-transplant contexts as well, such as prior to resection of large masses in native kidneys. This procedure is safe and effective, with an estimated 5% incidence of incomplete embolization, coil migration, or groin hematoma [8]. Many patients experience symptoms after embolization, such as pain or nausea, but these are typically mild and self-limited. [8] Of note, some failed allografts are thrombosed, and the absence of blood flow through the transplant renal artery, therefore, obviates the need for angioembolization. This highlights the utility of ultrasound during the workup of these patients, as assessment of blood flow through the allograft will guide management.

Immunosuppression Management

Immunosuppression is usually stopped after transplant nephrectomy, especially in the setting of early failure. This decision must consider a patient's prospect for re-transplantation. A highly sensitized patient awaiting re-transplant may be continued on low-dose immunosuppression after transplant nephrectomy. This is to prevent further sensitization due to the small amount of remaining allograft tissue after nephrectomy. Even if no kidney parenchyma is left behind, the proximal portions of the donor renal artery and vein remain anastomosed to the recipient iliac vessels.

Outcomes

Transplant nephrectomy is a major procedure with the potential for significant blood loss, injury to the iliac vessels, wound infections, sepsis, and cardiovascular complications. Rates of morbidity after the procedure range from 4 to 82% [9]. The effect of transplant nephrectomy on survival is uncertain and difficult to determine from observational studies. Some studies have reported improved survival among patients with a failed allograft who underwent transplant nephrectomy [10]. Another study reported increased mortality risk when nephrectomy was performed for early graft loss but decreased mortality when performed for late graft loss (beyond 1 year) [1]. Finally, nephrectomy may be associated with increased allosensitization [1, 9].

Summary

After the failure of a kidney allograft, transplant nephrectomy is often performed, though this decision must weigh many potential risks and benefits. Transplant nephrectomy is the most commonly performed for early allograft failure and symptoms associated with a failed allograft, but malignancy is an important, albeit less common, indication for nephrectomy as well. The operation can be challenging with the potential for significant blood loss, and preoperative angioembolization of the transplant renal artery can be considered to minimize the potential for blood loss. The decision to continue immunosuppression after transplant nephrectomy varies by patient and provider and must consider their prospect for re-transplant and any potential risk for allosensitization.

References

1. Johnston O, et al. Nephrectomy after transplant failure: current practice and outcomes. Am J Transplant. 2007;7(8):1961–7.
2. Griffith JJ, et al. Solid renal masses in transplanted allograft kidneys: a closer look at the epidemiology and management. Am J Transplant. 2017;17(11):2775–81.
3. Agarwal G, Mannon RB. Post-transplant lymphoproliferative disorder in a kidney transplant recipient. Clin J Am Soc Nephrol. 2019;14(5):751–3.
4. Neschis DG, et al. Intraoperative coil embolization reduces transplant nephrectomy transfusion requirement. Vasc Endovasc Surg. 2007;41(4):335–8.
5. Yeast C, et al. Use of preoperative embolization prior to transplant nephrectomy. Int Braz J Urol. 2016;42(1):107–12.
6. Al-Geizawi SM, et al. Role of allograft nephrectomy following kidney graft failure: preliminary experience with preoperative angiographic kidney embolization. J Nephrol. 2015;28(3):379–85.
7. Garcia-Padilla PK, et al. Renal graft embolization as a treatment for graft intolerance syndrome. Transplant Proc. 2020;52(4):1187–91.
8. Schwartz MJ, et al. Renal artery embolization: clinical indications and experience from over 100 cases. BJU Int. 2007;99(4):881–6.
9. Gómez-Dos-Santos, V., et al., The failing kidney transplant allograft. Transplant nephrectomy: current state-of-the-art. Current urology reports, 2020. 21(1).
10. Ayus JC, et al. Transplant nephrectomy improves survival following a failed renal allograft. J Am Soc Nephrol. 2010;21(2):374–80.

Chapter 70
Graft Failure in the Elderly

Anadil Faqah and M. Yahya Jan

Introduction

With improvement in immunosuppression therapies, kidney graft survival has significantly improved. As a result, more elderly kidney transplant recipients present with advanced chronic kidney disease and graft failure. During their post-transplant course, they may develop additional medical comorbidities, especially cardiovascular, that preclude them from re-transplantation and make them suboptimal candidates for dialysis. Frailty and age-related functional status changes also add to the complexity of these patients, requiring evaluation of goals of care and advanced care planning.

Case

A 72-year-old male with a history of End-Stage Kidney Disease (ESKD) due to diabetic nephropathy status post deceased donor kidney transplantation 10 years ago is seen in follow-up at the Kidney Transplant Clinic. Over the years, his creatinine has trended up, and his kidney biopsy 3 years ago showed chronic allograft nephropathy (CAN). Since his transplant, he has had an NSTEMI that required Percutaneous Intervention (PCI) and resulted in systolic heart failure. He also has had a left below-knee amputation due to a non-healing ulcer. His labs show a slowly creeping creatinine at 6.7 mg/dL and a BUN of 79 mg/dL. He has lost 20 lbs. recently and is here to discuss his worsening kidney failure.

A. Faqah · M. Y. Jan (✉)
Indiana University School of Medicine, Indianapolis, IN, USA
e-mail: myjan@iu.edu

© The Author(s), under exclusive license to Springer Nature Switzerland AG 2022
F. Aziz, S. Parajuli (eds.), *Complications in Kidney Transplantation*,
https://doi.org/10.1007/978-3-031-13569-9_70

Question 1

Which of the following is the most important assessment during this patient visit:

A. Evaluation of upper extremities for dialysis access.
B. Explaining how creatinine and BUN can rise when kidney function is poor.
C. Discuss repeat transplant evaluation.
D. Assessment of his frail functional status, encouraging him to discuss his future goals in light of this and referral to palliative medicine clinic.

The correct answer is D.

Dialysis access planning is an integral part of every advanced CKD patient who is anticipated to need dialysis in the coming 6–12 months. However, it is crucial to prioritize discussions about the patient's understanding of their overall health and the challenges they might encounter while on dialysis. This is especially important for those elderly patients on dialysis before transplant to explain how it will be different now with added comorbidities and reduced functional status (Fig. 70.1). Trending kidney function and explaining pathophysiological mechanisms are a part of nephrology practice; however, patients should be explained what it means in non-medical jargon and should be a part of the initial conversations about disease understanding. Those elderly patients who may qualify for re-transplantation should be referred; however, this should be based on a thorough review of recent past medical history, especially cardiovascular comorbidities since transplant. In patients such as the one discussed in this patient, the most critical next step is an assessment of frailty and independence in ADLs and IADLs to base their future goals. Palliative medicine consultation should be sought for longitudinal follow-up of these goals and discuss any setbacks that may come up along the way.

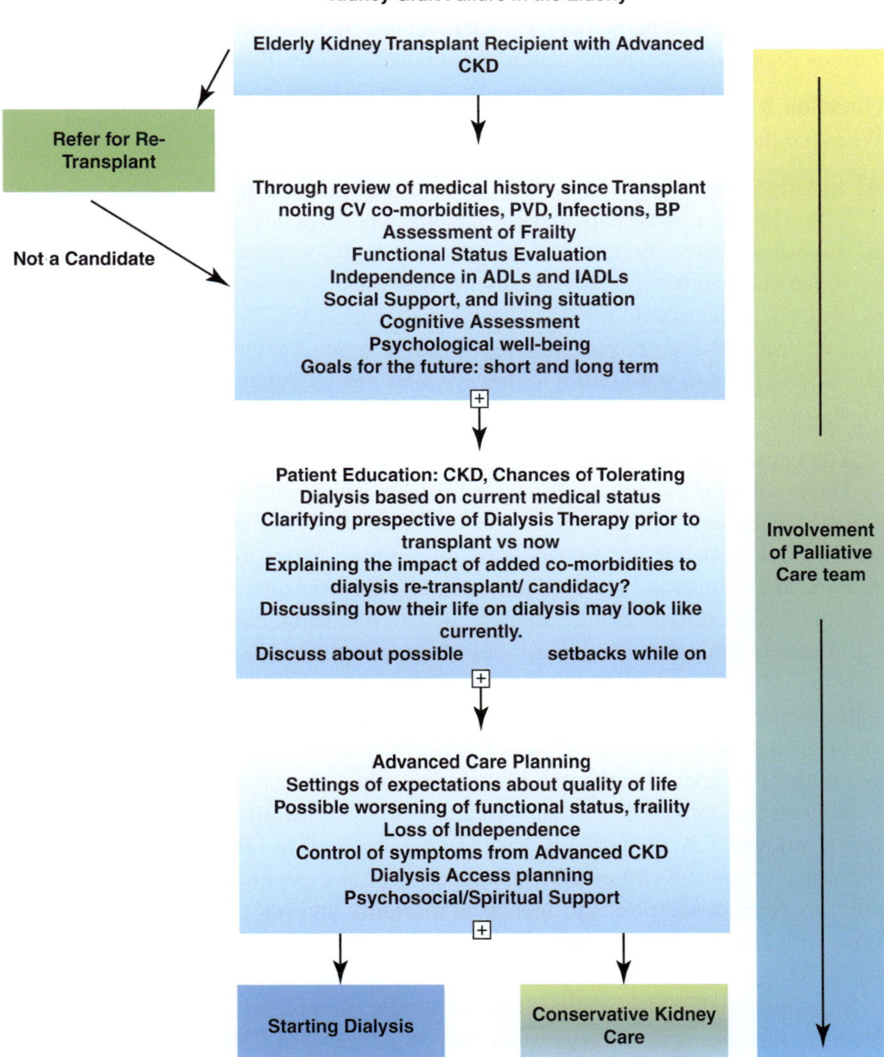

Fig. 70.1 Assessment of failing allograft

Further History

The patient informs you that despite having a prosthesis to his leg, he cannot perform some of his activities of daily living independently and is no longer driving. He also feels short of breath after minimal exertion. His wife passed away last year and given all the changes he had tried to adjust to, his mood is low, and he feels despondent. He hopes to be evaluated for a repeat transplant, though he understands his health has recently declined significantly. He recalls a challenging experience adjusting to life with hemodialysis, where he had to be in and out of the hospital for various issues, dialysis being a significant burden on his lifestyle.

Question 2

Which of the following is true pertaining to this patient?

A. Elderly patients who return to dialysis after graft loss have a higher mortality rate when compared with dialysis patients who have never received a transplant.
B. Elderly patients who return to dialysis after graft loss have a lower mortality rate when compared with dialysis patients who have never received a transplant.
C. Elderly patients who return to dialysis after graft loss have a similar mortality rate compared to dialysis patients who have never received a transplant.
D. Elderly patients who return to dialysis after graft loss have an unknown mortality rate compared to dialysis patients who have never received a transplant.

The correct answer is A.

The number of patients returning to Dialysis After Graft Loss (DAGL) has consistently increased over the past 20 years. This has been attributed to improved graft survival due to better immunosuppression regimes, better management of comorbidities, and an overall increased number of kidney transplants performed globally. Patients with DAGL constitute about 5–10% of incidental dialysis patients per year [1]. There is some recent evidence [2] of improved and possibly comparable survival in DAGL patients compared to transplant naïve patients although those deemed high risk (i.e., >65 years of age) were excluded from these analyses. Patients in this cohort also experience a sudden and significantly increased hazard of death (threefold higher) compared to the risk of mortality while on dialysis [3]. This is true for patients on the transplant waitlist who are on dialysis awaiting their first transplant having a lower risk of mortality than those compared to DAGL, highlighting the difference in age and comorbidity profile of these two populations [4]. On the other hand, more evidence points to increased mortality and poor quality of life among those with DAGL, with mortality highest in the first 12 months following graft failure [5, 6].

Significant risk factors include cardiovascular disease, which accounts for most deaths in this group(8), diabetes status(4), poor control of CKD parameters including anemia, mineral bone disease, poor nutritional status, and lack of permanent access [4, 7, 8]. Although no consensus definition of frailty has been agreed upon, generally, it refers to a decreased functional reserve to deal with health challenges and has long been accepted as a predictor of poor outcomes among elderly patients who initiate dialysis. A study done in the United Kingdom reported that only 10% of those with advanced CKD (including those with a kidney transplant) had discussed end-of-life care issues, while two-thirds regretted their decision to start dialysis [9]. The first step is identifying those at high risk, i.e., the elderly, those with diabetes, and cardiovascular comorbidities. Once identified from their clinical history, determination of their functional status and exploration of their goals of care are the next most important step, often in consultation with the palliative medicine team.

Discussion

According to the USRDS Annual Data Report(ADR) 2020 [10], the expected remaining lifetime in years for patients with ESKD who are 65–69 years old is 4.8 years for men and 4.9 years for women. This is significantly lower than the expected remaining lifetime of 16.3 years for men and 18.7 years for women among the general population without ESKD. Elderly patients returning to dialysis after graft failure remain a distinct group of patients who pose unique challenges for clinicians. Among KTRs older than 65 years of age, frailty, medical comorbidities, especially cardiovascular disease, poor functional status, loss of independence, and time on the transplant waitlist, most of these individuals do not qualify as candidates for repeat transplantation. In this scenario, they are left with the option to go back on dialysis or choose to pursue conservative kidney care, often in collaboration with palliative medicine teams.

Frailty is an important clinical parameter that should be assessed and recognized in this subset of individuals, as it has been shown to correlate with mortality [11]. Also, frailty is closely related to cognitive decline, falls, dialysis access failure, and poor quality of life.

Conversations related to care goals with a failing kidney graft and poor functional status are stressful both for patients and physicians [12]. From a physician's perspective, barriers to these conversations include a perception of a time-consuming process and increased reliance on specific numbers from clinical investigations. For patients facing this scenario, recall of past experience with dialysis or transplant several years ago when they had better functional status provides a comparison far detached from reality leading to unrealistic hopes and expectations about their future health. To add to this, the uncertainty about how a patient's life may look like on dialysis adds to the difficulty of approaching these discussions promptly, often delaying them to a point where patients end up in the hospital either too sick to pursue them or leaving the burden on family members or caregivers. Early conversations with patients about goals of care, prognosis, and end of life have led to care consistent with patient wishes.

Elderly patients with graft failure who are likely not to do well based on the risk factors mentioned above should be referred to the palliative medicine team promptly. In addition, they should be informed in detail about the potential benefits of pursuing dialysis, such as prolonging life, and improvement in symptoms of uremia, volume overload, etc. and how likely are they going to achieve these with the accompanying risks of hospitalizations for complications of dialysis such as access malfunction, infections, acute illnesses, and worsening frailty which may require placement in a nursing home. Specific details on how their life may look on dialysis, e.g., a significant amount of time lost in traveling to and from dialysis units three times a week, and symptoms from dialysis treatment itself such as post-dialysis fatigue, dizziness, cramping, etc. should be provided. Early referral of such elderly patients with graft failure to the palliative medicine team is a key intervention that nephrologists should recognize.

References

1. Marcén R, Teruel JL. Patient outcomes after kidney allograft loss. Transplant Rev (Orlando). 2008;22(1):62–72.
2. Mourad G, Minguet J, Pernin V, et al. Similar patient survival following kidney allograft failure compared with non-transplanted patients. Kidney Int. 2014;86(1):191–8.
3. Kaplan B, Meier-Kriesche HU. Death after graft loss: an important late study endpoint in kidney transplantation. Am J Transplant. 2002;2(10):970–4.
4. Rao PS, Schaubel DE, Jia X, Li S, Port FK, Saran R. Survival on dialysis post-kidney transplant failure: results from the scientific registry of transplant recipients. Am J Kidney Dis. 2007;49(2):294–300.
5. Kabani R, Quinn RR, Palmer S, et al. Risk of death following kidney allograft failure: a systematic review and meta-analysis of cohort studies. Nephrol Dial Transplant. 2014;29(9):1778–86.
6. Perl J, Zhang J, Gillespie B, et al. Reduced survival and quality of life following return to dialysis after transplant failure: the dialysis outcomes and practice patterns study. Nephrol Dial Transplant. 2012;27(12):4464–72.
7. Brar A, Markell M, Stefanov DG, et al. Mortality after kidneyallograft failure and return to dialysis. Am J Nephrol. 2017;45(2):180–6.
8. Gill JS, Abichandani R, Kausz AT, Pereira BJ. Mortality after kidney transplant failure: the impact of non-immunologic factors. Kidney Int. 2002;62(5):1875–83.
9. Muthalagappan S, Johansson L, Kong WM, Brown EA. Dialysis or conservative care for frail older patients: ethics of shared decision-making. Nephrol Dial Transplant. 2013;28(11):2717–22.
10. System USRD. In: Bethesda MD, editor. 2020 USRDS annual data report: epidemiology of kidney disease in the United States. National Institutes of Health, National Institute of Diabetes and Digestive and Kidney Diseases; 2020.
11. Lee SY, Yang DH, Hwang E, et al. The prevalence, association, and clinical outcomes of frailty in maintenance dialysis patients. J Ren Nutr. 2017;27(2):106–12.
12. Schell JO, Cohen RA. A communication framework for dialysis decision-making for frail elderly patients. Clin J Am Soc Nephrol. 2014;9(11):2014–21.

Chapter 71
Posttransplant Aortoiliac Aneurysms

Zaid Al-Dahabrah and Preethi Yerram

Introduction

Vascular complications are frequently seen in kidney transplant recipients and can contribute to morbidity and mortality in this patient population. Some of the vascular complications that may be seen include renal artery stenosis, renal artery thrombosis, renal artery aneurysm, renal vein thrombosis, and arteriovenous fistula [1]. In recent years, the frequency of aortoiliac aneurysms requiring surgical management has been rising due to the number of renal transplant recipients surviving later into life and transplants being offered to older patients [2].

Case

A 44-year-old man with a congenital solitary left kidney progressed to ESKD secondary to biopsy-proven membranoproliferative glomerulonephritis (MPGN) Type I. He was started on hemodialysis (HD) in 2002. The patient's past medical history is also significant for hypertension and hypothyroidism. He had a 60-pack year smoking history but was not a current user.

Z. Al-Dahabrah (✉)
Division of Nephrology, Department of Medicine, University of Missouri-Columbia, Columbia, MO, USA

P. Yerram
Division of Nephrology, Department of Medicine, University of Missouri-Columbia, Columbia, MO, USA

Nephrology Section, Harry S Truman VA Hospital, Columbia, MO, USA
e-mail: yerramp@health.missouri.edu

© The Author(s), under exclusive license to Springer Nature Switzerland AG 2022
F. Aziz, S. Parajuli (eds.), *Complications in Kidney Transplantation*,
https://doi.org/10.1007/978-3-031-13569-9_71

The patient received a three antigen-mismatched, deceased donor kidney transplant (DDKT) in 2004. Cold ischemic time was 5.5 h, and anastomosis time was 90 min. Pt received induction with anti-thymocyte globulin (ATG) 1.5 mg/kg daily for 4 days. His immediate postoperative period was complicated by a slow rise in creatinine but did not require dialysis. The patient was discharged with a serum creatinine of 6.7 mg/dL that eventually trended down to a baseline of 1.8–2 mg/dL. The patient was discharged on tacrolimus, mycophenolate mofetil, and a tapering prednisone dose. A kidney biopsy was done approximately 1 year after his transplant due to worsening proteinuria concerning recurrent MPGN. However, it showed nonspecific findings.

The patient did well for the next several years without any allograft complications, and his serum creatinine remained in the 2.0–2.6 mg/dL range while continuing on the triple-drug immunosuppressive regimen.

In 2018, 14 years after his transplant, the patient presented to the hospital complaining of pelvic discomfort and inability to void and was noted to have a serum creatinine of 8.26 mg/dL compared to 4.07 mg/dL noted 4 months prior.

CT abdomen showed a huge aneurysmal sac arising from the left internal iliac artery measuring up to 12 cm, which occupied most of the false pelvis, causing mass effect on the urinary bladder (Fig. 71.1). This aneurysm was appreciated in 2003 during the pre-transplant evaluation process, but it was smaller.

Question 1

What is the most common presentation of iliac artery aneurysms?

A. Fever.
B. Pelvic pain.
C. Asymptomatic.
D. Anemia.

The correct answer is C.

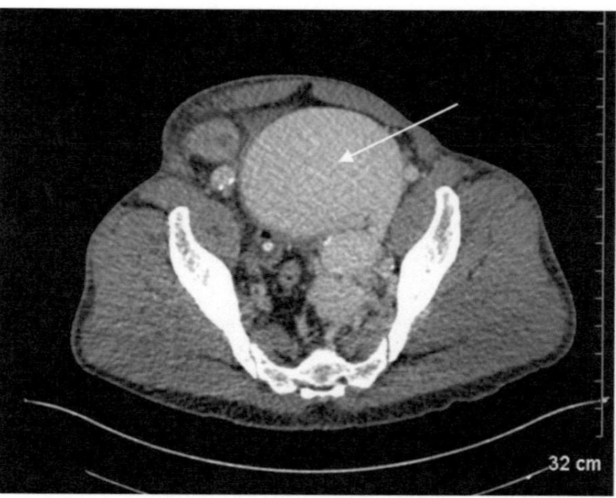

Fig. 71.1 a 12 cm large aneurysmal sac arising from left internal iliac artery (white arrow)

The majority of aneurysms are found incidentally and are asymptomatic [3]. However, patients with aneurysms can present with the following signs and symptoms: fever, anemia, ipsilateral limb ischemia, high blood pressure, compression of nearby organs, a decline in graft function, and bleeding due to rupture [1].

Subsequent Clinical Course

A percutaneous nephrostomy tube was inserted with improvement in creatinine to 3.44 mg/dL. The patient was seen by urology and vascular surgery and was not deemed a surgical candidate at that time. He was eventually discharged to be followed up in the outpatient clinic. His serum creatinine progressively worsened for the next 2 years, trending up to 6.66 mg/dL, but he did not have uremic symptoms and did not require dialysis.

The patient was readmitted in 2020 with COVID-19 infection and acute kidney injury (AKI) with serum creatinine up to 8.69 mg/dL. Repeat abdominal imaging showed further enlargement of the known saccular aneurysm of the left internal iliac artery compared to 2018 (Fig. 71.2). The patient eventually required hemodialysis (HD) initiation during this admission and was discharged on maintenance HD.

The patient subsequently underwent elective open surgical aneurysmal repair in October 2020 with improvement in serum creatinine to 3–3.5 mg/dL and was able to come off of maintenance dialysis. The patient continues to be dialysis-free and is undergoing evaluation for another kidney transplant.

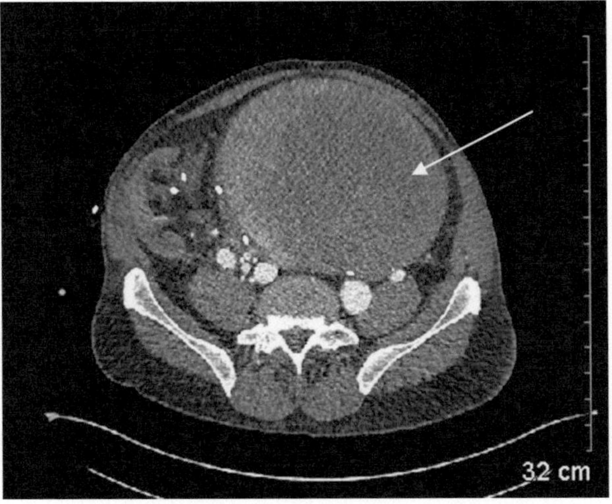

Fig. 71.2 Further enlargement of saccular aneurysm compared to previous CT study in 2018 (white arrow)

Question 2

Which one of the following is considered one of the indications for aneurysmal repair?

A. Size more than 0.5 cm.
B. Asymptomatic aneurysms that are found incidentally.
C. Aneurysms that are present for at least 3 years.
D. Infection.

The correct answer is D.

Indications for repair: Infection, aneurysms being symptomatic, larger than 2.5 cm in size, and progressive increase in size with risk of rupture [1, 4].

Discussion

Our patient had a substantial left internal iliac aneurysm with a significant mass effect on the transplanted kidney that contributed to his AKI and the need for renal replacement therapy. Once the aneurysm was repaired, his allograft function recovered, suggesting the significant mass effect the aneurysm had on the transplanted kidney.

The incidence of arterial pseudoaneurysm post-renal transplantation has been noted to be less than 1% [5]. It is crucial to recognize the development of posttransplant pseudoaneurysms because they are liable to acutely rupture, leading to significant hemorrhage [6]. Recent studies have demonstrated an increased incidence of aneurysm growth and rupture in transplant patients with devastating complications, thus making close surveillance critical in this population [7, 8].

The vast majority of iliac artery aneurysms (IAAs) are true aneurysms that are caused by arterial wall degeneration. In contrast, a pseudoaneurysm is caused by iliac artery dilation. It can happen as a consequence of para-anastomotic graft failure following a prior aortic graft repair [9], a vascular insult from penetrating mechanisms (gunshot, knife), or iatrogenic injury during pelvic surgeries [10, 11].

IAAs have also been linked to Behcet's disease [12], fibromuscular dysplasia [13], Takayasu's arteritis, and other connective tissue disorders [14]. Rarely, aneurysms may get infected. Organisms that have been isolated include Salmonella, Staphylococcus aureus, Klebsiella, and Candida [15].

Therapeutic options for repair include open surgical repair, administration of thrombin percutaneously under ultrasound guidance, and endovascular repair [2, 16].

Open surgical repair typically involves surgical removal of the aneurysm and arterial reconstruction via patch angioplasty, re-anastomosis, or allograft auto-transplantation [2]. Our patient had a sizeable expanding aneurysm with mass effect causing allograft dysfunction and required open surgical repair. He is currently being evaluated for a second kidney transplant and remains off dialysis, but with chronic kidney disease stage 4.

There is generally a lack of data regarding vascular complications post kidney transplantation. They are usually considered surgical emergencies when they are present and prompt recognition/intervention is indicated. Our patient had a chronic presentation of a left internal iliac artery aneurysm that enlarged over time, causing allograft dysfunction that was subsequently managed with open surgical repair and improved graft function.

References

1. Janho KE, Shishani JM, Habboub HK. Endovascular repair of renal artery aneurysm in a transplanted kidney. Oman Med J. 2019;34(2):169–71.
2. Reber PU, Vogt B, Steinke TM, Patel AG, Kniemeyer HW. Surgery for aortoiliac aneurysms in kidney transplant recipients. J Cardiovasc Surg. 2000;41(6):919–25.
3. Bracale UM, Carbone F, del Guercio L, Viola D, D'Armiento FP, Maurea S, et al. External iliac artery pseudoaneurysm complicating renal transplantation. Interact Cardiovasc Thorac Surg. 2009;8(6):654–60. https://doi.org/10.1510/icvts.2008.200386.
4. Busato CR, Utrabo CA, de Sousa WF, Gomes RZ, Hosoume JK, Hoeldtke E, et al. Renal artery aneurysm in a transplanted kidney: ex vivo graft repair and reimplantation. J Vasc Bras. 2009;8(1) https://doi.org/10.1590/S1677-54492009000100013.
5. Fleshner NE, Johnston KW. Repair of an autotransplant renal artery aneurysm: case report and literature review. J Urol. 1992;148:389.
6. Donckier V, De Pauw L, Ferreira J, et al. False aneurysm after transplant nephrectomy. Transplantation. 1995;60:303.
7. Englesbe MJ, Wu AH, Clowes AW, Zierler RE. The prevalence and natural history of aortic aneurysms in heart and abdominal organ transplant patients. J Vasc Surg. 2003;37:27–31.
8. Gang S, Rajapurkar M. Vascular complications following renal transplantation. J Nephrol Ren Transplant. 2009;2(1):122–32.
9. Bacharach JM, Slovut DP. State of the art: management of iliac artery aneurysmal disease. Catheter Cardiovasc Interv. 2008;71:708.
10. Appel N, Duncan JR, Schuerer DJ. Percutaneous stent-graft treatment of superior mesenteric and internal iliac artery pseudoaneurysms. J Vasc Interv Radiol. 2003;14:917.
11. Ijaz S, Geroulakos G. Ruptured internal iliac artery aneurysm mimicking a hip fracture. Int Angiol. 2001;20:187.
12. Kalko Y, Basaran M, Aydin U, et al. The surgical treatment of arterial aneurysms in Behçet disease: a report of 16 patients. J Vasc Surg. 2005;42:673.
13. Atsuta Y, Inaba M, Goh K, et al. Isolated iliac artery aneurysm caused by fibromuscular dysplasia: report of a case. Surg Today. 2003;33:639.
14. Crivello MS, Porter DH, Kim D, et al. Isolated external iliac artery aneurysm secondary to cystic medial necrosis. Cardiovasc Intervent Radiol. 1986;9:139.
15. Woodrum DT, Welke KF, Fillinger MF. Candida infection associated with a solitary mycotic common iliac artery aneurysm. J Vasc Surg. 2001;34:166.
16. Buimer MG, van Hamersvelt HW, Adam Van der Vliet J. Anastomotic pseudoaneurysm after renal transplantation; a new hybrid approach with graft salvage. Transpl Int. 2012;25(7):e86–8.

Chapter 72
Dialysis-Associated Steal Syndrome (DASS)

Abindra Sigdel and Prabesh Aryal

Introduction

Dialysis-associated steal syndrome (DASS) is an ischemic complication associated with hemodialysis access creation. Failure to diagnose and treat in a timely fashion may lead to loss of digits or an entire hand in a worst-case scenario. Although DASS diagnosis is easy, management of this condition could be complicated and frequently requires surgical intervention.

Patient History

A 62-year-old female presented with left finger numbness and pain 1-month following left brachiocephalic fistula creation. Past medical history was significant for a deceased donor kidney transplant 7 years ago. Due to deteriorating allograft function, the patient is expected to start dialysis soon. The patient states that the symptoms started about a week after creating the fistula and have only mildly progressed since. Her pain has been under control with the occasional use of Tylenol. On examination, the left arm incision is clean and dry, and the fistula has easily palpable thrill. Her fingers appear cool to touch. The left radial pulse is weaker compared to the right side. The radial pulse improves upon compression of the fistula. No digital ulcers or gangrene were present on examination.

A. Sigdel (✉)
Division of Vascular Surgery and Endovascular Therapeutics, University of Louisville School of Medicine, Louisville, KY, USA
e-mail: abindra.sigdel@louisville.edu

P. Aryal
Internal Medicine, Hurley Medical Education, Flint, USA

© The Author(s), under exclusive license to Springer Nature Switzerland AG 2022
F. Aziz, S. Parajuli (eds.), *Complications in Kidney Transplantation*,
https://doi.org/10.1007/978-3-031-13569-9_72

Question 1

What is the likely cause of the patient's symptoms?

A. Diabetic polyneuropathy.
B. Dialysis-Associated Steal Syndrome (DASS).
C. Ischemic Monomelic Neuropathy (IMN).
D. Raynaud's disease.

The correct answer is B.

Dialysis-Associated Steal Syndrome (DASS) is a condition where the patient develops ischemic symptoms of the hand after the creation of arteriovenous access in the involved extremity. A weak pulse that augments on compression of access is a common finding on a patient with DASS. Ischemic Monomelic Neuropathy (IMN) usually presents within hours of access creation, and the hand usually remains warm with normal pulse examination. Raynaud's disease usually occurs in a younger female, and it typically presents with reversible ischemia of the hand, unlike DASS, where symptoms remain persistent.

The patient was started on hemodialysis 2 months later through the existing fistula. The patient complains of increasing pain in her hand, causing her to stay awake during nighttime. The pain gets unbearable during dialysis. She has been unable to complete her routine 4 h dialysis session due to excruciating hand pain. The hand has been weak, and she has had trouble grasping objects with her left hand. Examination reveals easily palpable thrill over the fistula and barely palpable radial pulse. Her fingers are cool to touch and mildly cyanotic at the tips. She has a very weak grasp on her left hand. The radial pulse augments substantially upon compression of the fistula. Based on the current wait times, the patient has been listed for another kidney transplant but is not expected to receive one in the next 3–4 years. Duplex of the fistula shows that the fistula is patent, no stenosis is identified in the brachial artery, and volume flow of the brachial artery just proximal to anastomosis is 1000 mL/min.

Question 2

What is the most appropriate management at this time?

A. Continue conservative management.
B. Prescribe narcotic pain medicine.
C. Nerve conduction studies.
D. Vascular surgery consult for possible surgical intervention.

The correct answer is D.

This patient's symptoms have progressed significantly. Currently, she has stage III disease. The fistula volume flow is within the normal range. Vascular surgery service should be immediately consulted for possible surgical intervention. Appropriate treatment for this stage of DASS is a revascularization procedure with DRIL or Proximalization of Arterial Inflow (PAI). Both procedures are effective in reversing ischemic symptoms while maintaining the existing access. Continuation of conservative treatment or narcotic pain medicine alone is not an appropriate treatment at this stage because ongoing ischemia might lead to irreversible damage to the hand. Nerve conduction studies are usually valuable to rule out neuropathies. In this patient, symptoms are quite typical of steal syndrome; therefore, nerve conduction study findings will not make any difference in the management.

Discussion

Dialysis-associated steal syndrome (DASS) commonly refers to the ischemic complications of the hand following the creation of vascular access in the same extremity. DASS incidence varies widely in the published literature, with clinically significant DASS requiring surgical intervention reported somewhere between 1 and 8% [1]. DASS results when the portion of arterial flow diverts to the low resistance bed (the arteriovenous access) from the high resistance bed (the distal extremity) [2]. Incidence of DASS is variable for different types of accesses. An overwhelming majority of DASS is seen with the brachial artery-based access. DASS is extremely uncommon with radial artery-based hemodialysis access [3].

Risk factors for DASS include female sex, diabetes, hypertension, coronary artery disease, tobacco use, and age older than 60 [1, 4, 5].

Clinical Presentation

Though physiological steal occurs in up to 90% of cases, most remain asymptomatic. The spectrum of symptoms ranges from cool, painless hands to major gangrene leading to loss of the hand. Paresthesia, finger numbness, and hand pain are the most common symptoms. Symptoms usually tend to worsen during a hemodialysis session. Though weak or absent distal pulses are commonly observed, the presence of a normal pulse does not rule out the diagnosis of DASS.

The following four-stage classification of symptoms [6] helps accurately stratify the severity of DASS. This staging system is also helpful in formulating the management plan in patients with DASS.

Stage I Pale/livid hand and/or cool hand without pain.
Stage IIa Tolerable pain during exercise and/or during dialysis.
Stage IIb Intolerable pain during exercise and/or during dialysis.
Stage III Rest pain or loss of motor function.
Stage IVa Limited tissue loss, the potential for preservation of hand function.
Stage IVb Irreversible tissue loss, significant hand function is lost.

Symptoms can also be classified according to the timing of onset following the access placement.

Acute: Within hours of access placement.

Subacute: Within hours–1 month.
Chronic: > 1 month.

Ischemic Monomelic Neuropathy (IMN): IMN is a distinct clinical entity often regarded as a variant of DASS. It is caused by focal nerve ischemia, and the symptoms usually occur immediately after the fistula placement. This condition presents predominantly neurologic symptoms with minimal to absent vascular symptoms. All three nerves of the hand and forearm are involved resulting in profound pain, paresthesia, numbness, and weakness of the hand. The hand is usually warm with a good capillary refill and normal pulse examination.

Evaluation

History and physical exam: A thorough evaluation of the patient helps diagnose and stage the severity of the steal. On examination, the type and location of the access should be determined. Palpation of the fistula and distal pulse should be performed. Motor and sensory examination of the hand should be routinely performed in patients presenting with steal symptoms. The likelihood of DASS is very high in a patient presenting with ischemic symptoms following access creation if the symptom is partially or completely relieved upon compression of the arteriovenous access.

Though the diagnosis of steal syndrome is often straightforward, some of the differential diagnoses are Raynaud's disease, compressive neuropathies like carpal tunnel syndrome, cervical spondylosis, and different types of arthritis.

The following diagnostic tests can be used to confirm the diagnosis of DASS.

Arterial duplex: A duplex examination of the inflow artery will reveal any stenosis of the artery proximal or distal to the anastomosis. The volume flow of the access should be obtained, and the access categorized as low volume (<600 mL/min), normal volume (600–1500 mL/min), and high volume (>1500 mL/min).

DBI: Digital pressure of < 60 mmHg or a DBI < 0.4 in a patient with arteriovenous (AV) access is highly associated with hand ischemia [7].

Digital waveform: Doubling of amplitude in response to compression of AV access is indicative of DASS.

Angiography: Helps identify the arterial disease of the feeding artery. This is mostly utilized in the treatment of DASS rather than the diagnosis of DASS.

Nerve conduction evaluation: Occasionally utilized to determine the severity of neurological damage. It could be helpful to rule out compressive neuropathies.

Management

Prevention of DASS is the best approach. Every attempt should be made to identify the patients at risk of DASS prior to creating access. Some common strategies to prevent DASS are:

1. Preoperative correction of arterial lesions.
2. Avoidance of brachial artery as the inflow vessel. Always look for the possibility of using radial artery, as DASS is uncommon with radial artery-based accesses.
3. Limiting arterial inflow: Avoid making sizeable arterial anastomosis. Usually, a 4 to 6 mm long arterial anastomosis is adequate to maintain enough volume flow. If required to use a graft, consider using the tapered AV grafts.

Despite all carefulness, DASS still occurs in some groups of patients. Though ligation of access promptly and effectively reverses the ischemic symptoms, the need for new access and the possibility of steal with the new access make this approach less than ideal. Therefore, the guiding principle in the management of DASS involves reversing ischemic symptoms while preserving access.

The management of DASS is individualized according to the stage of the disease at presentation.

State I/IIa: Nonoperative management.
Stage IIb/III/IVa: Surgical intervention. The type of surgery is based on access volume flow.
Stage IVb: AV access ligation.

Stage I and IIa should be managed with close monitoring, hand warming, physical therapy, vasodilators, and reducing antihypertensive medications. If the symptoms do not resolve or continue to escalate, surgical intervention should be considered.

Patients with Stage IIb/III/IVa need surgical intervention to correct the flow pattern. All these patients should undergo flow volume measurement as the type of surgical procedure is primarily based on the volume flow of the access.

Low flow volume (<800 mL/min): Correction of arterial stenosis within the feeding artery may be all that is required. If no such lesions are identified, two revascularization procedures are widely utilized in cases of low or normal flow (800–1500 mL/min) flow steal. Proximalization of arterial inflow (PAI) and Distal Revascularization Interval Ligation (DRIL) procedures are commonly utilized interventions in this group of patients. PAI involves moving the inflow from the distal brachial artery to the proximal brachial artery at least 5 cm proximal to the existing anastomotic site [8].

Distal Revascularization Interval Ligation (DRIL) procedure (Fig. 72.1) involves brachial artery bypass from proximal brachial artery/axillary artery to distal brachial artery past the arteriovenous anastomosis. The intervening segment of the brachial artery between two anastomoses is then ligated to prevent reversal of flow proximally. This procedure is very effective in reversing symptoms while maintaining long-term patency of access [9]. DRIL procedure is considered the procedure of choice in patients with DASS.

High volume flow (>1500 mL/min): Banding and Revision Using Distal Inflow (RUDI) are two popular surgeries in cases of high flow steal patients. Banding can be accomplished using open or catheter-based techniques. Banding of the access involves constricting the access outflow, thereby increasing the resistance in the venous outflow tract, which effectively reduces flow through the access and diverts the blood to the forearm and hand. Intraoperative flow volume measurement can aid

Fig. 72.1 DRIL Procedure for DASS

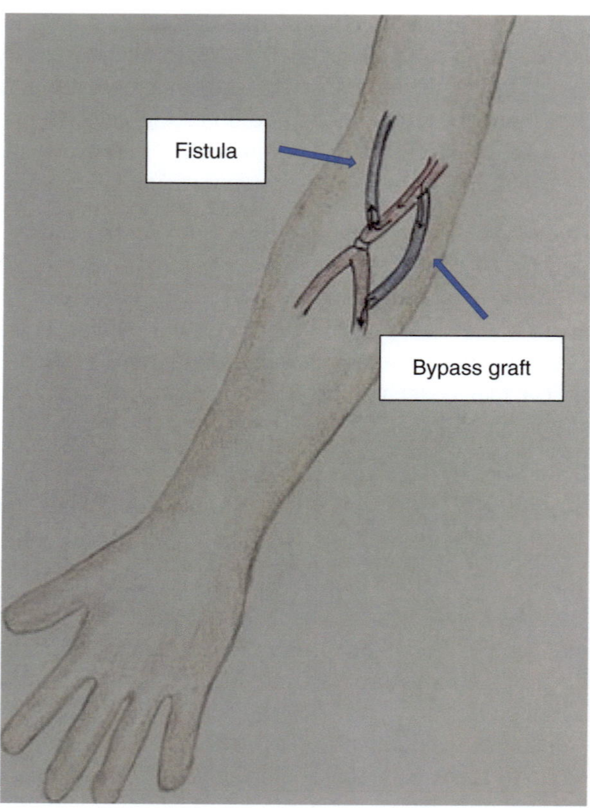

in the precise degree of flow reduction in the access, the procedure also known as "Precision Banding."

RUDI procedure involves ligating the access and moving the anastomosis from the brachial artery to the proximal radial or ulnar artery [10]. By moving the inflow to the small-diameter artery, RUDI increases the resistance and decreases the flow into the fistula.

In any patient with severe ischemic symptoms or IMN, immediate AV access ligation should be performed to prevent loss of digits, hands, or irreversible neurological damage of the hand.

References

1. Beathard GA, Spergel LM. Hand ischemia associated with dialysis vascular access: an individualized access flow-based approach to therapy. Semin Dial. 2013;26(3):287–314.
2. Mohamed AS, Peden EK. Dialysis-associated steal syndrome (DASS). J Vasc Access. 2017;18(Suppl 1):68–73.
3. Zanow J PM, Petzold K. Diagnosis and differentiated treatment of ischemia in patients with arteriovenous vascular access. Vascular Access for Hemodialysis VII 2001:201.

4. Gupta N, Yuo TH, Gt K, Dillavou E, Leers SA, Chaer RA, et al. Treatment strategies of arterial steal after arteriovenous access. J Vasc Surg. 2011;54(1):162–7.
5. DeCaprio JD, Valentine RJ, Kakish HB, Awad R, Hagino RT, Clagett GP. Steal syndrome complicating hemodialysis access. Cardiovasc Surg. 1997;5(6):648–53.
6. Morsy AH, Kulbaski M, Chen C, Isiklar H, Lumsden AB. Incidence and characteristics of patients with hand ischemia after a hemodialysis access procedure. J Surg Res. 1998;74(1):8–10.
7. Schanzer A, Nguyen LL, Owens CD, Schanzer H. Use of digital pressure measurements for the diagnosis of AV access-induced hand ischemia. Vasc Med. 2006;11(4):227–31.
8. Zanow J, Kruger U, Scholz H. Proximalization of the arterial inflow: a new technique to treat access-related ischemia. J Vasc Surg. 2006;43(6):1216–21. discussion 21
9. Kordzadeh A, Parsa AD. A systematic review of distal revascularization and interval ligation for the treatment of vascular access-induced ischemia. J Vasc Surg. 2019;70(4):1364–73.
10. Minion DJ, Moore E, Endean E. Revision using distal inflow: a novel approach to dialysis-associated steal syndrome. Ann Vasc Surg. 2005;19(5):625–8.

Index

© The Editor(s) (if applicable) and The Author(s), under exclusive license to
Springer Nature Switzerland AG 2022
F. Aziz, S. Parajuli (eds.), *Complications in Kidney Transplantation*,
https://doi.org/10.1007/978-3-031-13569-9

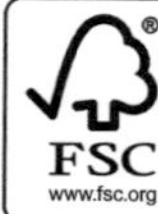

MIX
Papier aus verantwortungsvollen Quellen
Paper from responsible sources
FSC® C105338

If you have any concerns about our products,
you can contact us on
ProductSafety@springernature.com

In case Publisher is established outside the EU,
the EU authorized representative is:
Springer Nature Customer Service Center GmbH
Europaplatz 3, 69115 Heidelberg, Germany

Printed by Libri Plureos GmbH
in Hamburg, Germany